Recent Advances in
CRITICAL CARE MEDICINE

IAIN McA. LEDINGHAM MD(Hons) FRCS(Ed) FRCP(Glas) FIBiol FRSE
Professor of Intensive Care, University Department of Surgery; Chairman, Intensive Therapy Unit, Western Infirmary, Glasgow

Recent Advances in
CRITICAL CARE MEDICINE

EDITED BY

IAIN McA. LEDINGHAM

NUMBER THREE

CHURCHILL LIVINGSTONE
EDINBURGH LONDON MELBOURNE AND NEW YORK 1988

CHURCHILL LIVINGSTONE
Medical Division of Longman Group UK Limited

Distributed in the United States of America by
Churchill Livingstone Inc., 1560 Broadway, New York,
N.Y. 10036, and by associated companies, branches and
representatives throughout the world.

First published 1988

ISBN 0 443 032157
ISSN 0143 344X

Cataloguing in Publication Data is available from the
British Library

Library of Congress Catalog Card No. 77–30001

Printed in Great Britain at The Bath Press, Avon

Preface

Intensive care is presently undergoing a phase of rapid transformation as a consequence of increasing commitment to bedside research and development. During earlier times emphasis was appropriately placed upon the establishment of policies and procedures for patient care that could be modified in the light of new technological and therapeutic advances — often direct from the laboratory. The emergence of a variety of clinical scoring systems and the development of machines and methods specifically designed for intensive care have resulted in a better understanding of acute physiological dysfunction and, in some disease states, evidence of a reduction in morbidity and mortality. This third volume of *Recent Advances in Critical Care Medicine* reflects the foregoing changes.

The opening chapter originates from one of the centres most closely associated with the development of clinical scoring systems. The APACHE II system is being evaluated on a world-wide scale and, as separate disease categories are investigated, it becomes increasingly possible to envisage such a system being employed for individual patients. Present limitations prevent the use of this system to determine admission policy but sequential assessment over three to five days is increasingly accepted as an accurate indicator of the likelihood of success of further treatment. The three respiratory chapters deal with the continuing growth areas of weaning from mechanical ventilation, acute or chronic respiratory failure and status asthmaticus. In spite of a variety of technological innovations there is no good evidence that any of the new weaning procedures, although often simpler to use, are more effective than traditional techniques. The importance of prevention of acute respiratory failure in patients with chronic pulmonary disorders is emphasised and, in the case of asthma, a better evaluation of severity on the part of patients, relatives and medical practitioners is essential if potential life-threatening complications are to be avoided. Under-treatment rather than over-treatment in the early stages seems to be a common fault.

Sedation and analgesia were covered in the previous volume of this series but such major changes in attitude and practice have occurred in the ensuing four years that a further update was considered important. Essentially, adequate sedation is no longer deemed to require prolonged unconsciousness, and a variety of techniques is available to achieve patient comfort. Disseminated intravascular coagulation is seen less frequently than formerly in the modern intensive care unit but diagnosis remains a problem and treatment continues to be non-specific, the main component as always being elimination of the underlying cause. Of the various topics within the cardiovascular field, right ventricular dysfunction has emerged as one of the most fascinating and challenging. Techniques are now available for early detection of this disturbance and improved understanding of the pathophysiological mechanisms is leading to more rational and effective use of vasoactive drugs.

Infection continues to be of importance to intensive care specialists and the first of two chapters devoted to this subject reviews the sepsis syndrome and its complex metabolic disturbances, often associated with the onset of progressive organ failure. Emphasis is placed on physiological and biochemical support, buying time for the process to cure itself. The therapeutic problems highlighted in this account underscore the importance of prophylaxis, one aspect of which may be the importance of the gut in the aetiology of multiple organ failure. In this regard, the possibility of reducing the incidence of the sepsis syndrome by using a prophylactic regimen of enterally administered non-absorbed antibiotics is discussed in the context of Gram-negative infection. The first group to report this technique in general intensive care reviews present achievements and speculates on possible future trends.

Previous editorial practice in the *Recent Advances* series has been to include one or two contributions dealing with research developments and in the present volume some aspects of thermoregulation after injury, and endogenous opioids in shock of relevance to intensive care, are described. The dependence of 'flow' phase changes on stimulated macrophages is discussed and attention is drawn to the challenge of identifying the stimuli which trigger the 'flow' phase. In spite of the excitement generated by the early publications it seems that endogenous opioids are not the primary cause of shock and agents such as naloxone have not proved beneficial to cardiovascular function in a significant or sustained fashion. Nevertheless, the use of selective opiate antagonists, partial agonists, or thyrotrophin releasing hormone may prove to be of future therapeutic value in shock.

The concluding chapter describes and evaluates the plethora of new techniques in the management of acute renal failure. While the final place of a number of these techniques remains to be determined there is no doubt that major advances have been made in this aspect of intensive care. Clearly, the future implications of these advances in the overall management of the patient suffering from acute renal failure will be of interest to the intensive care and renal physician alike.

I wish to record my gratitude to all the authors who have contributed to this volume and, as always, it is a pleasure to record my thanks to the publishers and printers for their continuing support and forbearance when competing commitments have interfered with arranged production schedules.

Contributors

JULIAN F. BION MRCP FFARCS
Senior Lecturer in Anaesthetics and Intensive Care, University of Birmingham;
Honorary Consultant Anaesthetist, Queen Elizabeth Hospital, Birmingham,
England

ROGER C. BONE MD
Professor and Chairman, Department of Internal Medicine; Chief, Pulmonary and
Critical Care Medicine, Rush Medical College, Chicago, USA

FRANK R. CERRA MD
Associate Professor of Surgery, University of Minnesota, Minneapolis, USA

MICHAEL D. J. DONALDSON MB BS MRCP FFARCS
Research Registrar, St Bartholomew's Hospital, London, England

JOHN D. DUCAS MD FRCP (C)
Assistant Professor of Medicine, Department of Medicine, Section of Cardiology,
University of Manitoba, Canada

CHARLES J. HINDS MB BS MRCP FFARCS
Consultant and Senior Lecturer, Department of Anaesthesia; Director, Intensive
Care Unit, St Bartholomew's Hospital, London, England

KAJ A. JØRGENSEN MD
Physician-in-Chief, Department of Medicine and Hemodialysis, Fredericia Hospital,
Denmark

WILLIAM A. KNAUS MD
Professor and Director, ICU Research, The George Washington University Medical
Center, Washington DC, USA

DIETER LANGREHR MD
Professor of Anaesthesia, University of Groningen, The Netherlands

IAIN McA. LEDINGHAM MD(Hons) FRCS(Ed) FRCP(Glas) FIBiol FRSE
Professor of Intensive Care, University Department of Surgery; Chairman, Intensive
Therapy Unit, Western Infirmary, Glasgow, Scotland

FRANCOIS LEMAIRE MD
Professor of Intensive Care, Paris XII University Department of Intensive Care,
Henri Mondor Hospital, Creteil, France

RODERICK A. LITTLE
MRC Trauma Unit, Stopford Building, University of Manchester, England

D. REIS MIRANDA MD PhD
Director, Intensive Care Unit, Department of Surgery, University Hospital,
Groningen, The Netherlands

VICTOR PARSONS MA DM FRCP
Physician, King's College Hospital; Nephrologist, Dulwich Renal Unit, London,
England

CLAUDE PERRET FCCP
Head of the Intensive Care Service, Department of Medicine, University Hospital,
Lausanne, Switzerland

RICHARD M. PREWITT MD FRCP(C)
Associate Professor, Departments of Medicine and Pharmacology; Manitoba Heart
Foundation Research Professor; Head, Section of Cardiology, Health Sciences
Centre, Winnipeg, Manitoba, Canada

MICHAEL R. SILVER MD
Assistant Professor of Medicine; Fellow, Division of Pulmonary and Critical Care
Medicine, Rush Medical College, Chicago, USA

PETER G. M. WALLACE MB ChB FFARCS
Consultant Anaesthetist, Western Infirmary, Glasgow; Honorary Clinical Lecturer,
University of Glasgow, Scotland

JACK E. ZIMMERMAN MD
Professor and Director, ICU Research, The George Washington University Medical
Center, Washington DC, USA

Contents

1. Prediction of outcome from critical illness

William A. Knaus   Jack E. Zimmerman

Few specialties are influenced more by outcome prediction than critical care medicine. Each day, critical care physicians decide which patients should be admitted to an ICU and how vigorously to treat them. Such decisions are ultimately based on outcome predictions, i.e. the need or potential benefit of ICU treatment. Unfortunately, there are few systematic clinical observations that reduce the uncertainty inherent in such decision making.

Over the past three decades, rapid advances in diagnostic and therapeutic technology have rarely been rigorously evaluated to define their specific value for patient care. Instead, philosophy, logic, and pragmatism have dictated that many new technologies and the patients who might benefit from them be concentrated within ICUs. It is, therefore, not surprising that a recent NIH Consensus Development Panel found that evidence of effectiveness is equivocal for a large proportion of ICU admissions (NIH Consensus, 1983). This panel also found that at virtually every level of critical care practice — from the decision to insert a pulmonary artery catheter to selecting patients for care — decision making is characterised by controversy, dissension, and uncertainty.

While physicians remain uncertain about the best way to treat critical illness, patients and society have become increasingly concerned over the economic, social, and personal costs of current practices. In the United States, ICU care accounts for a major and rapidly growing proportion of medical costs. There is also concern that the ICU is a place where the human consequences of illness are obscured by an unyielding dedication to treatment in the face of a poor prognosis.

The theme of this chapter is that a clearer understanding of the factors determining patient outcome will improve our ability to evaluate intensive care, its many unique therapies, and that such understanding will eventually improve the treatment of critically ill patients. Because there is substantial confusion about the methods and goals of outcome prediction, the factors influencing outcome will first be briefly discussed within a conceptual framework. We will then review our recent efforts to improve outcome prediction for both groups of critically ill patients and individuals.

DETERMINANTS OF OUTCOME

When an acutely ill individual is admitted to an ICU, there are four patient-related and two treatment factors that will influence his/her outcome (Table 1.1).

Type of disease
A careful, objective, and reproducible method for describing disease is the foundation of any attempt to predict outcome. This is because, inherent in our labelling of disease,

1

we incorporate knowledge of the disease's aetiology when it is known and, for many diagnoses, such improved information leads to better treatment (Wagner et al, 1986).

Disease labelling should be natural. It should recognise the basic mechanism or aetiology of the disease and the major organ systems involved, i.e. septic shock has an infectious aetiology and primarily involves the cardiovascular system. This concept of labelling disease using aetiology and organ system has recently been reviewed (Gonnella et al, 1984). Their approach meets two other important criteria for a good disease classification system. First, it is exhaustive, e.g. all potential ICU patients can be classified. Secondly, it is disjointed implying that a patient will always be classified into one category; thus a patient with septic shock has an infectious aetiology involving the cardiovascular system. A major limitation to this approach and one that is especially important for ICU admissions is an inability to classify patients with more than one primary disease. The ICU, for example, may treat a patient with leukaemia who develops septic shock which is linked to an intra-abdominal abscess. How should the patient be classified?

Table 1.1 Factors influencing outcome

Patient factors	Treatment factors
Type of disease	Type of therapy
Physiologic reserve	Application of therapy
Severity of disease	Timing
Response to therapy	Process

First, it is important to keep in mind what outcome one is trying to predict. If interested in immediate outcome from intensive care, then the diagnosis of septic shock may be sufficient. If one is concerned with hospital or longer term outcome, then including information about the patient's leukaemia would be appropriate. The more precisely one can identify the disease, the more accurate the final prognosis. The value of this increased precision, however, must be balanced against the need to group patients into categories for analysis. Too limited a definition of disease will mean that too few patients are available for statistical analysis. Too broad a characterisation will make analysis meaningless for clinical comparison.

Researchers and clinicians reporting prognostic information on ICU patients should ensure that disease description incorporates both aetiology and system. Beyond this, disease description should be as well defined as possible without becoming overly restrictive. As experience with such work increases, we will gain knowledge about natural disease groupings that will lend themselves to prognostic stratification.

Physiologic reserve

The ability to survive an acute illness is also related to a patient's condition before he or she became acutely ill. Previous analyses have documented the independent impact of advanced chronologic age on the ability to recover from an acute illness for patients treated in an ICU (Scheffler et al, 1982). This is most likely due to the decrease in physiologic function of many major organ systems that accompanies ageing (Kenney, 1982). Therefore, any attempt to predict outcome should include information on patient age.

It is also widely recognised, although less well documented, that chronic health problems that are independent of patient age also decrease the probability of survival. Chronic disease (e.g., severe emphysema or cirrhosis) probably decreases the ability to respond to acute insults by limiting the physiologic response, thus making recovery to independent function impossible. Unfortunately, we do not yet have objective, reliable methods for measuring the exact physiologic impact of chronic organ system dysfunction on physiologic reserve. We must use relatively crude definitions of these important measures of co-morbidity. Nevertheless, while these measures may not be as precise as we would like, it is important to consider them within the overall analysis as one important source of variation in outcome.

Severity of disease
Severity can be defined in different ways, although most previous attempts have focused on the extent of injury. For trauma patients, the *extent* of injury has been defined by the Injury Severity Scoring system (ISS) (Baker et al, 1974). ISS assigns points to major anatomic regions depending on the type and extent of injury. Higher ISS scores are associated with increasing severity of injury. For patients with acute burns, the burn index measures severity by taking into account the extent of surface area involved by third degree burns (Feller et al, 1980). The larger the surface area burned, the greater the severity of the burn.

Another approach to defining severity is to assess the impact of disease or injury on *function*. For example, the level of neurologic function is the major determinant for assessing severity of acute head injury using the Glasgow Coma Score (Teasdale & Jennett, 1974). The Glasgow Coma Score assigns points to the best performance of motor, verbal, and conscious acts with a lower score indicating increased neurologic impairment and severity of injury.

Each of these severity measurement systems are correlated with hospital mortality rates and have proved useful in discovering relationships concerning treatment and outcome. Each, however, is limited in the amount of variation in outcome it can explain and the type of patients for whom it is applicable. Because of these limitations, there have been recent efforts directed at methods of measuring severity that would be useful in many different diagnoses.

These efforts are focused primarily on physiologic measurements. Defining and describing severity using physiologic measurements is useful since functional abnormalities are common to many acute diseases and the extent of derangement represents an objective, reproducible way of measuring severity. Which physiologic measures to use and how to decide on the importance or weight of each one are important decisions. There are two major ways this can be done.

The first method involves selection of physiologic variables before patient study. Selection and weighting is based on past studies and expert opinion. This is the approach used in the trauma score (Champion et al, 1981), and in the acute physiology score of the APACHE and APACHE II severity of disease classification systems (Knaus et al, 1981, 1985).

A second method is to collect physiologic information on groups of acutely ill patients as they are treated. At the conclusion of treatment, the characteristics or physiologic patterns of survivors and non-survivors can be contrasted. The physiologic measures are then given weights based on how often specific physiologic values were associated with survivors versus non-survivors. This is the method used by, among others, Shoe-maker and colleagues (1979), Siegel et al (1971), and more recently by Teres et al (1982) and Lemeshow et al (1985). In the case of the Shoemaker and Siegel studies, the results of the investigations are aimed at guiding and improving the treatment of individual patients. The work of Teres and Lemeshow is more oriented toward risk stratification of groups.

In principle, both methods of severity measurement are correct. A few precautions, however, should be kept in mind. First, the computer selection approach requires testing or validation in two independent groups of patients — the group from which the physiologic variables and weights were first obtained and then a second independent validation group. Second, if the objective of severity measurement is to predict the outcome of patients by estimating their relative risk of death prior to treatment, neither method should rely extensively on physiologic or other information collected over time. This confuses severity measurement with response to treatment.

Response to therapy

The variation in outcome we can now account for using information available before treatment is limited by our incomplete understanding of the patient factors that deter-mine outcome. One way to increase precision is to use information obtained after we have begun to treat the patient. From the works of Shoemaker, Siegel, and others, we have evidence that there may be important variations in the physiologic response of patients who will survive versus those who will die. Although the exact pattern and consistency of these results are not yet clear, including information on response to treatment is an important element in predicting outcome.

Many of the principles used to describe disease and severity also apply to estimating prognosis based on an individual patient's response to treatment. The information used should emphasise objective physiologic data rather than the type of therapy since not all patients are treated in the same way. For example, prognostic estimates based on the number of days a patient remains on a ventilator require that all patients with that diagnosis be admitted to ICUs and ventilated for a specific period before a prognostic estimate can be made (Schuster & Marion, 1983). It also assumes that all potentially reversible causes of respiratory failure, such as fluid overload, have been identified and properly treated. Although such studies provide useful informa-tion, they impose obvious restrictions on this method of defining outcome.

A less restrictive method would be to combine an exact description of the patient's diagnosis with dynamic physiologic evidence of individual response, such as the number and extent of other organ system failures. How soon in the course of treatment such analyses provide a prognosis is critical in determining their usefulness. Studies that provide prognostic estimates only for patients that have failed extensive therapy are not very useful in reducing the unnecessary economic or human costs of intensive care, but such retrospective studies may provide important clues for prospective research.

Type, use, and timing of therapy

Not all patients are treated in the same way and at the same time. For example, Jennett has demonstrated substantial differences in the use of specific treatments for head trauma patients depending on the hospital and country as well as changes in the use of treatments at one centre over time (Jennett, 1984). Studies that compare variations in the type, skill, and timing of medical interventions are also beginning to provide information on how widely medical practice varies at different institutions.

These variations in 'standard' medical practice makes it mandatory to closely examine treatment variations when discussing outcome from acute illness. In ICU outcome studies, the type and amount of treatment can best be measured with the Therapeutic Intervention Scoring System (TISS) (Keene & Cullen, 1983).

Information on the timing and process of treatment is also essential when assessing patient outcome. This is because variations in the skill and timing of medical care influence prognosis. Timing of therapy, specifically the interval from onset of the illness to the initiation of treatment, should be carefully recorded. The process or skill of care is much more difficult to measure but should also be considered as a possible explanation for variations in outcome unexplained by patient or treatment factors. As we make progress in these areas, we should become more precise in our understanding of these critical but currently elusive factors.

The use of outcome prediction in the assessment of group risk

Using the concepts just reviewed, we have recently completed work on a severity of disease classification system aimed at providing an estimate of the pre-treatment risk of death for the type of acutely ill patients treated in ICUs. The APACHE II (Acute Physiology and Chronic Health Evaluation) severity of disease classification system is designed to be used to risk or prognostically stratify individual patients so that different therapies or treatment programmes can be more accurately compared (Knaus et al, 1985). It does this by combining information on the risk factors of acute physiologic derangement, age, and chronic health status into a cardinal index number, a score which varies from 0–50, with a greater score indicating a higher risk of death. Because the APACHE II classification system has special relevance for patients treated in intensive care units, its design will be briefly described.

The APACHE II system uses a point score based on the worst, e.g., most abnormal, value of 12 routine physiologic measurements, age, and previous health status obtained during the initial 24 hours of intensive care to provide a general measure of severity of disease. The 12 physiologic measures were obtained from the 34 used in the original APACHE system (Knaus et al, 1981). Clinical judgment, established physiologic relationships, and a variation of the nominal group process were used to pick these physiologic variables. Information on each of the 12 measurements is needed to evaluate a patient with APACHE II. They make up the Acute Physiology Score (APS). The APS score is combined with points provided for increased age and a poor chronic health status to obtain the final APACHE II score. The exact format and scoring of the APS and APACHE II are given in Figure 1.1.

The approach taken by APACHE II has been tested and validated by determining prospectively that admission APACHE II scores for patients treated in a number of ICUs correlate with subsequent hospital mortality rates. Figure 1.2 shows the relationship between admission APACHE II scores, major diagnosis, and hospital death rates for 5030 ICU patients treated at 13 US medical centres. This figure illustrates that, when combined with information on a patient's disease, APACHE II scores provide a reliable method for estimating group outcome among ICU patients.

To make the estimates derived from APACHE II scores as independent of therapy

PHYSIOLOGIC VARIABLE	HIGH ABNORMAL RANGE					LOW ABNORMAL RANGE			
	+4	+3	+2	+1	0	+1	+2	+3	+4
TEMPERATURE – rectal (°C)	≥41°*	39°-40.9°*		38.5°-38.9°*	36°-38.4°	34°-35.9°	32°-33.9°*	30°-31.9°*	≤29.9°*
MEAN ARTERIAL PRESSURE – mm Hg	≥160	130-159	110-129		70-109		50-69		≤49
HEART RATE (ventricular response)	≥180	140-179	110-139		70-109		55-69	40-54	≤39
RESPIRATORY RATE – (non-ventilated or ventilated)	≥50	35-49		25-34	12-24	10-11	6-9		≤5
OXYGENATION: A-aDO₂ or PaO₂ (mm Hg) a. FIO₂ ≥ 0.5 record A-aDO₂	≥500	350-499	200-349		<200				
b. FIO₂ < 0.5 record only PaO₂					PO₂ >70	PO₂ 61-70		PO₂ 55-60	PO₂ <55
ARTERIAL pH	≥7.7	7.6-7.69		7.5-7.59	7.33-7.49		7.25-7.32	7.15-7.24	<7.15
SERUM SODIUM (mMol/L)	≥180	160-179	155-159	150-154	130-149		120-129	111-119	≤110
SERUM POTASSIUM (mMol/L)	≥7	6-6.9		5.5-5.9	3.5-5.4	3-3.4	2.5-2.9		<2.5
SERUM CREATININE (mg/100 ml) (Double point score for acute renal failure)	≥3.5	2-3.4	1.5-1.9		0.6-1.4		<0.6		
HEMATOCRIT (%)	≥60		50-59.9	46-49.9	30-45.9		20-29.9		<20
WHITE BLOOD COUNT (total/mm3) (in 1,000s)	≥40		20-39.9	15-19.9	3-14.9		1-2.9		<1
GLASGOW COMA SCORE (GCS): Score = 15 minus actual GCS									
Ⓐ Total ACUTE PHYSIOLOGY SCORE (APS): Sum of the 12 individual variable points									
Serum HCO₃ (venous-mMol/L) [Not preferred, use if no ABGs]	≥52	41-51.9		32-40.9	22-31.9		18-21.9	15-17.9	<15

Ⓑ AGE POINTS:
Assign points to age as follows:

AGE(yrs)	Points
≤44	0
45-54	2
55-64	3
65-74	5
≥75	6

Ⓒ CHRONIC HEALTH POINTS
If the patient has a history of severe organ system insufficiency or is immuno-compromised assign points as follows:
a. for nonoperative or emergency postoperative patients — 5 points
or
b. for elective postoperative patients — 2 points

DEFINITIONS
Organ insufficiency or immuno-compromised state must have been evident prior to this hospital admission and conform to the following criteria:

LIVER: Biopsy proven cirrhosis and documented portal hypertension; episodes of past upper GI bleeding attributed to portal hypertension; or prior episodes of hepatic failure/encephalopathy/coma.

CARDIOVASCULAR: New York Heart Association Class IV.

RESPIRATORY: Chronic restrictive, obstructive, or vascular disease resulting in severe exercise restriction, i.e., unable to climb stairs or perform household duties; or documented chronic hypoxia, hypercapnia, secondary polycythemia, severe pulmonary hypertension (>40mmHg), or respirator dependency.

RENAL: Receiving chronic dialysis.

IMMUNO-COMPROMISED: The patient has received therapy that suppresses resistance to infection, e.g., immuno-suppression, chemotherapy, radiation, long term or recent high dose steroids, or has a disease that is sufficiently advanced to suppress resistance to infection, e.g., leukemia, lymphoma, AIDS.

APACHE II SCORE

Sum of Ⓐ + Ⓑ + Ⓒ

Ⓐ APS points _____
Ⓑ Age points _____
Ⓒ Chronic Health points _____

Total APACHE II _____

Fig. 1.1   The APACHE II severity of disease classification system. (From Knaus et al, 1985a.)

as possible, scoring should be done on the patient's admission to the ICU and the current system requires data obtained within the initial 24 hours of ICU admission. Perhaps APACHE II scores at a specific point in time, such as ICU admission, would be more accurate than scoring based on the most abnormal value over 24 hours? In preliminary testing, this has not been verified. Since point-in-time scores are also more susceptible to bias, we urge users to follow our original definitions.

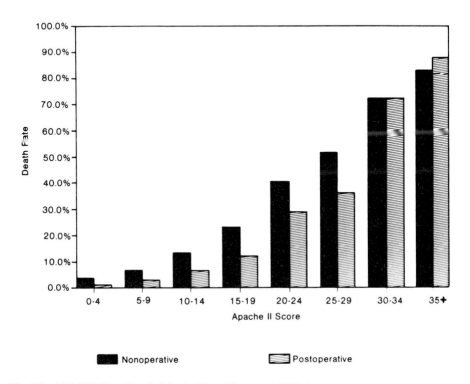

Fig. 1.2   APACHE II and hospital death. (From Knaus et al, 1985a.)

Once information on APACHE II scores and disease are obtained, they are entered into an equation to compute an estimated risk of death for an individual patient. This equation requires careful recording of the exact nature of each patient's disease. The equation uses patient information from 5030 ICU patients treated at 13 major medical centres in the US. The 13 centres are broadly representative of tertiary care ICU practices in the US. As experience with the APACHE II system increases, patient information from other centres and countries will be added. As the number of patients with specific diagnostic problems increases, separate analysis will be done for individual diseases.

What are the potential uses of this system? One example was recently provided by gastrointestinal surgeons, who were concerned with the difficulties in interpreting results of treatment studies for acutely ill patients with intra-abdominal infection (Meakins et al, 1984). Reported mortalities ranged from 0–90% and no method of relating patient outcome to prior risk existed. This made it impossible to evaluate the incremental value of new or existing treatments. How was it possible to know whether a new antibiotic treatment regimen or a different surgical approach influenced outcome?

To remedy the situation, they have incorporated the APACHE II system with an anatomical classification of intra-abdominal infections (Dellinger et al, 1985). Their system classifies patients into narrow mortality risk groups (i.e., <10%, 10–20%, >90%, etc.). This stratification allows more precise outcome comparisons by examining patients within each range or by estimating pre-treatment death rates. Similar methods could be applied to other diagnoses since the principles used in APACHE II appear to apply to a broad variety of diagnoses including ARDS (Montgomery et al, 1985). By helping to answer the question of whether the control and treatment groups were similar, risk stratification can improve the precision of clinical research.

APACHE II can also be useful for clinicians who are not engaged primarily in research. The ability to risk stratify ICU patients should allow ICU's to compare their outcome results with others. This can improve the clinical practice of intensive care by helping to identify practices that improve patient outcome as opposed to those that are non-productive.

In 1982, for example, we published a study comparing the outcome of acutely ill patients treated in French and American ICUs using our original APACHE system (Knaus et al, 1982). For patients with severe gastrointestinal disorders, the French hospital death rate was significantly greater than we predicted on the basis of the US experience. At the time we completed the study, we were uncertain why this variation occurred. It has been recently suggested that some of this variation in outcome was from different indications for surgery in the two countries for patients suffering from acute pancreatitis, one of the common diagnoses in our study (Smadja et al, 1984).

We are now completing other international comparisons in Australia, Denmark, and New Zealand. We have found that, while the patient selection criteria vary among these countries (in New Zealand, for example, elderly patients and those suffering from chronic diseases are not admitted to ICUs with the same frequency as in the US), the APACHE II approach to risk stratification appears to work well. Using this system along with information on the patients' disease and major organ system involvement, we were able to compare and contrast the performance of intensive care in these countries. We have found that the time when acutely ill patients are admitted to one hospital in Denmark may be substantially influencing the quality of care. Within our Australian survey, we have found variations in outcome that appear to be related to the degree of coordination of care among the ICU teams. Using the experience from these studies, we feel we are close to being able to apply these predictive techniques to intensive care units worldwide. Such comparisons would not only help us to determine how important are variations in the coordination of ICU staffs, they could also lead to improvements in our basic understanding of how various patient and medical care factors influence outcome from a severe illness. Until now, isolating various aspects of care has been difficult since so much of the variation in patient outcome has been unaccounted for by traditional methods of prediction or prognostic stratification. Using a combination of disease description and APACHE II scoring, however, it is possible to reduce variation from patient factors so that the influence of other variables may be more apparent.

The best example of how such an approach can be used to determine the value of specific aspects of intensive care comes from a recent analysis of performance we completed of 5030 ICU patients at the 13 US hospitals that participated in our national validation of APACHE II.

We first risk stratified each hospital's ICU patients by their individual risk of death using diagnosis, indication for ICU treatment, and APACHE II score, all determined within 24 hours of ICU admission. Using the group experience as the standard, the number of patients that would have died at each hospital was then predicted and compared to the actual death rate.

We found that one hospital performed significantly better (p. < 0.0001) than all others with 41 actual but 69 predicted deaths. Of the 13 hospitals, another's performance was significantly inferior with 58% more deaths than expected (52 actual versus 33 predicted, p < 0.0001). These variations in performance were found within specific diagnoses, for medical admissions alone, as well as for medical and surgical patients combined (Knaus et al, 1986).

This variation in performance appeared most related to the interaction and coordination of each hospital's intensive care unit staff rather than the administrative structure of the unit, the amount of unique ICU treatment used, or the hospital's teaching status. These results suggest that, like surgery, outcome from intensive care may now be substantially influenced by the skill of its practitioners — specifically, how well they work together in the treatment of acutely ill patients. These findings also suggest that good intensive care does save lives!

The use of outcome prediction for individuals
To accomplish outcome predictions for individuals, we must first recognise that the factors determining outcome for groups of patients and for individual patients are identical. Scientifically, there is no distinction between the objectives of group versus individual prediction; but there are the possible implications of the findings and the current state of our predictive science. When we speak about individuals, the precision of our predictions must be great and the confidence we have in these estimates must be high. There are two ways to increase confidence: by improving our predictive techniques and by increasing the number of patients studied.

At our current level of understanding, prognostic estimates based on information available *prior to treatment* enable us to confidently estimate risk in only limited groups of patients regardless of the numbers studied. We are, therefore, frequently obligated to treat many patients in order to determine their response to therapy. Once we have this additional information, however, our estimates of outcome become more accurate.

We have recently completed an analysis to illustrate this point. By using the data obtained from our 5815-patient 13-hospital study — specifically, the number and type of organ system failures that developed in 2719 of these patients according to objective definitions of failure for the following five major organ systems (cardiovascular, respiratory, renal, haematologic, neurologic) — we were able to obtain estimates of hospital mortality (Fig. 1.3) (Knaus et al, 1985b).

These estimates demonstrate that mortality increases directly with the number and duration of organ system failure. These estimates were obtained from a sufficient number of patients and in a form so that they can be confidently applied to the treatment of future patients and used as reference data for future studies aimed at improving on this record.

Number of OSF		Day of Failure						
		1st	2nd	3rd	4th	5th	6th	7th
1	Percent Mortality*	22%	31%	34%	35%	40%	42%	41%
	No. Deaths	450	261	204	159	142	118	80
	No. Patients	2070	847	607	455	356	279	195
2	Percent Mortality*	52%	67%	66%	62%	56%	64%	68%
	No. Deaths	239	147	103	118	96	78	56
	No. Patients	458	219	156	191	171	122	82
≥3	Percent Mortality*	80%	95%	93%	96%	100%†	100%†	100%†
	No. Deaths	152	70	50	50	38	33	32
	No. Patients	191	74	54	52	38	33	32

*To calculate confidence level: 95% confidence level (±2 standard deviation [std. dev.])

1 std. dev. = $\sqrt{N\,P\,Q}$
N = total number; P = percent death rate; Q = $1 - P$

For a patient with ≥3 OSF on the 4th day of OSF,
N = 52, P = .96, Q = .04; therefore, 1 std. dev.
= 1.4 and 1.4/52 = 2.7%, so ±2 std. dev. = 96% ±5.4%.

Therefore, the next patient to have ≥ 3 OSF on the 4th day
of OSF has a projected death rate from 90.6 to 100%.
(Use of poisson distribution yields equivalent results).

† Survival unprecedented with maximal statistical probability of survival of 10%
(with 95% confidence).

Projections are based on 2,719 patients from 13 hospitals.

Fig. 1.3 Hospital mortality according to number and duration of organ system failure. (From Knaus et al, 1985b.)

In a related study, Bion and his colleagues from the Clinical Shock Study Group of the Western Infirmary in Glasgow used an approach similar to APACHE II to also estimate outcome for patients who had failed to respond to initial treatment efforts (Bion et al, 1985). They studied a group of 50 critically ill patients transported between hospitals by a mobile ICU team. They used a slightly modified version of our APACHE II score, termed the sickness score, as indication of physiological status and patient risk at four different points in time: when the shock team first arrived at the outlying hospital to pick up the patient, after they had completed their initial evaluation and resuscitation, when they returned to the Western Infirmary, and then 24 hours later (Fig. 1.4).

The results indicate that, in this sample of critically ill patients, those who have a high degree of persistent physiologic instability despite the best care possible at the referring hospital (time point one)—a condition roughly equivalent to persistent multiple organ system failure—may not benefit from later, more aggressive efforts at treatment.

We believe future such studies that combine physiologic assessment techniques with precise descriptions of disease and other patient risk factors could improve the quality and compassion of intensive care. They could help us avoid what Professor Jennett has called the vicious cycle of commitment when future therapy is initiated—not because of its expected value but only because past therapy has failed (Jennett, 1985). They could also assist us in improving future treatment through a more precise assessment of which new techniques improve outcome.

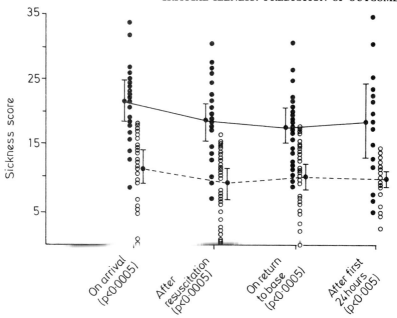

Fig. 1.4 Individual sickness scores, mean values and confidence intervals during resuscitation and transport of survivors (○) and non-survivors (●). From Bion et al (1985).

SUMMARY AND CONCLUSION

This chapter has presented a conceptual approach to the prediction of outcome in critical illness and has reviewed our recent experience with this model in the comparison of intensive care units and in prediction of outcome for patients with multiple organ system failure. These early results are encouraging. They suggest there may be some underlying consistent relationships between acute physiologic abnormalities and risk of death. When information on these physiologic abnormalities are combined with precise descriptions of disease and other patient risk factors such as age and chronic health status, we have the beginnings of a scientifically valid and reproducible approach to prediction. These new scientific capabilities could improve our ability to document the value of intensive care in modern medicine and thereby improve its performance. Some of the findings from these investigations may challenge many of our traditional beliefs, such as the superiority of teaching versus non-teaching hospitals (Knaus et al, 1986), but they may also bring us closer to the truth about the power of our science.

The availability of expanded information on the probability of success from advanced medical care will raise other new questions. How do we begin to incorporate knowledge and information concerning outcome risks and benefits (which will become increasingly available because of computers and large data bases) into the diagnosis and treatment of critically ill patients? The complexity of modern intensive care and the amount of information currently available frequently makes it impossible for one individual to use personal intuitive judgment to decide on the course of treatment. Often, the best course of action will only become apparent only through a careful balancing of prognostic information with ethical, moral, and legal considerations.

But most critical care professionals would emphasise that even the best prognostic facts concerning a patient do not tell what should be done in a particular situation. A course of action must also be influenced by values, particularly the patient's values, along with those of the society in which he lives. This is one major challenge that those of us in critical care face in the years ahead. How do we incorporate the factual information within a moral system that best fits the ideals of medical practice in our respective countries? Only by facing this challenge directly will we be able to maintain control over the practice of our specialty and its future.

REFERENCES

Baker S P, O'Neil B, Haddun W, Long W B 1974 The injury severity score: a method for describing patients with multiple injuries and evaluating emergency care. Journal of Trauma 14: 187–196

Bion J F, Edlin S A, Ramsay G et al 1985 Validation of a prognostic score in critically ill patients undergoing transport. British Medical Journal 291: 432–434

Champion H R, Sacco W T, Carnazzo A J 1981 Trauma score. Critical Care Medicine 9: 672–676

Dellinger E P, Wertz M J, Meakins J L, Solomkin J S, Allo M P, Howard R J, Simmons R L 1985 Surgical infection stratification system for intra-abdominal infection: multicenter trial. Archives of Surgery 120: 21–29

Feller I, Tholen D, Cornell R G 1980 Improvements in burn care, 1965 to 1979. Journal of the American Medical Association 244: 2074–2078

Gonnella J S, Hornbrook M C, Louis D Z 1984 Staging of disease: a case-mix measurement. Journal of the American Medical Association 251: 637–644

Jennett B 1984 Outcome of intensive therapy for severe head injuries: an inter-center comparison. In: Parillo J E, Ayres S M (eds) Major issues in critical care medicine. Williams & Wilkins, Baltimore, Md,

Jennett B 1985 Inappropriate use of intensive care. British Medical Journal 289 (6160): 1709–1711

Keene A R, Cullen D J 1983 Therapeutic Intervention Scoring System: update 1983. Critical Care Medicine 11: 1–3

Kenney R A 1982 Physiology of Aging: A Synopsis. Chicago Year Book Medical Publishers, Chicago

Knaus W A, Draper E A, Wagner D P, Zimmerman J E 1985a APACHE II: a severity of disease classification system for acutely ill patients. Critical Care Medicine 13: 818–829

Knaus W A, Draper E A, Wagner D P, Zimmerman J E 1985b Prognosis in acute organ system failure. Annals of Surgery 202(6): 685–692

Knaus W A, Draper E A, Wagner D P, Zimmerman J E 1986 Evaluation of outcome from intensive care in major medical centers. Annals of Internal Medicine 104: 410–418

Knaus W A, LeGail J R, Wagner D P et al 1982 A comparison of intensive care in the U.S.A. and France. Lancet ii: 642–646

Knaus W A, Zimmerman J E, Wagner D P et al 1981 APACHE — acute physiology and chronic health evaluation: a physiologically based classification system. Critical Care Medicine 9: 591–597

Lemeshow S, Teres D, Pastides H, Aurinin J S, Steingrub J S 1985 A method for predicting survival and mortality of ICU patients using objectively derived weights. Critical Care Medicine 13: 519–525

Meakins J L, Solomkin J S, Allo M D et al 1984 A proposed classification of intra-abdominal infections: stratification of etiology and risk for future therapeutic trials. Archives of Surgery 119: 1372–1378

Montgomery A B, Stager M A, Carrico C T, Hudson L D 1985 Causes of mortality in patients with the adult respiratory distress syndrome. American Review of Respiratory Diseases 132: 485–489

NIH Consensus Development Conference Statement 1983 Journal of the American Medical Association 250: 798–804

Scheffler R M, Knaus W A, Wagner D P, Zimmerman J E 1982 Severity of illness and the relationship between intensive care and survival. American Journal of Public Health 72: 449–454

Schuster D P, Marion J M 1983 Precedents for meaningful recovery during treatment in a medical intensive care unit: outcome in patients with hematologic malignancy. American Journal of Medicine 75: 402–408

Shoemaker W P, Chang P, Czer L 1979 Cardiovascular monitoring in post-operative patients. Critical Care Medicine 7: 237–241

Siegel J H, Goldwyn R M, Friedman H P 1971 Patterns and process in the evaluation of human septic shock. Surgery 70: 232–240

Smadja C, Bismuth H 1984 Pancreatites aigues ne crotiques: pour une restriction oes indications operatures. Gastroenterologie Clinique et Biologique 8: 536–540

Teasdale G, Jennet B 1974 Assessment of coma and impaired consciousness: a practical scale. Lancet ii: 81–84

Teres D, Brown R B, Lemeshow S 1982 Predicting mortality of intensive care patients: the importance of coma. Critical Care Medicine 10: 86–94

Wagner D P, Knaus W A, Draper E A 1986 Physiologic abnormalities and outcome from acute disease. Archives of Internal Medicine 146: 1389–1396

2. Weaning from mechanical ventilation

Francois Lemaire

INTRODUCTION

Many important studies concerning weaning from mechanical ventilation (MV) were conducted during the sixties. The most commonly used criteria for predicting the success or failure of weaning were the maximum negative inspiratory airway pressure, minute ventilation, maximum voluntary minute ventilation and vital capacity (Sahn & Lakshminarayan, 1973, Sahn et al, 1976). The usefulness of these criteria has been questioned on the grounds that they were developed from studies of patients weaned after short-term ventilation, often post-operatively, and do not necessarily apply to patients ventilated for weeks or months (Fiastro et al, 1986; Morganroth et al, 1984). In addition to the duration of MV, another problem is the increasing number of older and more seriously ill patients admitted to the ICU for MV, in whom the problems associated with resumption of spontaneous breathing present a major challenge.

Several new modes of ventilation, some mixing spontaneous and mechanical breaths, have been described within the last 10 years. All of these modes can be used during weaning (CPAP, IMV, SIMV, MMV, inspiratory pressure support, etc.). Whether or not these techniques can facilitate weaning is unclear. Since overviews of the subject of weaning have recently been published (Browne, 1984; Weisman et al, 1983) this chapter will concentrate upon recent physiological observations and therapeutic approaches, including haemodynamic changes during weaning, new modes of mechanical ventilation and the inspiratory work of breathing.

GAS EXCHANGE AND HAEMODYNAMIC CHANGES DURING WEANING

When a patient starts to breathe spontaneously after days or weeks of mechanical ventilation, the resultant change in respiratory status induces an alteration in haemodynamic performance. Gilbert (1974) described these respiratory alterations during the first hours off the ventilator in eight COPD patients. Respiratory rate (RR) increased from 13 to 25/min and tidal volume fell from 700 to 300 ml. PaO_2 decreased while $PaCO_2$ increased. Table 2.1, which summarizes a number of published clinical reports, illustrates that $PaCO_2$ invariably increases during the first attempts at weaning from MV. After weaning, hypercarbia results from chronic alveolar hypoventilation in COPD patients, due to an increased work of breathing and the larger ventilatory dead space caused by the increased respiratory rate (shallow breathing). Hypoxaemia can result from increased venous admixture due to increased $\dot{V}/\dot{Q}$ imbalance and often atelectasis. Dantzker et al (1982) studied nine patients in the process of weaning from MV after open heart surgery. Reduced minute ventilation from 10.4 to 6.2 l/min induced an increase in $PaCO_2$ from 39 to 48 mm Hg. No major change occurred in

Table 2.1

Author year (No of patients)	Patients		PaO_2		$PaCO_2$		$\dot{Q}s/\dot{Q}$		CI		SAP		PAOP		$\dot{V}O_2$	
			CV	SV	CV	SV	CV	SV	CV	SV	CV	SV	CV	SV	CV	SV
Beach, 1973 (37)	Post op cardiac surgery	A	258	242	31	37			3.7	4.4	88	93			166	185
Wolff, 1975 (38)	Post op cardiac surgery	B	241	250	29	34			3.2	2.6	90	93			205	171
		NW	304	195	38	45	10	12	2.5	2.1			23	24	136	129
		W	327	295	36	42	11	11	2.7	2.9					137	150
Delooz, 1976 (41)	Post op cardiac surgery	NW	183	180	34	41	13	26	2.2	2.6	76	84	15	17	260	248
		W	181	200	31	38	9	8	2.3	2.5	75	85	10	11	268	286
Kennedy, 1977 (20)	Miscellaneous	NW			40	52	17	20					6	8		
		W			36	43										
Hastings, 1980 (18)	Post op cardiac surgery				40	45			5.7	6.0					246	235
Mathru, 1982 (20)*	Post op cardiac surgery	C	122	116	38	39	8	9	2.2	2.8	98	93	8	12		
		D	114	118	37	39	9	8.4	2.6	2.1	101	85	16	21		
Nikki, 1982 (9)	AMI		70	73	36	40	26	26	2.25	2.60	81	87	20	23	121	132
Räsänen, 1984 (12)	AMI		110	95	33	38	8	12	2.8	2.8	80	86	15	20	162	151
Bergeret, 1986 (4)	COPD + LVF	NW	86	54	46	68			2.8	2.8	80	86	15	20	162	151
		W	91	74	46	51			2.6	3.4	72	79	13	14	163	178
Downs, 1977	Post op cardiac surgery		88	91	29	43	13	14	4.98	5.63	88	95	75	94		

A = increase in CI; B = decrease in CI; C = LVEDP < 16 mm Hg; D = LEVDP > 16 mm HC; (*) = IMV 2/min; W = weaner; NW = non weaner; AMI = acute myocardial infarction; LVF = left ventricular failure; CV = controlled mechanical ventilation; SV = spontaneous ventilation; QS/QT = venous admixture; CI = cardiac index; SAP = systemic arterial pressure; PAOP = pulmonary artery occluded pressure; $\dot{V}O_2$ = oxygen consumption.

the distribution of $\dot{V}/\dot{Q}$ ratios. The shunt was not altered significantly (from 17.9 to 19.9%) and the dead space not at all (from 0.37 to 0.37). The $\dot{V}/\dot{Q}$ ratio corresponding to the peak blood flow was slightly shifted from 1.0 to 0.69 due to reduced ventilation in the presence of an unchanged cardiac output.

Withdrawal of mechanical ventilation during weaning modifies intra-thoracic pressures. Mechanical ventilation is delivered under positive pressure, thereby increasing the mean pleural pressure. Conversely, spontaneous inspiration decreases the airway and pleural pressures. In addition, any airway obstruction — circuit and ventilator resistance when the patient breathes via a demand-valve, bronchospasm and/or laryngeal oedema after extubation — increases the expiratory pressure, but also amplifies the inspiratory swings, leading to a more negative intra-thoracic pressure. Obviously, any major modification of pleural pressure will influence pulmonary haemodynamic values and cardiac output.

Table 2.1 shows that when patients are disconnected from MV cardiac output usually increases by 10–20% (Beach et al, 1973; Deloon, 1976; Downs, 1977, Hastings et al, 1980). Several factors cause this increase of cardiac index:

1. Increased *oxygen consumption* due to activation of respiratory muscles, especially in patients with COPD
2. *Sympathetic discharge:* Kennedy et al (1977) reported that during spontaneous breathing, urinary norepinephrine excretion increased from 2.35 to 3.64 μg per 24 hours. Urinary catecholamine excretion was greater in weaners than in non-weaners.
3. *Hypercarbia:* a positive linear relationship has been repeatedly observed between $PaCO_2$ and cardiac output (Kelman & Prys-Roberts, 1967). However, in some clinical studies the change in $PaCO_2$ and cardiac output are not closely related, suggesting that hypercarbia is not the only factor involved.
4. Increase in *venous return*, due to a lowered pleural pressure.

Several authors believe that the increase in cardiac output is beneficial during weaning, supplying increased metabolic need (Delooz, 1976; Wolff & Gradel, 1975). In the series of Wolff and Gradel (1975), patients who weaned successfully had an increase of cardiac index from 2.7 to 2.9 l/min. Conversely, a reduced mean CI (from 2.5 to 2.1 l/min) predicted a failure of weaning. Similarly, Kennedy found the largest increase of catecholamine excretion was associated with successful weaning (Kennedy et al, 1977).

In patients mechanically ventilated for an acute episode of left ventricle insufficiency, resumption of spontaneous breathing may lead to acute left ventricular failure. Mathru et al (1982), in a study of patients with poor ventricular reserve (LVEDP > 16 mm Hg and ejection fraction (EF) < 0.6), showed that the introduction of IMV (six mechanical breaths/minute) decreased CI from 2.6 to 2.1 l/min and systemic blood pressure from 101 to 85 mm Hg. The pulmonary arterial occlusion pressure (PAOP) increased from 16 to 21 mm Hg. Nikki et al (1982) showed that shifting from IPPV at 12/min to IMV in nine patients ventilated for pulmonary oedema following a myocardial infarction improved the PaO_2 and $P\bar{v}O_2$, increasing the CI from 2.25 to 2.60 l/min. Another study by this same group (Räsänen et al, 1985) suggested that weaning of these patients should be done at 5 to 15 cm H_2O CPAP. Chin et al (1985) studied the right and left haemodynamic patterns in 30 patients with pre-existing cardiac disease during a trial of weaning. They showed that the PAOP increased slightly but significantly while left ventricular end-diastolic (LV ED) volume remained unchanged, suggesting a fall in LV compliance due to ischaemia.

We recently examined a group of four patients with COPD and pre-existing left heart failure (mostly of ischaemic origin) in whom weaning from MV was especially difficult. Attempts to allow the patients to breathe on their own invariably led to hypercapnia, an increased cardiac output and elevated systemic arterial pressure (Bergeret et al, 1986). The PAOP increased from 14 to 33 mm Hg (Figure 2.1) while

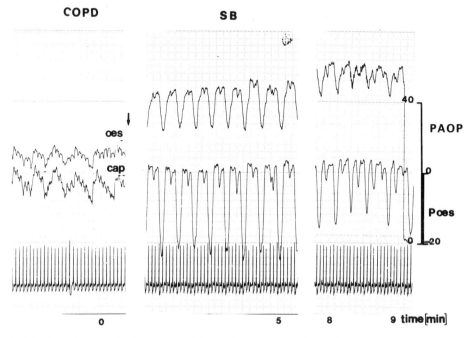

Fig. 2.1 Oesophageal and pulmonary arterial occluded pressures during a trial of weaning in a patient with COPD and ischaemic heart disease. During controlled mechanical ventilation (left of the figure) oesophageal pressure (Poes) is slightly positive during inspiration and end-expiratory pulmonary artery occluded pressure (PAOP) is 12 mm Hg. Then the patient is disconnected from the ventilator (arrow). After 5 minutes of mechanical ventilation, mean Poes is negative and end-expiratory PAOP is 42. After 8 minutes it goes up to 46. All pressures are given in mm Hg; time 0 corresponds to mechanical ventilation.

the right atrial pressure increased from 8.5 to 11 mm Hg. Within a few minutes, reconnection to the ventilator became necessary. After one week of treatment of left heart failure (vasodilator and diuretics), weaning was possible in three of these four patients and PAOP did not increase during spontaneous breathing.

TIMING OF WEANING: CRITERIA

Weaning from MV should be started only when a patient is able to sustain unassisted ventilation (Sahn et al, 1976). He must be in a steady state, i.e. not obviously infected, shocked or agitated etc. When the reason for intubation and mechanical ventilation is a bacterial pneumonia, this must be first treated. Similarly, a pneumothorax, central respiratory depression (narcotics overdose, etc.), acute heart failure or systemic sepsis must be treated before weaning is contemplated. Table 2.2 gives the criteria that

Table 2.2 Usual criteria for weaning

Tidal volume (Vt)	> 5 ml/kg
Vital capacity	> 10–15 ml/kg
Functional residual capacity	$> 50\%$ of predicted
Max inspiratory force	> -25 cm H_2O
Respiratory rate	< 35/min
Vent/min ($\dot{V}E$)	< 10 l/min
Dead space (VD/Vt)	< 0.55–0.60
PaO_2 (FIO$_2$:0.4)	< 60 mm Hg
P(A − a)O$_2$:(FIO$_2 < 1.0$)	< 300 mm Hg
$\dot{Q}S/\dot{Q}T$	< 0.10–0.20
pH	> 7.30
$PaCO_2$ ↑ after disconnection	< 8 mm Hg

have been proposed to predict the success of weaning. These criteria are simple to collect, as they are measured routinely on patients in the ICU. The most reliable weaning criteria are the maximum inspiratory force, minute ventilation (MV), maximal voluntary ventilation and vital capacity (VC). Each has been studied in a large series of patients. Sahn and Lakshminarayan (1973) assessed the predictive values of these criteria on 100 consecutive patients. Seventy-six patients had an MV less than 10 l/min, could voluntarily double their MV and could exert a negative peak airway pressure during blocked inspiration of at least 30 cm H_2O: each was successfully weaned. Browne et al (1972) showed that successful weaning for 24 hours could be achieved in 25 patients when the mean negative inspiratory force was −34 cm H_2O and the mean VC 16 ml/kg body weight. The other criteria are less useful: functional residual capacity is not measured routinely, dead space only indicates the level of hyperventilation and hypoxaemia can usually be corrected by increasing FIO$_2$.

These conventional weaning criteria have not been extensively tested after prolonged mechanical ventilation. Morganroth et al (1984) found them unhelpful in predicting successful weaning in 11 patients ventilated for a mean duration of 50 days ±28. These authors developed both a ventilator score (using FIO$_2$, PEEP level, static and dynamic compliances, minute ventilation and the triggered respiratory rate) and an 'adverse factor' score taking into account heart rate, blood pressure, temperature, CVP or PAOP, level of consciousness, ability to communicate, emotional state, etc. A high ventilator score predicted respirator dependency, while the adverse factor score assessed the number or degree of underlying medical problems. The maximum value of both summed scores was 150. All patients at the onset of successful weaning scored less than 60. While such scores are cumbersome for routine use, they provide strong evidence that after prolonged ventilation successful weaning requires more than simply ventilatory performance. Fiastro et al (1986) showed recently that measurements of the work of breathing were better predictors of successful weaning than the conventional criteria in a group of patients requiring long-term ventilatory support.

THE MODALITIES OF WEANING

T-Piece

The most commonly used means of weaning consists of connecting the tracheal tube to a humidified, O_2 enriched gas mixture, under ambient pressure. The excess work of breathing due to the circuit is minimal. This mode is routinely used in all patients by some physicians, and by others for patients after surgery and/or for weaning patients with COPD. It needs close monitoring and surveillance by trained personnel.

CPAP

This is a most effective means of weaning in cases of alveolar instability, e.g. during the recovery period from ARDS, and/or with atelectasis or superinfection of the lungs. CPAP maintains the lungs inflated and prevents end-expiratory alveolar collapse. In a controlled study of patients with acute respiratory failure, Feeley et al (1975) showed that in the treated group (15 patients) 5 cmH$_2$O CPAP prevented the increase of $(A - a) PO_2$ ($+10$ mm Hg) which occurred in the control group (13 patients) not receiving PEEP.

Recently, Räsänen et al (1985) studied the effects of increasing levels of CPAP in 14 patients after acute myocardial infarction complicated by circulatory and respiratory failure. CPAP improved arterial blood oxygenation, and, in patients with left ventricular dysfunction, increased the stroke work index. A beneficial effect of CPAP on left heart function, as demonstrated experimentally by Robotham et al (1978), suggests that weaning of patients with left heart failure should be done with CPAP.

Moreover, there is evidence that weaning should always be done with 5 to 8 cm H$_2$O CPAP. Quan et al (1981) showed that the PaO$_2$ and FRC were improved in 12 patients at CPAP 5 cm H$_2$O when compared with patients breathing air via the endotracheal tube. These results as well as those of Feeley et al (1975), suggest that glottic function, bypassed by an endotracheal tube, may be beneficially restored by applying a minor degree of CPAP. More recently, Khan et al (1983) showed that a similar effect could be obtained by using a ventilator with the IMV mode set at zero, probably due to an 'auto-PEEP' effect (Pepe & Marini, 1982; Rossi et al, 1985).

Intermittent mandatory ventilation (IMV)

This was proposed as a ventilatory mode to reduce the intra-thoracic pressure when employing high level PEEP. Shortly thereafter IMV was employed for weaning from MV. Downs et al, in 1974 showed that the mean duration of ventilation was 21 hours in 12 patients using IMV compared to 38 hours in a control group of 12 patients ventilated in a controlled mode. It was argued later, however, that the two groups were poorly matched and that no conclusion should be drawn from this study (Petty, 1975). Many subsequent investigators, comparing IMV with other modes, have failed to find any difference in the mean duration of weaning (Hastings et al, 1980; Muir et al, 1982) (Table 2.3). Indeed, Shachter et al (1981) reported in 1976 that the introduction of IMV into their institution nearly doubled the duration of mechanical ventilation.

Despite the lack of evidence that IMV shortens the weaning period, IMV is extensively used in the majority of ICUs. The reasons are that IMV is easy to employ, allows monitoring to be provided via the ventilator (respiratory rate, tidal volume,

Table 2.3 Weaning: CMV (T-piece) versus IMV

Author	Year	Journal	Patients	Mode	No.	Duration	Study
Downs	1974	*Archives of Surgery*	Post-operative & ARF	CMV IMV	12 12	38 hours 21 hours	Prospective
Cullen	1975	*Archives of Surgery*	Flail chest	CMV IMV	15 16	19 days 5 days	Retrospective
Hastings	1980	*Anaesthesiology*	Uncomplicated post-operative patients	CMV IMV	10 8	150 min 169 min	Prospective
Shaster	1981	*Journal of the American Medical Association*	ICU patients	CMV IMV	58 77	17 days 36 days	Retrospective
Prakash	1982	*Chest*	Uncomplicated cardiac surgery	CMV IMV	15 13	— —	Prospective
Hoang	1983	*European Society Pneumology*	Flail chest	CMV IMV	21 22	18 days 7 days	Retrospective

minute ventilation), and needs fewer trained personnel than weaning via a T-piece. The problem with IMV is that it requires the patient to breathe via the ventilator circuit (tubing, humidifier, demand-valve), which increases the work of breathing (see below). Improved demand-valves with lower resistance will probably further increase the use of IMV.

Mandatory minute ventilation (MMV)

In this mode, the minute volume is predetermined and the expired minute ventilation ($\dot{V}E$) is monitored. If the patient is unable to spontaneously breathe sufficiently to meet the required $\dot{V}E$, the ventilator starts delivering mechanical breaths (CPU1, Ohmeda, Figure 2.2) or provides increasing pressure support (Veolar, Hamilton,

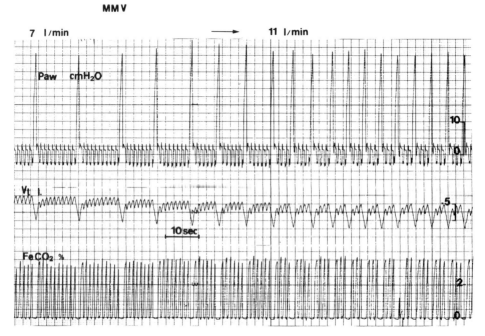

Fig. 2.2   Mandatory minute ventilation (MMV) in a spontaneously breathing patient with the *Ohmeda CPU1*. Patient Vt is 250 ml and mechanical Vt is 750. When the mandatory minute volume is 7 l/min, the machine respiratory rate is 5 l/min. When this mandatory volume is increased to 11 l/min, the machine respiratory rate is automatically and progressively doubled. The CPU1 adjusts the mandatory minute volume by altering the expiratory time, thus the mechanical respiratory rate, the pre-set Vt remaining unchanged. Paw = airway pressure; Vt = tidal volume; $FeCO_2$ = fraction of expired CO_2.

Figure 2.3). Therefore, the preset MMV is always delivered to the patient. Although the MMV mode is provided by several ventilators (Ohmeda CPU1, Hamilton Veolar, Engström Erica, Dräger Eva), its value as a technique for weaning has not yet been reported. In 1979, Higgs and Evans reported a patient with myasthenia gravis who was successfully weaned using MMV. Employing MMV we assessed the effects of increasing parenteral caloric intake upon the patients' ability to breathe spontaneously (Laaban et al, 1985). We noted that the more calories the patients received, the more they breathed spontaneously. However, three patients with COPD experienced hypercapnea. During this study, we found MMV easy to implement and well accepted

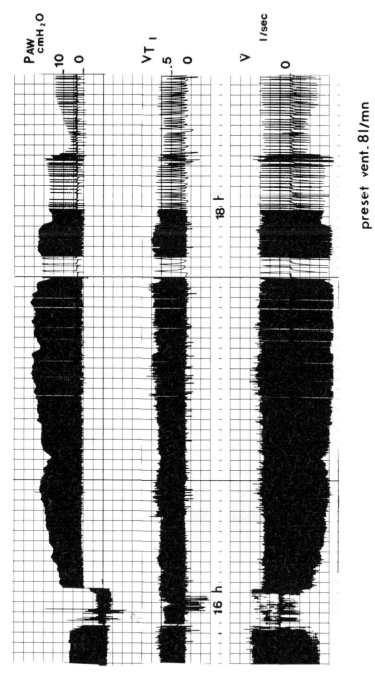

Fig. 2.3 Mandatory minute ventilation using the *Hamilton Veolar*. Two hours strip chart record of airway pressure (Paw), tidal volume (Vt) and instantaneous gas flow (V̇) (inspiration above the zero line and expiration under the zero line). To fit the preset minute ventilation of 8 l/min, a varying level of inspiratory assistance is added to the ventilator circuit. With this technique, the patient controls the rate of breathing and the ventilator modulates the size of each tidal breath.

by the patients. We then tried to define those patients most likely to benefit from MMV ventilation. We found MMV was most useful for patients with wide fluctuations of their level of consciousness (for example, after excessive sedation, anaesthesia or acute cerebral disease) or during recovery from respiratory muscle paralysis due to neuromuscular disease (myopathy, myositis, Guillain-Barré syndrome, etc.). In all these diseases, when mechanical ventilation is prolonged and the weaning process may take weeks or even months, MMV may provide a useful tool, but this remains to be proven.

Pressure support
Inspiratory pressure support (IPS) is a new modality of assisted ventilation, designed to increase the volume of spontaneous breaths. With IPS, a supplemental gas flow is delivered to the patient during inspiration via a demand valve, thereby producing a positive inspiratory pressure at a pre-set value. Increasing the level of this inspiratory airway pressure up to 20–30 cm H_2O increases the tidal volume (Figure 2.4) and

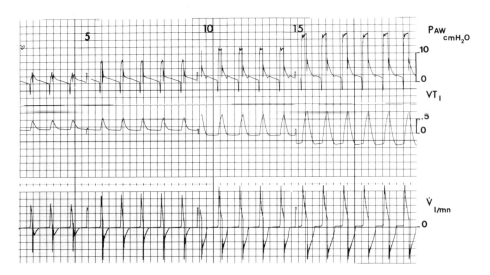

Fig. 2.4   Pressure support with the Siemens Servo 900 C (model study). Same legends as Figure 2.3, 5, 10 and 15 cm H_2O IPS are applied to a lung model. Respiratory rate is unchanged but tidal volume increases from 350 to 1250 ml. Note that increased tidal volumes are obtained through higher inspiratory flow rates.

reduces respiratory frequency (Macintyre, 1986). We reported recently (Brochard et al, 1987) that during their weaning phase in eight spontaneously breathing patients, an IPS of 10 cm H_2O increased the Vt by 20%, and prevented deterioration of blood gas tensions. Similarly Fahey et al (1985) compared the oxygen cost of breathing with CPAP and IPS at 5 cm H_2O in twelve patients with COPD. They showed that the O_2 cost of breathing was significantly reduced with IPS, since the O_2 consumption was 171 ml/min during controlled ventilation, 232 ml/min with CPAP, but only 190 ml/min with IPS (+5 cm H_2O). It is likely that the pressure support ventilation mode will be useful during prolonged and difficult weaning, but this also remains to be established.

RESPIRATORY WORK OF BREATHING

When a patient breathes through a tracheal tube the respiratory work of breathing is increased. If, additionally, he breathes via any of the possible modes delivered by a ventilator, the work load imposed upon the respiratory muscles is even greater. Each time a patient is ventilated with any of these modes (CPAP, IMV, SIMV, MMV), the expected benefits have to be balanced against an increased work of breathing.

Respiratory circuit

First, the endotracheal tube — especially with an outside diameter of less than 8F — reduces the airway lumen and increases the airway resistance. When the patient is connected to the ventilator, he breathes through the tubing, humidifier and demand valves, all components of the breathing circuit which have been shown to be highly resistive.

Demand-valves

No demand-valve has yet been proven to be as effective at minimizing inspiratory work load as the continuous flow system (CFS). Gibney et al (1982) compared the inspiratory work of breathing (WOB) done by eight normal volunteers breathing spontaneously via two demand-valves (Puritan Bennett MA2 and Bournes Bear I) and two free flow circuits. They showed that the WOB with the CFS was half that with the demand-valves. Similar findings have been published by Christopher et al (1985) and OpTholt et al (1982) measuring the gradient of airway pressure necessary to open demand-valves, and by Katz et al (1985), using a lung model to compute the inspiratory WOB as $PAW \times Vol$. Why are demand-valves so inefficient? The main reason is the inherent mechanical delay between the triggering signal (decrease in airway pressure, change of flow pattern) and the opening time of the demand-valve (Iotti et al, 1985). Thus, the patient initially breathes against a closed valve, and the airway and oesophageal pressures markedly decrease, increasing the work done by the respiratory muscles. Ward et al (1985) suggested that the inspiratory WOB expended during the respiratory cycle was determined by the early negative inspiratory airway pressure. Another limitation to demand valve performance is that they limit the maximum inflow of gas to between 60 and 140 l/min, which at times may be less than the peak inspiratory flow rate. Finally, the square waveform of inspiratory flow that is delivered by most demand-valves may also be a limitation, since the spontaneous flow waveform is sinusoidal. Again, at mid-inspiration, the gas flow rate may be insufficient for the patient's requirements.

Expiratory valves

Most commercially available expiratory valves can also be a source of increased airway resistance as demonstrated recently by Marini et al (1985). Using a model of passive and active exhalation, they showed that the added expiratory work due to a mushroom resistor valve was comparable to the excess work due a 5 mm diameter endotracheal tube. The scissors valves opened reluctantly at the beginning of each expiration, producing high pressures before release. Spring-loaded valves were found to be prohibitively resistive and unsuitable for clinical use.

Auto-PEEP

In COPD patients, a supplementary inspiratory threshold load is added by the 'auto-PEEP' effect: Pepe and Marini (1982) showed in three patients that occlusion of the expiratory port at the end of expiration provided evidence of a residual positive airway pressure even when the PEEP valve was set to zero. This positive pressure indicated that the emptying of lung volume was incomplete due to reduced elastic recoil. Shallow breathing, a frequent occurrence during weaning, enhances this mechanism due to a reduced expiratory time. Subsequently, Rossi et al (1985) showed that auto-PEEP — which they called 'intrinsic' PEEP — was present in 10 of 14 patients and ranged from to 2 to 7.5 cm H_2O. It is clear that auto-PEEP markedly increases the inspiratory elastic WOB, since inspiratory flow can start only after contraction of inspiratory muscles has decreased the airway pressure to subatmospheric level. Pepe and Marini proposed that weaning of patients with auto-PEEP would be facilitated by IMV, and Rossi et al suggested that CPAP would reduce their inspiratory effort.

WOB AND MODES OF VENTILATION

T-piece
Spontaneous ventilation through a T-piece minimally increases the respiratory WOB, since the added dead space is small and airway resistance depends only upon the diameter and length of the tracheal tube.

CPAP
Some recent reports have suggested that breathing through a CPAP system decreases the respiratory WOB. In sixteen spontaneously breathing patients recovering from an episode of acute respiratory failure, Katz and Maks (1985) showed that a mean of 9 cm H_2O CPAP increased both lung compliance and tidal volume, reducing both the respiratory rate and the work of breathing. These results contrast with those of Gherini et al (1979) who measured an increased WOB when a CPAP mask was applied to young athletes. In these volunteers with normal lungs, the expiratory resistance increased the FRC well above the volume of the relaxed thoracic cage, thereby leading to less efficient diaphragmatic contractions. In contrast, when the FRC is below normal, which is likely to occur in ARF, lung distension becomes advantageous, restoring the lung volume to normal and placing the diaphragmatic musculature in an optimal distending position.

The assist control mode of ventilation should reduce the patient's WOB, since the majority of the inspiration is mechanically supported. Previous mention was made that this hypothesis has been challenged (Marini et al, 1985).

Pressure support
Providing a spontaneously breathing patient with a supplementary inflow of gas should minimize the resistance to breathing via the airway, tubing and demand-valve. Using a lung model, Macintyre (1986) measured 'muscle' WOB during increasing levels

of IPS. He reported that ventilatory 'muscle' work per minute was reduced with IPS, especially at levels of pressure support above 20 cm H_2O (Figure 2.5).

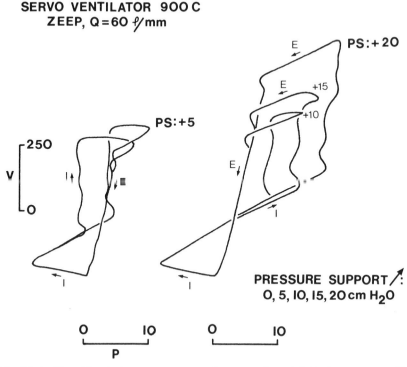

SERVO VENTILATOR 900 C
ZEEP, Q = 60 ℓ/mm

PS:+20
+15
+10
PS:+5
250
V
0

PRESSURE SUPPORT:
0, 5, 10, 15, 20 cm H_2O

0   10   0   10
P

Fig. 2.5 Work of breathing during pressure support (by means of a model). P: airway pressure, V: lung volume. Increasing the pressure support level from zero to 20 increases the tidal volume from 550 to 1000 ml. The work of breathing made by the 'patient' is the area PAW × Vol under the zero line. The area right of the atmosphere pressure corresponds to work done by the machine. However, in patients, only the work computed by using the oesophageal pressure can indicate the work done by the patient.

In eight patients recovering from ARF (see above) we measured blood gases, Vt and transdiaphragmatic pressure (Pdi) to estimate the force developed by the diaphragm at an IPS level of 10 cm H_2O (Brochard et al, 1987). We demonstrated that spontaneously breathing patients had a significantly higher Vt, and a reduced Pdi, suggesting reduced diaphragmatic work (Figure 2.6). In two of these patients, we measured a reduced diaphragmatic EMG, despite an increased Vt and better alveolar ventilation.

Demand valves of modern ventilators provide low levels of inspiratory assistance — even when inspiratory pressure support levels are set to zero — raising the airway pressure throughout inspiration to the atmospheric, or end-expiratory level. Since the WOB is computed as the P-V area, measuring PAW with these ventilators provided a very low WOB (Katz et al, 1985). In fourteen patients resuming spontaneous breathing after prolonged mechanical ventilation, we compared the inspiratory WOB done with a demand-valve (CPU1, Ohmeda) and an 'assisted one' (Siemens, Servo 900 C) (Lemaire et al, 1986). The WOB computed using the PAW was reduced by nearly half that when the Servo was used. By using the oesophageal pressure for complications,

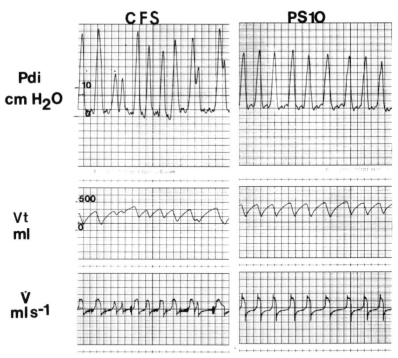

Fig. 2.6 Pressure support (PS). A spontaneously breathing patient is placed under a continuous flow system (CFS) and a pressure assistance of 10 cm H₂O (Siemens Servo C). Tidal volumes (Vt) are increased and more regular with IPS, and transdiaphragmatic pressure is reduced, suggesting a decrease of the diaphragm work load.

WOB was similar with both ventilators. However, the tidal volume was slightly but significantly increased with the Siemens Servo 900 C.

REFERENCES

Beach T, Millen E, Grenvik A 1973 Hemodynamic response to discontinuance of mechanical ventilation. Critical Care Medicine 1: 85–90

Bergeret S, Abrouk F, Brun-Buisson C, Lemaire F 1986 Vasodilator treatment and diuretics ease weaning from mechanical ventilation of patients with COPD and associated left heart failure. (Abstract) Intensive Care Medicine 12 (suppl): 200

Brochard L, Pluskwa F, Lemaire F 1987 Improved efficiency of spontaneous breathing with inspiratory pressure support. American Review of Respiratory Disease 136: 1111–1115

Browne D R G, Pontoppidan H, Chiang H 1972 Physiological criteria for weaning patients from prolonged artificial ventilation. Abstract of scientific papers, annual meeting of the American Society of Anesthesiologists, Boston: 69–70

Browne D R G 1984 Weaning patients from mechanical ventilation. Intensive Care Medicine 10: 55–58

Chin W D N, Cheung H W, Driedger A A, Cunningham D G, Sibbald W 1985 Assisted ventilation in patients with preexisting cardiopulmonary disease. Chest 88: 503–511

Christopher K L, Neff T A, Bowman J L, Eberle D J, Irvin C G, Good J T 1985 Demand and continuous flow intermittent mandatory ventilation systems. Chest 87: 625–630

Dantzker D, Cowenhaven W M, WIlloughby W J, Kirsh M M, Bower J S 1982 Gas exchange alteration association with weaning from mechanical ventilation. Chest 82: 674–677

Delooz H H 1976 Factor influencing successful discontinuance of mechanical ventilation after open heart surgery: a clinical study of 41 patients. Critical Care Medicine 4: 265–270

Downs J B, Derkins H M, Modell D H 1974 Intermittent mandatory ventilation. Archives of Surgery 105: 519–523

Downs J B, Douglas M E, Sanfelippo P M, Stanford E, Hodges M R 1977 Ventilatory pattern, intrapleural pressure and cardiac output. Anesthesia and Analgesia 56: 88–94

Fahey P J, Vanderwarf C, David A 1985 Comparison of O_2 cost of breathing during weaning with CPAP versus pressure support ventilation. American Review of Respiratory Disease 131 (suppl II); 131: 130

Feeley T W, Saumarez R, Klick J M, McNabb T G, Skillman J J 1975 Positive end expiratory pressure in weaning patients from controlled ventilation. Lancet i: 725–728

Fiastro J F, Campbell S C, Shon B Y, Habib M P 1986 Comparison of standard weaning parameters and mechanical work of breathing in mechanically ventilated patients. American Review of Respiratory Disease 133 (suppl): A122

Gherini S, Peters R M, Virgilio R W 1979 Mechanical work on the lungs and work of breathing with PEEP and CPAP. Chest 76: 251–256

Gibney R T N, Wilson R S, Pontoppidan H 1982 Comparison of work of breathing on high gas flow and demand valve continuous positive airway pressure systems. Chest 82: 692–695

Gilbert R 1974 The first few hours off a respirator. Chest 65: 152–157

Hastings P R, Bushnell L S, Skillman J J, Weintraub R M, Hedley-Whyte J 1980 Cardio-respiratory dynamics during weaning with IMV versus spontaneous ventilation in good risk cardiac-surgery patients. Anesthesiology 53: 429–431

Henry W C, West G A, Wilson R S 1983 A comparison of the O_2 cost of breathing between a continuous flow CPAP system and a demand-flow CPAP system. Respiratory Care 28: 1273–1281

Higgs B D, Evans J C 1979 Use of mandatory minute ventilation in the peri operative management of a patient with myasthenia. British Journal of Anaesthesiology 51: 1181–1183

Iotti G, Braschi A, Locatelli A, Bellinzona G 1985 Respiration spontanée au cours de la ventilation artificielle, importance de la resistance des valves. Presse Medecale 14: 165

Katz J A, Kraemer R W, Gjerde G E 1985 Inspiratory work and airway pressure with continuous positive airway pressure delivery systems. Chest 88: 519–526

Katz J A, Marks J D 1985 Inspiratory work with and without CPAP in patients with acute respiratory failure. Anesthesiology 63: 598–607

Kelman G R, Prys-Roberts C 1967 Circulatory influences of artificial ventilation during nitrous anesthesia in man: the relative influence of mean intra-thoracic pressure and arterial CO_2 tension. British Journal of Anesthesia 39: 533–542

Kennedy S K, Weintraub R W, Skillman J J 1977 Cardiorespiratory and sympatho adrenal responses during weaning from controlled ventilation. Surgery 82: 233–240

Khan F A, Mukherji R, Chitkara R, Juliano J, Iorio R 1983 Positive airway pressure in patients receiving intermittent mandatory ventilation at zero rate. Chest 84: 436–438

Laaban J P, Lemaire F, Baron J F, Trunet P, Harf A, Bonnet J L, Teisseire B 1985 Influence of caloric intake on the respiratory mode during mandatory minute ventilation. Chest 87: 67–72

Lemaire F, Rieuf P, Rauss A, Ben Lakhal S 1986 A clinical comparison of the work of breathing through demand-valve systems. American Review of Respiratory Disease 133 (suppl): A121

Macintyre N R 1986 Respiratory function during pressure support ventilation. Chest 89: 677–683

Marini J J, Culver B H, Kirk W 1985 Flow resistance of exhalation valves and positive end expiratory pressure devices used in mechanical ventilation. American Review of Respiratory Disease 131: 850–854

Marini J J, Capps J S, Culver B H 1985 The inspiratory work of breathing during assisted mechanical ventilation. Chest 87: 612–618

Mathru M, Rao T L K, El Etr A A, Pifarre R 1982 Hemodynamic response to changes in ventilatory patterns in patients with normal and poor left ventricular reserve. Critical Care Medicine 10: 423–426

Morganroth M L, Morganroth J L, Petty T L 1984 Criteria for weaning from prolonged mechanical ventilation. Archives of Internal Medicine 144: 1012–1016

Muir J F, Aubry P, Levi-Valensi P 1982 Deux techniques de sevrage du respirateur (avec et sans IMV). Revue Francaise Maladie Respiratoires 10: 131–141

Nikki P, Rasanen J, Tahvanainen J, Makelainen A 1982 Ventilatory pattern in respiratory failure arising from acute myocardial infarction. Critical Care Medicine 10: 75–78

OpTholt T B, Hall M W, Bass J B, Allison R C 1982 Comparison of changes in airway pressure during CPAP between demand valve and continuous flow devices. Respiratory Care 27: 1200–1207

Pepe P E, Marini J J 1982 Occult positive end expiratory pressure in mechanically ventilated patients with airflow obstruction. American Review of Respiratory Disease 126: 166–170

Petty T L 1975 IMV versus IMC (editorial). Chest 67: 630–631

Quan S F, Falltick R T, Schlobohm R M 1981 Extubation from ambient or expiratory positive airway pressure in adults. Anesthesiology 55: 53–56

Rasanen J, Vaisanen I T, Heikkila J, Nikki P 1985 Acute myocardial infarction complicated by left ventricular dysfunction and respiratory failure. Chest 87: 158–162

Robotham J L, Lixfeld W, Holland L, McGregor D, Bryan A C, Rabson J 1978 Effects of respiration on cardiac performance. Journal of Applied Physiology 44: 703–709

Rossi A, Gottfried S B, Zocchi L, Higgs B D, Lennox S, Calverley P M A, Begin P, Grassino A, Milic-Emili J 1985 Measurement of static compliance of the total respiratory system in patients with acute respiratory failure. American Review of Respiratory Disease 131: 672–677

Sahn S A, Lakshminarayan S 1973 Bedside criteria for discontinuation for mechanical ventilation. Chest 63: 1002–1005

Sahn S A, Lakshminarayan S, Petty T L 1976 Weaning from mechanical ventilation. Journal of the American Medical Association 235: 2208–2212

Schachter E N, Tucker D, Beck G J 1981 Does intermittent mandatory ventilation accelerate weaning. Journal of the American Medical Association 246: 1210–1214

Ward M E, Corbeil C, Gibbons W, Newman S, Macklem P T 1985 Role of initiating inspiratory effort in determining the work of breathing during mechanically assisted ventilation. American Review of Respiratory Disease 131 (suppl): A131

Weisman I M, Rinaldo V E, Rogers R M, Sanders M H 1983 Intermittent mandatory ventilation. American Review of Respiratory Disease 127: 641–647

Wolff G, Gradel E 1975 Haemodynamic performance and weaning from mechanical ventilation following open heart surgery. Intensive Care Medicine 1: 99–104

3. Acute respiratory failure and chronic obstructive pulmonary disease

Michael R. Silver   Roger C. Bone

INTRODUCTION

In the last decade the incidence of acute respiratory failure (ARF) has climbed dramatically (Pontoppidan et al, 1972). Several significant advances have diminished the short-term mortality for patients with chronic obstructive pulmonary disease (O'Donohue et al, 1970; Rogers, 1972). Recently there has been a trend toward controlled oxygen therapy with decreasing endotracheal intubation, less invasive monitoring techniques as well as the institution of therapy to prevent the progression of chronic obstructive pulmonary disease (COPD). In the following sections we define COPD and respiratory failure and discuss the pathophysiology in patients with these conditions. An approach to management of patients with COPD and ARF is presented and their prognosis is summarised.

DEFINITION

Acute respiratory failure, chronic respiratory failure (CRF) and chronic obstructive pulmonary disease (COPD) are physiologic conditions for which agreement on definitions is lacking. Acute respiratory failure in individuals without COPD has been defined as a decrease in p_aO_2 greater than predicted from age and inspired oxygen concentration *combined* with an increase in the pCO_2 above 50 mm Hg (Pontoppidan et al, 1972). Defining ARF by using a specific p_aO_2 value and p_aCO_2 (usually greater than 50 mm Hg) (Murray, 1979) has some validity in defining a homogeneous study population but little role in the management of the individual patient. Patients who are not chronically hypercapnic usually develop ARF after the appearance of the adult respiratory distress syndrome (ARDS). They have primarily a failure of oxygenation and only in later stages develop CO_2 retention characteristic of the above definition of ARF. Detailed discussion of these patients has been extensively reviewed elsewhere (Balk & Bone, 1983; Bell et al, 1983; Hudson, 1981; Francis, 1983) and will not be discussed in this chapter.

Clinically, chronic respiratory failure represents either a forced expiratory volume in 1 second (FEV_1) less than 2 litres/min or hypercapnia with a near normal pH. This means a new equilibrium has been reached between hypoventilation and metabolic buffering. Other definitions that use specific arterial blood gas values ($p_aO_2 < 75$ mm Hg, %sat < 93% and/or $p_aCO_2 > 47$ mm Hg) (Ciba Guest Symposium, 1959) seem to have some theoretical basis (Kawakami et al, 1982). The chronic elevation of p_aCO_2 above 45 mm Hg occurs when respiratory muscle strength is less than 30% of predicted (Braun et al, 1983).

Most patients with CRF also have chronic obstructive pulmonary disease. COPD has been defined as a nonspecific change in lung parenchyma and bronchi that may lead to emphysema and intermittent or permanent airflow obstruction (Snider, 1983). This definition incorporates earlier definitions of both bronchitis (non-neoplastic disorder of structure or function from infectious or non-infectious processes) (ACCP, ATS, 1975) and emphysema (anatomic alterations of lung with an increase of airspaces distal to non-respiratory bronchi with destruction of lung) (Snider, 1983). Recently, authors have begun using the term 'airflow limitation' rather than airflow obstruction to describe the loss of elastic recoil in emphysematous lung (22nd Aspen Lung Conference, 1980; Macklen & Permutt, 1979).

PHYSIOLOGY

COPD is associated with impaired gas exchange in the lung, changes in the mechanical property of the lungs that increases the load on respiratory muscles, and changes in the geometry of the lung due to hyperinflation (Sykes et al, 1976). Moderate degrees of $\dot{V}/\dot{Q}$ mismatch will cause hypoxemic respiratory failure, however as mismatch worsens hypercapnic respiratory failure will occur (West, 1979). The $\dot{V}/\dot{Q}$ mismatch occurs secondary to several processes seen in COPD, namely vascular obliteration, chest wall abnormalities, destruction and obstruction of ventilatory units, or change in intrathoracic pressure (Bone, 1981).

Central to the understanding of ARF is an understanding of respiratory muscle fatigue. Fatigue can be defined as inability of muscles to maintain an expected force, while muscle weakness or failure is the inability to develop expected force. Simply stated, fatigue results from an imbalance of respiratory muscle strength, load, efficiency as well as energy supply (Roussos et al, 1979). The pressure developed at a given level of electrical excitation is dependent on the velocity of contraction (Bellemare & Grassino, 1982; Roussos & Macklem, 1977; Farkas & Roussos, 1982; Grassino et al, 1978; Gross et al, 1973; Bigland & Lippold, 1954; Goldman et al, 1978), which is proportional to muscle length, inspiratory flow and geometry of the chest (Goldman et al, 1978; Kim et al, 1979). Two reviews of respiratory muscle function and fatigue have been published (Roussos & Macklem, 1982; Roussos, 1985).

Muscle strength can be expressed by graphing muscle tension vs. muscle length (Dantzker, 1985) (Fig. 3.1). Inspection of this curve reveals that at smaller resting muscle lengths, less force is generated, i.e. hyperinflation results in less muscle force (Roussos & Macklem, 1977). In emphysema, compensation for this occurs by a shortening of muscle fibre length and is represented by a shift of the curve to the left. This is accomplished by sarcomere shortening as well as by a decrease in their total number. The result is to give a normal force/tension curve in animal models when expressed as a percentage of length rather than absolute length (Farkas & Roussos, 1982). Because lung volume affects muscle work, measurement of muscle fatigue is dependent on the lung volume at the time the study is conducted (Roussos et al, 1979) as well as the velocity of shortening and type of muscular contraction i.e., miometric, pleometric or isometric (Juan et al, 1984).

The ability to predict the onset of muscle fatigue in patients with COPD would be extremely useful. Experimentally the onset of muscle fatigue can be predicted by examining the tension-time index. This index is the product of respiratory frequency and the area under the curve obtained when the diaphragmatic pressure vs. duration of inspiration is graphed. The result is the average pressure/minute the respiratory

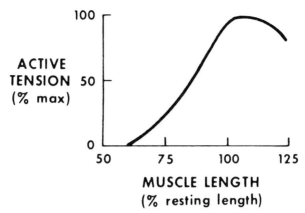

Fig. 3.1 The length–tension relationship. As the resting length is shortened, there is a sharp decrease in the tension that it can develop. (From Rochester D F, Braun N M T 1978 The respiratory muscles. Basics of Respiratory Disease 6:1.)

muscles generate — values greater than 0.13–0.15 predicting the onset of muscle fatigue (Bellemare & Grassino, 1982; Juan et al, 1984). Other measurements to predict the onset of fatigue include quantification of the measured to maximal transdiaphragmatic pressure (greater than 40% predicts fatigue (Roussos & Macklem, 1977)), the inspiratory time as a percent of time spent in the inspiratory phase (Grassino & Macklem, 1984; Bellemare & Grassino, 1983), and the amount of ventilatory effort expressed as a percent of the MVV (Freedman, 1970; Leith & Bradly, 1976).

Recently, the electromyogram (EMG) has been used to predict the onset of fatigue. EMG's may be obtained from the abdominal surface over the diaphragm (easily obtainable, technically difficult), by placement of oesophageal leads (relatively easy and reproducible) or by diaphragmatic insertion (most accurate, potentially dangerous). Two EMG patterns of fatigue have been described. One is seen in response to high frequency (60–110 Hz) stimulation and the other type is seen with low frequency (10–30 Hz) stimulation. High frequency fatigue has a recovery period of minutes, while low frequency fatigue may require hours to days for recovery (Dantzker, 1985). Another approach is to measure the shift in power spectral density. With fatigue there is reported to be a shift from high-frequency to low-frequency power density before clinically detectable fatigue appears (Lindstrom et al, 1970).

There are several mechanisms by which the diaphragm resists fatigue. Blood flow to the diaphragm increases exponentially with the work it performs (Robertson et al, 1977). Extraction also increases until maximal extraction is obtained, at which point blood flow continues to increase (Roberts et al, 1977; Rochester & Bettini, 1976). In addition, oxygen content of the blood in patients with chronic hypoxia is increased by secondary erythrocytosis. With exercise, there appears to be a shift of the oxyhaemoglobin dissociation curve that favours oxygen unloading (Van der Elst & Kreukniet, 1982).

The high oxidative capacity of the diaphragm helps it to resist fatigue. Normal composition of the diaphragm muscle is 76% red fibre, high oxidative muscle of which two thirds is slow twitch-fatigue resistant and one third is fast twitch-fatigue resistant. Only 24% is white fibre, low oxidative fast twitch-fatiguable muscle (Lieberman et al, 1973). The alternation of the diaphragm and intercostal muscles in performing the work of breathing is another mechanism by which the diaphragm resists fatigue (Roussos & Macklem, 1977; Dantzker, 1985).

The transition from chronic respiratory failure to acute respiratory failure is marked by an increase in the p_aCO_2. Carbon dioxide retention in ARF occurs not because of a decrease in ventilatory drive but because of either increased production or an increase in the percent of dead space ventilation (Vd/Vt) (Aubier et al, 1980a). Oxygen administration during COPD has been shown to increase Vd/Vt (Cotes et al, 1963; Rodman et al, 1962; Lee & Read, 1967) and increase the area in the lung with a high $\dot{V}/\dot{Q}$ (Bone, 1981; Wagner et al, 1977). It also increases the inhomogeneity of $\dot{V}/\dot{Q}$ distribution within the lung (Aubier et al, 1980b). An acute increase in p_aCO_2 has been shown to reduce the normal unfatigued diaphragm force generated as well as producing EMG's consistent with fatigue seen with resistive breathing. Unfortunately, an acute decrease in p_aCO_2 has no notable effect on diaphragmatic function (Grassino & Macklem, 1984). This increase in fatiguability is thought to be mediated by a decrease in the pH (Aubier et al, 1980). The decrease in pH decreases the affinity of troponin for calcium (Katz & Hecht, 1969), increases the binding of calcium to the sarcoplasmic reticulum (Nakamaru & Schwartz, 1972) and decreases the rate of glycolysis and thus ATP regeneration (Hermansen, 1981).

Patients with COPD have other disturbances in physiology when compared with normal patients. One of these differences is an abnormal ventilatory pattern. Although minute ventilation is normal, COPD patients have an increase in the respiratory rate and a decrease in tidal volume. In ARF these patients further increase their respiratory rate as their tidal volume falls (Aubier et al, 1980). This results in a marked increase in inspiratory pressure and flow which markedly increases the work of breathing.

Abnormal renal physiology has been noted in patients with clinically stable hypercapnic COPD. Many of these patients have increased levels of plasma renin (PRA), aldosterone (PA) and arginine vasopressin (AVP). The increase in PRA and PA result in impaired sodium handling and oedema formation while the increase in AVP leads to reduced free water clearance and hyponatremia (Farber et al, 1975, 1977, 1982, 1984). PRA, PA and AVP all increase in response to hypoxia or hypercapnia (Anderson et al, 1978; Sutton et al, 1977; Weitzman, 1979) with hypoxia being the largest stimulus to AVP secretion (Farber et al, 1984). Why some individuals with severe COPD have normal levels of PRA, PA and AVP and others do not still is unclear.

MANAGEMENT

Perhaps no aspect of management is more important than the recognition and treatment of the factors responsible for the development of ARF. As many as 55% of patients with CRF and ARF are thought to have acute infections as the cause of their deterioration (Burk & George, 1973). *Haemophilus influenzae* and *Streptococcus pneumoniae* are two of the most common bacterial pathogens in individuals with chronic bronchitis and pneumonia. The diagnosis of pneumonia can be difficult in patients with severe COPD especially in those patients with an abnormal baseline chest radiograph. Furthermore, patients with chronic bronchitis often have purulent sputum, making detection of a change difficult. A recent study comparing tetracycline with placebo found no objective or subjective difference in patients with an exacerbation of chronic bronchitis (Nicotra et al, 1982), however this study probably did not have enough patients to show a positive result if there was really a difference. Other studies have documented the superiority of sulfa/trimethoprim over tetracycline (Somner, 1972; Huddy et al, 1973). Whether or not an infection is documentable, most clinicians use antibiotics whenever the possibility of a concurrent infection is seriously entertained. The choice of antibiotics must be made on an individual case basis depending on the severity of illness, sensitivity pattern in the community and available culture data. Cephalosporins and aminoglycosides are all valid choices in special situations, but for most patients, sulfa/trimethoprim or possibly tetracycline will suffice for the patient with respiratory failure associated with an exacerbation of chronic bronchitis.

Left ventricular failure is a common precipitator of ARF in patients with COPD. Because of this, diuretic agents are frequently administered to patients with ARF. Diuretics do not change exercise tolerance or left ventricular ejection fraction in patients with COPD unless left ventricular failure is present as well (Mathur et al, 1984). When they must be used, it is preferable to use potassium sparing diuretics because of the tendency toward hypokalaemia in patients with COPD (Hill, 1986). Recognition and aggressive treatment of CHF in patients with COPD and ARF is important. A summary of the changes in right and left ventricular function occurring with COPD has been published (Robotham, 1981). There is also available an excellent review of the non-invasive assessment of cardiac function in patients with acute and chronic respiratory failure (Berger & Matthay, 1981).

Assessment of blood volume status in patients with COPD and ARF is important. Frequently, an accurate non-invasive assessment is hampered by a baseline abnormal radiograph, chronic lung disease with abnormal auscultory findings and/or concurrent right-sided heart failure from cor pulmonale. In these cases, insertion of a flow directed pulmonary artery catheter (e.g. Swan–Ganz catheter) may provide useful information. Pulmonary artery pressure, pulmonary vascular resistance and cardiac output can be measured. However, the interpretation of accurate measurements has increasing complexity in the patient with COPD and ARF because of the wide variations in pleural pressure that often exists in these patients. Thus, these values should be interpreted cautiously in this clinical situation. Mixed venous oxygen content can be measured and total oxygen consumption computed. Appropriate use of the above information should allow the clinician to safely maximise cardiac output and therefore oxygen delivery without elevating pulmonary artery pressures or precipitating pulmonary oedema. There are complications associated with the catheter insertion (pneumothorax, haemothorax, ventricular arrhythmias, infective endocarditis, septicaemia from an indwelling catheter, rupture of pulmonary artery and perforation of ventricle) which can be minimised by the site of insertion, duration of monitoring and skill of operator. Most serious complications are rare and frequent complications (i.e., ventricular arrhythmias) are usually transient and rapidly reversible. Even so, some risk remains and because of this we do not advocate routine insertion of a pulmonary artery catheter in patients with ARF and COPD.

Other factors that can exacerbate COPD and lead to ARF are hypophosphatemia, malnutrition and body position. Decreases in serum phosphate can decrease oxygen delivery to tissues secondary to the shift of the oxyhaemoglobin dissociation curve. It may also increase the infection rate secondary to attenuated phagocytosis, bacterial killing and chemotaxis of polymorphonuclear cells (Craddock et al, 1974). Perhaps the most disastrous effect is on the diaphragm, where hypophosphatemia causes decreased contractility and as a result may interfere with weaning (Farber et al, 1977, 1982). Total parental nutrition has been shown to increase inspiratory muscle strength in normal patients (Kelly et al, 1984). While starvation weakens muscle strength (Anona & Rochester, 1982), the institution of hyperalimentation may exacerbate ARF because of the associated hypophosphatemia and increased CO_2 production (Covelli et al, 1981). It should be remembered that patients who present with ARF and COPD are relatively malnourished compared with individuals not in ARF (Driver et al, 1982). However, consumption of sufficient calories to produce an increase in body mass may cause an even greater increase in CO_2 production and impair weaning. We recommend a cautious approach to nutritional support especially near the time of weaning.

Normal individuals show a slight (6.5%) fall in vital capacity when changing position from standing to supine. Patients with obstructive disease tend to have a greater fall than patients with restrictive disease. Both these groups of patients tend to have greater falls in vital capacity by changing position than normal patients (Allen et al, 1982). As individuals go from standing to sitting to semi-recumbent to supine there is a marked fall in expiratory reserve volume (ERV) with a modest fall in functional residual volume (FRC); residual volume (RV) remains unchanged (Boren et al, 1966).

Management of the patient with ARF compounding CRF should also include optimising existing lung function and preventing any further deterioration. Subcutaneous heparin will significantly reduce the incidence of pulmonary embolism (Dingleton et al, 1981) and titration of antacids to neutralise gastric acidity will prevent stress ulceration (Khan et al, 1981; Prieke et al, 1980). The use of cimetidine or ranitidine, if gastric acid is effectively neutralised, may be as efficacious as antacids. The diagnosis of pulmonary embolism should be suspected in patients with CRF who have an acute decrease in the p_aCO_2 and p_aO_2 (Lippmann & Fein, 1981). In some patients with chronic hypercapnic respiratory failure, decreased carbohydrate intake combined with effective dieting may improve oxygen saturation, decrease resting heart rate, reduce ectopic ventricular contractions and decrease arterial carbon dioxide tension (Tirlapur & Mir, 1984). Yearly flu vaccines may reduce the incidence of viral upper respiratory tract infections due to influenza that precipitate ARF in the patient with CRF. Pneumovax administration has been the subject of some debate. Several recent articles offer contrasting views and conflicting recommendations (Bolan et al, 1986; Susk & Riegelman, 1986; Williams & Moser, 1986). An accompanying editorial (La Force & Eickhoff, 1986) offers some prudent advice, namely, patients hospitalised with pneumonia regardless of their underlying lung condition should probably receive pneumovax.

Oxygen therapy
A drug recently advocated in the treatment of ARF and COPD is oxygen (Campbell, 1964; King et al, 1973). In the hypoxaemic patient with CRF and ARF increasing the p_aO_2 to levels of 55 mm Hg significantly increase the oxygen content of the blood by virtue of the oxyhaemoglobin dissociation curve. A potential complication is an increase in the p_aCO_2 in patients with chronic hypercapnia. This may occur by several

mechanisms: the reestablishment of perfusion to poorly ventilated areas; the decrease in CO_2 binding to haemoglobin in the presence of increased amounts of oxyhaemoglobin (the Haldane effect (Luft et al, 1981; Christiansen et al, 1914)); and the suppression of respiratory drive (Aubier et al, 1980). The signs of CO_2 retention, such as stupor and coma (Campbell & Fabbis, 1966; Campbell, 1964; Warrell et al, 1970; Hutchinson et al, 1964), must be watched for during oxygen therapy. It may be possible to predict which patients in ARF will significantly retain CO_2 (Fig. 3.2, Bone et al, 1978). Two delivery systems of controlled oxygen therapy are nasal cannula and Venti-mask.

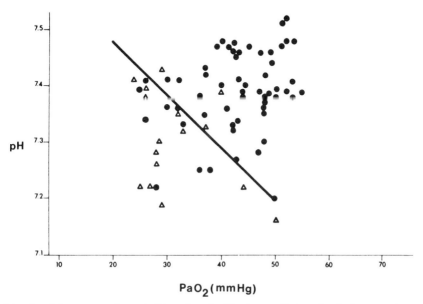

Fig. 3.2   Arterial oxygen tension and pH on admission blood gases. Patients developing somnolence on controlled oxygen therapy were in general severely hypoxemic or had a combination of moderate hypoxemia and acidosis. The graph demonstrates the importance of hypoxemia and acidosis as risk factors for carbon dioxide narcosis on controlled oxygen therapy. The line separating high from low risk patients was found by discriminant analysis (pH = 7.66–0.00919 PO_2). Closed circles, intubated patients; open triangles, non-intubated patients. (From Bone R C, Pierce A K, Johnson R L, Jr. 1978 American Journal of Medicine 65: 869.)

In the patient with COPD, CO_2 retention and normal resting hypoxaemia we recommend the Venti-mask system over the nasal cannula. The Venti-mask allows accurate control of inspired FIO_2 and this can be crucial in the patient with hypoxic drive and respiratory distress. Although the nasal cannula is more comfortable, the inspired oxygen concentration is significantly affected by the pattern of breathing i.e., nose vs. mouth, rate, tidal volume etc. Approximately 30 minutes after initiating oxygen therapy in the patient with COPD and ARF it is desirable to obtain an arterial blood gas measurement. If CO_2 retention is not observed we may repeat the measurement several hours later, even if there is no clinical deterioration, in patients we consider likely to retain carbon dioxide. If the arterial blood gas obtained 30 minutes after instituting oxygen therapy demonstrates significant CO_2 retention (greater than 6 mm Hg), the risk–benefit ratio of oxygen administration must be considered. Any time a patient's condition worsens, a careful reassessment of physiologic parameters (oxygenation, acid–base status, blood pressure, etc.) is essential. If improvement of the patient's oxygenation to levels approaching 90% saturation is crucial, then elective intubation may be necessary. This may occur in patients with COPD and ARF complicated by acute myocardial infarction, significant arrhythmia or an acute change in mental status. In all patients, especially the hypoxaemic patient with significant CO_2 retention from oxygen therapy, non-invasive monitoring of oxygen saturation by ear oximetry is an ideal continuous method of evaluating changes in arterial oxygen saturation.

Use of oxygen therapy for treatment of hypoxic CRF, with and without cor pulmonale, has been advocated (Petty et al, 1979; Abraham et al, 1968). In two well done studies with some differences in patient populations, oxygen therapy has significantly improved survival of patients with COPD (Nocturnal Oxygen Therapy Trial Group, 1980; MRC, 1981). The mechanism of improvement in patients without cor pulmonale remains unclear. It has been shown that oxygen therapy in these patients reduces pulmonary hypertension and ventricular arrhythmias as well as improves EEG function (Abraham et al, 1968; Flick & Block, 1979; Coccagna & Lugaresi, 1978; Brezinuva et al, 1979). In fact, a significant fall in mean pulmonary artery pressure after oxygen therapy may be predictive of improved survival (Timms et al, 1985). The danger of CO_2 retention exists in these patients as well. In a recent study (Goldstein et al, 1984), oxygen treatment of all patients with hypoxic respiratory failure resulted in an insignificant rise (less than 6 mm Hg) in p_aCO_2 in 80% of patients. Patients with early morning headaches and/or significant acute CO_2 retention with oxygen therapy are likely to have obstructive sleep apnea (Goldstein et al, 1984). Some authors believe oxygen therapy in sleep apnea may be potentially dangerous (Guilleminault et al, 1980). However, two studies have presented convincing evidence that nocturnal oxygen therapy may actually cure sleep apnea (Martin et al, 1982a; McNicholas et al, 1982), suggesting that the institution of oxygen therapy in patients with COPD and sleep apnea must be individualised. An excellent review of the effects of long term oxygen therapy in a variety of patients has recently been published (Anthonisen, 1983).

Bronchodilator and stimulant agents
Several other interventions in the treatment of ARF and CRF deserve mention. After many years of debate, a large multicentre trial has concluded that bronchodilator aerosol delivered via an intermittent positive pressure breathing (IPPB) machine is equivalent to medication delivered by nebuliser with regard to mortality, rate and duration of hospitalisation, change in lung function and effect on life quality (IPPB Trial Group, 1983). Although this study did exclude patients with resting hypoxaemia or restrictive disease, we do not recommend IPPB in the treatment of patients with CRF or ARF in the patient that does not require intubation.

Another drug frequently effective in ARF and CRF is theophylline (Bukowskyj et al, 1984). Methylxanthines are extremely effective in improving both cardiac and pulmonary function. Recent studies show that theophylline improves right and left ventricular ejection fraction in both normal patients and patients with COPD (Matthay et al, 1978). Methylxanthines have also been shown to improve diaphragmatic contractility in normal individuals (Aubier et al, 1981), in patients with COPD (Murciano et al, 1984) and in animals in ARF (Vires et al, 1984). An additive effect when combined with a beta-agonist has been documented in patients with COPD (Lamont et al, 1982). A recent study indicates that the improvement in diaphragmatic contractility and resistance to fatigue persists 7 and 30 days after treatment (Murciano et al, 1984). The authors suggest that this improvement is not through increased central stimulation.

Treated with theophylline, patients with COPD have also shown an improvement in forced vital capacity (FVC) and in the FEV_1 (Matthay et al, 1978; Alexander et al, 1980). One other study supporting the use of theophylline in patients with COPD has shown a decrease in the work of breathing while walking and a fall in lung resistance (Jenne et al, 1984). Several reviews summarise many of the therapeutic actions of theophylline (McFadd, 1985; Van Dellen, 1979; Hendeles & Weinberger, 1983).

Because of the fluctuations in theophylline levels seen in critically ill patients (Powell et al, 1978), close monitoring of theophylline is essential. The dosing formula recommended is (Jenne, 1984):

Intravenous Loading Dose = 6 mg/kg for patients not already receiving theophylline
Intravenous Maintenance Dose = 0.5 mg/kg/hr in healthy non-smoking adults

We suggest modifying the maintenance dose by the following factors in the presence of the stated conditions:

Healthy smokers	1.6 × maintenance
Critically ill patients	0.8 × maintenance
Drugs such as cimetidine, erythromycin	0.5 × maintenance
Severe liver disease and	
Severe congestive heart failure	0.3 × maintenance

These guidelines will usually result in a theophylline level of 10–20 mg/l. A blood level should be obtained one hour after the maintenance dose is begun and the maintenance infusion adjusted to keep the blood level between 10–20 mg/l.

The use of beta-2 specific bronchodilators has been extremely effective especially when given by inhalation rather than orally. The most recent advance in inhaled bronchodilators is the documentation of significant reversibility with anticholinergic inhalants, greater than beta-agonists (Gross & Skorodin, 1984a). Atropine sulfate may be used in doses of 0.025 mg/kg every 4–8 hours (Pak et al, 1982). Although most anticholinergic drugs are not commercially available in the United States, within the next year several agents should be marketed. An article that reviews anticholinergic bronchodilators has just been published (Gross & Skorodin, 1984b).

Several other drugs have been tried in ARF. Corticosteroids have been shown (in doses of 0.5 mg/kg q6h) to improve airflow acutely when compared with placebo (Albert et al, 1980a,b). Naloxone has no effect in the treatment of ARF in a well designed randomised study (Montserrat et al, 1985). Doxapram has been used as a central stimulant of respiratory drive for 20 years and is effective when used in the appropriate patient (Moser et al, 1973). In doses of 0.5–1 mg/kg IV push, followed by a maintenance drip of 1–2 mg/min, it can stimulate patients with a suppressed respiratory drive secondary to anaesthesia, CO_2 narcosis or drug overdose. It is not a long-term solution for chronic hypoventilation.

Impending respiratory failure

Compared with normal patients, patients with COPD (with and without hypercapnia) have different breathing patterns (Burrows et al, 1966; Sorli et al, 1978). The phenomena of rapid, shallow breathing in patients with COPD is characteristic. Normal individuals attempt to minimise respiratory work and in patients with increased dead space and increased compliance (COPD) this should lead to slow deep breathing. The reasons why this does not occur include: the respiratory centre receiving impulses to increase respiratory drive; mechanical receptors in the lung and chest wall; and overworked respiratory muscle under disadvantageous length–tension conditions (Campbell & Howell, 1963; Ramsey, 1955, 1959; Levine, 1977, 1979).

Complaints of increased breathlessness, dyspnea, is sometimes used as a sign of impending respiratory failure. Unfortunately, this complaint is not associated with total O_2 consumption, change in minute ventilation or respiratory rate (Campbell et al, 1961, 1970). The sensation of dyspnea is thought to be secondary to 'length–tension' inappropriateness (Burki, 1980) and is not useful in predicting the onset of ventilatory failure.

Two physical signs sometimes seen in impending respiratory failure are dirhythmic breathing, sometimes termed respiratory alternans, and paradoxical abdominal motion (Sackner et al, 1984; Gilbert et al, 1979; Cohen et al, 1982). Seen in severely disabled and dyspneic patients with emphysema, dirhythmic breathing is thought to be a result of augmented respiratory drive coexisting with greatly increased respiratory mechanical impedance (Flemister et al, 1981). It appears to be a result of activating inspiratory muscles via two different central neural pathways whose influences converge on the medullary respiratory centre or on the respiratory muscle motor neuron. The result is a 'voluntary' attempt to take slow deep breaths (sleep abolished) and an 'involuntary' drive toward rapid, shallow breathing. The rapid shallow breathing is unaffected by consciousness, but will change with a change in p_aCO_2.

Mechanical ventilation

Despite optimal medical management, patients with COPD and ARF may require ventilatory support. Currently, the decision to intubate and mechanically ventilate the patient with ARF is solely a bedside judgment. As our sophistication improves, it may be possible to monitor routinely for respiratory fatigue and intervene before respiratory failure occurs. Presently arterial blood gas measurement associated with subjective clinical evaluation are the guides clinicians use for endotracheal intubation and mechanical ventilation.

Ideally, intubation should be performed by an experienced individual in a controlled setting. Although mechanical ventilation will decrease the work of breathing (Field et al, 1982), endotracheal intubation may be associated with a two to threefold increase in airway resistance (Sullivan et al, 1976). To minimise this effect, a large bore endotracheal tube (8 mm i.d.) should be inserted when possible (Demens et al, 1977).

Initially and during ventilatory support, checking for adequate alveolar ventilation and appropriate tube placement is extremely important. The occurrence of problems with either has been associated with increased morbidity and mortality (Zwillich et al, 1974). Cardiac monitoring is mandatory in the unstable patient with acute respiratory failure as these individuals have more arrhythmias than patients with acute myocardial infarction (Alcover et al, 1984; Holford & Mithoefer, 1973; Sideris et al, 1979).

In acutely ill patients intubated for ARF, we initially provide full respiratory support with high concentrations of inspired oxygen and the assist-control ventilator mode. After initial determination of arterial blood gases, we decrease the oxygen concentration to the level necessary to provide 90% saturation of haemoglobin. Significant loss of blood buffering capacity will impair weaning efforts. Tidal volumes of 7–10 ml/kg are usually appropriate and occasional sighs of 1.5–2 times tidal volume can be used.

Most important and frequently neglected is the use of appropriate inspiratory flow rates (Connors et al, 1981). Although the pattern of airflow delivery may be important (Dammann et al, 1978), incorrect adjustment of the inspiratory flow rate may have disastrous consequences. Ideally, for a given respiratory cycle, the ratio of inspiratory time to expiratory time should be 1:3. This allows for more complete air emptying in patients with chronic airflow limitation as well allowing time for venous return (Courhard et al, 1952). Care must be taken not to increase maximum airway pressure (P_{max}) excessively in an attempt to provide higher flow rates and shorten the inspiratory time.

Physiologic parameters in patients receiving mechanical ventilation should also be monitored. Gas exchange can be assessed by checking the respiratory rate and arterial blood gases. Daily chest radiographs are appropriate to detect complications. More sophisticated non-invasive monitoring equipment, such as end-tidal CO_2 monitors, ear oximeters, Co_2 monitors and recently the Respiragraph, are also available.

Other physiologic parameters that should be routinely monitored in patients with COPD and ARF are changes in pulmonary mechanics. Maximum airway pressure, tidal volume, minute ventilation and compliance can all be easily determined in patients receiving mechanical ventilation (Fallat, 1984). In the absence of on-line monitoring of flow rates, tracking the dynamic characteristic, which is defined as the tidal volume/(P_{max}) − PEEP) may be useful (Bone, 1976). Monitoring the peak pressure and static pressure over time can noninvasively lead to earlier detection of complications (Bone, 1976).

Weaning from mechanical ventilation

There is not a specific formula to determine when a patient no longer needs mechanical ventilation. As we have stated previously (Bone, 1980), weaning is truly an art. Prior to the discontinuation of mechanical ventilation, an attempt should be made to optimise all conditions which impact on weaning. Summarised recently by the mnemonic 'WEANS NOW' (Beaton & Bone, 1985), this includes consideration of the weaning tests, endotracheal tube size and patency, arterial blood gases, nutritional status, secretions, presence of neuromuscular disease, airflow obstruction and the degree of wakefulness. Reports have appeared of an inability to wean secondary to hypercapnia arising from carbohydrate feeding, so nutritional support must be tempered with good judgment (Dark et al, 1985).

There exist several schemes for evaluating when weaning should begin. Earlier reports used a resting minute ventilation (MV) less than 10 l/min, the ability to double the MV with a maximal voluntary ventilation (MVV) manoeuvre and the presence of a peak negative pressure on maximal inspiration (PNP) greater than $30\,cm\,H_2O$ to predict successfully who could safely have mechanical ventilation discontinued (Sahn & Lakshminaiayan, 1973). A much more sophisticated scoring system has recently been published. In this approach multiple factors, such as inspired oxygen content, positive end-expiratory pressure, static and dynamic compliance, ventilator delivered minute ventilation and machine triggered respiratory rate, are evaluated and a ventilator score is generated. This is combined with the adverse factor score which evaluates non-ventilator factors. These non-ventilator factors include heart rate, central venous pressure, temperature, arrhythmias, level of consciousness, emotional state, mobility, the quality and quantity of recreation, caloric intake, and the use of medications such as antibiotics, vasopressors, analgesics, sedative and steroids. This technique and other approaches to weaning have recently been reviewed (Morgan-noth et al, 1984; Nett et al, 1985). Regardless of the system used to assess the likelihood of weaning, there is no substitution for close observation while weaning.

Another approach has been to observe the patient during their first episode of spontaneous ventilation. Based on the number of the following six factors present (heart rate >120 or <70, respiratory rate >30, palpable scalene muscle retraction during inspiration, abdominal tensing during expiration, irregular respiratory rhythm with apnea of any duration, coma or any mental status that prevents a patient from performing a vital capacity manoeuvre) one can predict the likelihood of successfully terminating mechanical ventilation (Pardee et al, 1981). All patients with more than two of these factors were unable to wean from mechanical ventilation. A recent study of patients with COPD and ARF concluded that the work/litre of ventilation correlated with the mechanical properties of the lung and may be used as a guide for weaning (Fluery et al, 1985a).

There are several commonly used weaning modalities and a discussion of the different modes is available (Browne, 1984). Reviewed in depth (Luce et al, 1981; Weisman et al, 1983), intermittent mandatory ventilation (IMV) has been advocated for shortening the time a patient spends on a ventilator (Weaver et al, 1973, Downs et al, 1974). Recently, several authors have been critical of IMV as it may increase respiratory muscle work, thereby precipitating muscle failure and prolonging the need for mechanical ventilation (Williams, 1980; Gibney et al, 1981; Downs, 1978; Christopher et al, 1981, 1983).

Probably the most common form of weaning patients with COPD is intermittent T-piece trials. These trials of spontaneous breathing are performed for short periods of time with a gradual increase in the duration and number of daily trials. In the appropriate patient it may be possible to deflate the inflated endotracheal cuff to further decrease airway resistance and postpone the onset of muscular fatigue. Obviously this would not be prudent in patients at high risk for aspiration. Significant coughing after deflation of the cuff indicates probable aspiration and the cuff should be reinflated and left inflated throughout weaning.

Muscle training
Potentially one of the greatest tools to prevent ARF and facilitate weaning is inspiratory muscle training. It has been demonstrated that a comprehensive exercise programme combined with chest physical therapy, controlled oxygen and antibiotics does increase exercise tolerance in patients with severe airflow obstruction although no significant

changes in pulmonary function tests were observed (Petty et al, 1969). Other studies have shown that exercise training lowers pulmonary artery pressure at rest, increases p_aO_2 and decreases resting cardiac output (Pierce et al, 1964; Paez et al, 1967; Christie, 1968; Nicholass et al, 1970). Animal studies and studies in patients with cystic fibrosis, COPD, quadriplegia and normal lung function all show an increase in muscle strength and endurance with exercise training (Leith & Bradly, 1976; Lieberman et al, 1973; Pardee et al, 1981; Gross et al, 1978; Keens et al, 1977; Sunne & Pavis, 1982; Gross et al, 1981) and exercise has even facilitated weaning in some cases (Aldrich & Karpel, 1985). This is thought to occur by an increase in the percent of fatigue-resistant, high oxidative capacity muscle fibres in the diaphragm as well as an improved delivery of oxygen and nutrients (Lieberman et al, 1972; Keens et al, 1978; Holloszy & Booth, 1976). A more detailed discussion is available (Braun et al, 1983; Dantzker, 1985; Rochester & Campbell, 1979; Derenne et al, 1978).

There are three areas of controversy surrounding inspiratory muscle training. First, while it is generally agreed that 'deconditioning' occurs after the cessation of a training programme and that too much exercise can lead to muscle fatigue, the point at which useful exercise becomes counterproductive for the respiratory muscles is not clear. Second, it is thought that an improvement in endurance rather than strength is more useful (Dantzker, 1985), however, there may be occasions when an increase in maximum muscle tension is desirable. The third area of controversy is what type of exercise is most useful and which muscles should be trained. While most training programmes are directed at the respiratory system, it must be kept in mind that preferential training of one group of muscles may not be optimal (Bradley & Leith, 1978). Muscle work can be increased by resistive loading i.e., increasing the resistance that the muscles must overcome or by volume loading as occurs when breathing abnormally high concentrations of carbon dioxide in experimental situations. Which of these two methods of training is preferable is debatable.

Tracheostomy

Tracheostomy used to be performed early in the hospital course of patients on mechanical ventilation because of the high incidence of complication resulting from the high pressure endotracheal cuffs. With the newer high compliance, low pressure cuffs it has been shown that there is no greater incidence of tracheal complications with long term (21 days) endotracheal intubation then with early tracheostomy (Stauffer et al, 1981). Although ventilation through a tracheostomy tube is more comfortable than nasotrachael or oratracheal ventilation we do not advocate routine early tracheostomy unless it is clear that the patient will be ventilator dependent for greater than 3 weeks. Tracheostomy decreases the patients ability to clear secretions as well as deprives them of 'intrinsic' PEEP (Fleury et al, 1985b) after discontinuation of ventilation.

Patients with ARF and COPD who receive ventilatory support for long periods of time demonstrate decreased responsiveness to hypercapnia. This may be from aggressive use of diuretics leading to a contraction alkalosis with an increased serum bicarbonate level. Other possibilities include decreased respiratory drive and muscle atrophy. In a small study of patients with COPD and ARF, the patients who recovered their sensitivity to CO_2 6–10 hours after the discontinuation of mechanical ventilation did well. Those patients who did not recover their sensitivity either died or were pulmonary cripples (Amaka & Mureyasu, 1981).

Despite all attempts to wean patients, there is a group of patients with COPD and ARF who will need long-term ventilator support. We agree with a recent editorial (George, 1985) and support home health care for stable ventilator dependent patients.

PROGNOSIS

In ARF complicating COPD, the short-term survival is excellent (Martin et al, 1982b), while the long-term survival is not. This is in contrast to ARDS where the in-hospital mortality is high, but survivors have a normal life expectancy (Demling & Nerlich, 1983). The two-year mortality in patients with COPD who required intubation for treatment of ARF has been reported to be 66% (Gottlieb & Balchun, 1973). Without oxygen therapy the yearly mortality had been reported to be as high as 20–48% (Renzetti et al, 1966). In that study, VC, RV/TLC, FEV_1, arterial blood gases and degree of RVH were all accurate prognostic indicators. The presence of weight loss, radiographic evidence of emphysema or decreased DLCO signified decreased survival. The presence or absence of polycythaemia did not appear to affect survival.

Oxygen therapy clearly prolongs survival (Nocturnal Oxygen Therapy Trial Group, 1980; MRC, 1981). A recent study indicates that a change in pulmonary artery pressures over 6 months of oxygen treatment correlated with survival, both in patients with 12 hour and patients with continuous oxygen therapy (Timms et al, 1985). The presence of dirhythmic breathing in oxygen treated patients with CRF may portend a poor prognosis (Gilbert et al, 1977). A more recent study found that VC and p_aO_2 were good discriminators for survival, but FEV_1 and FEV_1/FVC were not. The authors reported a 4-year survival of 46%. Although hypoxia and hypercapnia are poor prognosticators, the worst prognostic factor appears to be the presence of right sided CHF and RVH (Mitchell et al, 1969; Neff & Petty, 1970). Although the presence of cor pulmonale has been thought to be one of the worst prognostic factors, this has been challenged by a recent study (Kawakami et al, 1983). This study suggests that impaired right heart function and elevated pulmonary artery pressures do not portend a poor outcome, unless they are associated with evidence of poor oxygen delivery as manifested by abnormal mixed venous oxygen content. If this is confirmed, it may be possible to stratify survival based on dynamic physiologic properties and institute treatment to reverse abnormal physiologic conditions.

CONCLUSIONS

The diagnosis of impending respiratory failure remains a difficult clinical assessment. Although physical signs, arterial blood gases and physiological studies are helpful, the decision to institute ventilatory support must be made by a clinician at the bedside. Optimal therapy involves prevention of the development of ARF as well as the identification and treatment of precipitating factors whenever possible. Short term survival remains good, however even with aggressive out-patient therapy long term survival remains poor. With a better understanding of pulmonary pathophysiology and advances in technology to monitor their changes, it may be possible to detect the initial onset of ARF in patients with COPD as well as improve patients long-term outlook.

REFERENCES

Abraham A S, Cole R B, Bishop J M 1968 Reversal of pulmonary hypertension in patients with chronic bronchitis. Circ Res 23: 147–157

ACCP–ATS Joint Commission on pulmonary nomenclature. ACCP, ATS 1975 Pulmonary term and symbols. Chest 67: 583–593

Albert R, Martin R, Lewis S 1980a Methylprednisolone improving chronic bronchitis with acute respiratory insufficiency. Chest 77: 314–315

Albert A K, Martin T R, Lewis S W 1980b Controlled clinical trial of methylprednisolone in patients with chronic bronchitis and acute respiratory failure. Ann Int Med 92(6): 753–758

Alcover I A, Henning R J, Jackson P L 1984 A computer-assisted monitoring system for arrhythmia detection in a medical intensive care unit. Crit Care Med 12: 888–892

Aldrich T K, Karpel J P 1985 Inspiratory muscle resistance training in respiratory failure. Am Rev Resp Dis 131(3): 461–462

Alexander M R, Dull W L, Kasik J E 1980 Treatment of chronic obstructive pulmonary disease with orally administered theophylline, a double-blind, controlled study. JAMA 244: 2286–2290

Allen S M et al 1982 Fall in vital capacity with posture. Brit J Dis Chest 79: 267–271

Amaha K, Mureyasu S 1981 Ventilatory response to carbon dioxide in patients after long-term ventilation for acute respiratory failure secondary to chronic obstructive lung disease. Crit Care Med 9(11): 796–800

Anderson R J, Pluss R C, Berns A S, Jackson J T, Arnold P E, Schrier R W et al 1978 Mechanisms of effect of hypoxia on renal water excretion. J Clin Invest 62: 769–777

Anthonisen N R 1983 Long-term oxygen therapy. Ann Int Med 99: 519–527

Arora N S, Rochester D F 1982 Respiratory muscle strength and MVV in undernourished patients. Am Rev Resp Dis 126(9): 5–8

Aubier M, Murciano D, Fournier M, Milic-Emili J, Pairente R, Derenne J P 1980a Central respiratory drive in acute respiratory failure of patients with chronic obstructive pulmonary disease. Am Rev Resp Dis 122: 191–199

Aubier M, Murciane D, Milic-Emili J et al 1980b Effects of the administration of oxygen on ventilation and blood gases in patients with chronic obstructive pulmonary disease during acute respiratory failure. Am Rev Resp Dis 122(5): 747–754

Aubier M, De Troyer A, Sampson M, Machlem P T, Roussos C 1981 Aminophylline improves diaphragmatic contractility. N Engl J Med 305: 249–252

Aubier M, Murciano D, Lecocouic Y, Viires N, Jacquens Y, Squarn D, Pariente R 1985 Effect of hypophosphotemia on diaphragm contractility in patients with acute respiratory failure. N Engl J Med 313(7): 420–424

Augisti A G, Jones A, Estopa R et al 1984 Hypophophatemia as a cause of failed weaning: The importance of metabolic factors. Crit Care Med 12: 142

Balk R, Bone R C 1983 The adult respiratory distress syndrome. Medical Clinics of North America 67(3): 685–701

Beaten N, Bone R C 1985 Criteria for weaning your patients from respirators. J of Resp Dis 6(4): 80–83

Bell R C, Coalson J J, Smith J D, Johanson W G 1983 Multiple organ system failure and infection in adult respiratory distress syndrome. Annals of Internal Medicine 99: 293–298

Bellemare F, Grassino A 1982 Effect of pressure and timing of contraction on human diaphragm fatigue. Journal of Applied Physiology 53: 1196–1206

Bellemore F, Grassino A 1983 Force reserve of diaphragm in patients with chronic obstructive pulmonary disease. J Appl Phys 55: 8

Berger H J, Matthay R A 1981 Noninvasive radiographic assessment of cardiovascular function in acute and chronic respiratory failure. Am J Cardiol 47: 950

Bigland B, Lippold O C J 1954 The relationship between force, velocity and integrated electrical activity in human muscles. Journal of Physiology (London) 123: 214–224

Bolan G, Broome C, Fachlam R R et al 1986 Pneumococcal vaccine efficacy in selected populations in the United States. Ann Int Med 104(1): 1–6

Bone R C 1976 Thoracic pressure-volume curves in respiratory failure. Crit Care Med 4: 148

Bone R C 1980 Treatment of respiratory failure due to advanced chronic obstructive lung disease. Arch Int Med 140: 1018–1021

Bone R C 1981 Acute respiratory failure and chronic obstructive lung disease: Recent advances. Medical Clinics of North America 65(3): 563–578

Bone R C, Pierce A K, Johnson R L 1978 Controlled oxygen administration in adult respiratory failure in chronic obstructive pulmonary disease. Am J Med 65: 896–902

Boren H G, Kory R L, Syner J C 1966 VA-Army Cooperative study of pulmonary function. Am J Med 41: 96–114

Bradley M E, Leith D E 1978 Ventilatory muscle training and the oxygen cost of sustained hyperpnea.

J Appl Phys 45: 885–892

Braun N M T, Faulkener J, Hughes R L, Roussos C, Sahgal V 1983 When should respiratory muscles be exercised. Chest 84(1): 76–84

Brezinuva V, Calverley D M A, Flenley P C, Townsend H R A 1979 The effect of long-term oxygen on the EEG in patients with stable ventilatory failure. Bull Eur Physiopath Res 15: 603–609

Browne D R 1984 Weaning from mechanical ventilation. Intensive Care Med 10: 55

Bukowskyj M, Nakatsu K, Munt P W 1984 Theophylline therapy reassessed. Ann Int Med 101(1): 63–73

Burk R H, George R B 1973 Acute respiratory failure in chronic obstructive lung disease. Arch Int Med 132: 865

Burki N K 1980 Dyspnea in chronic airway obstruction. Chest 77(2): sup 298–299

Burrows B, Saksena F B, Diener G F 1966 Carbon dioxide tension and ventilatory mechanics in obstructive lung disease. Ann Int Med 65: 685–700

Campbell E J M 1964 Management of respiratory failure. Brit Med J 2: 1328–1338

Campbell E J M, Fabbis T 1966 Mask and tent for providing controlled oxygen concentration. Lancet 1: 468

Campbell E J M, Howell J B L 1963 The sensation of breathlessness. Brit Med Bull 19: 36

Campbell E J M, Freedman S, Smith P S et al 1961 The ability of man to detect added elastic loading to breathing. Clin Sci 20: 223–231

Campbell E J M, Newsome D J 1970 Respiratory sensation. In: The Respiratory Muscles. Campbell E T M, Agostoni E, Newsome D T eds. Philadelphia, Saunders, p. 291

Christiansen J, Douglas C G, Haldane J S 1914 The absorption and dissolution of carbon dioxide by human blood. J Phys Clin (London) 48: 244

Christie D 1968 Physical training in chronic obstructive lung disease. Brit Med J 2: 150–151

Christopher K L, Good J T, Bowman J L et al 1981 Should chronic obstructive pulmonary disease patients be weaned by T piece or intermittent mandatory ventilation. A comparison of pressure and resistance in different systems. Chest 80: 381

Christopher H L, Neff T A, Bowman J L, Eberle D J, Irvin C G, Good S T 1985 Demand and continuous flow intermittent mandatory ventilation systems. Chest 87(5): 625–630

Ciba Guest Symposium 1959 Terminology, definition and classification of chronic pulmonary emphysema and related conditions. Thorax 14: 286–299

Coccagna G, Lugaresi E 1978 Arterial blood gas and pulmonary and systemic arterial pressure during sleep in chronic obstructive pulmonary disease. Sleep 1: 117–124

Cohen C A, Zagelbaum G, Gross D et al 1982 Clinical manifestations of respiratory muscle fatigue. Am J Med 73(3): 308–316

Connors A F Jr, McCaffres D R, Gray B A 1981 Effect of inspiratory flow rate on gas exchange during mechanical ventilation. Am Rev Resp Dis 124(5): 537–543

Cournard A, Motley H C, Werko C et al 1952 Physiological study of the effects of intermittent positive breathing on cardiac output in man. J Appl Phys 152: 162–174

Covelli H D, Black J W, Olsen M S et al 1981 Respiratory failure precipitated by high carbohydrate load. Ann Int Med 95(5): 579–581

Cotes J E, Piza Z, Thomas A T 1963 Effects of breathing oxygen upon cardiac output, heart rates, ventilation, systemic and pulmonary blood pressure in patients with chronic lung disease. Clin Sci 25: 305–321

Craddock Y, Yawata L, VanSonten S et al 1974 Acquired phagocyte dysfunction: A complication of the hypophosphatemia of parental hyperalimentation. N Engl J Med 290: 1403–1407

Dammann J F, McAsian T C, Maffeo C J 1978 Optimal flow pattern for mechanical ventilation of the lung. The effect of sine vs. square wave for flow pattern with and without end inspiratory pressure on patients. Crit Care Med 6(5): 693–310

Dantzker D R 1985 Respiratory muscle function and fatigue. In: Critical Care: A comprehensive approach. Ed. R. C. Bone. Park Ridge, Il: ACCP, pp. 48–59

Dark P S, Pingleton S K, Kerby G R 1985 Hypercapnia during weaning. A complication of nutritional support. Chest 88(1): 141–143

Demers P R, Sullivan M T, Paliottz J 1977 Airflow resistance of endotracheal tubes. JAMA 237(13), 1362

Demling R H, Nerlich M 1983 Acute respiratory failure. Med Clin North Am 63(2): 337–355

Derenne J-D H, Macklem P T, Roussos C 1978 The respiratory muscles: mechanics, control and pathophysiology. Am Rev Resp Dis 118: 119–133, 373–390, 581–601

Downs J B 1978 Inappropriate application of intermittent mandatory ventilation. Chest 78: 897

Downs J B, Perkins H M, Modell J M 1974 Intermittent mandatory ventilation: An evaluation. Arch Surg 109: 519–523

Driver A G, McAlevy M T, Smith J L 1982 Nutritional assessment of patients with chronic obstructive pulmonary disease and acute respiratory failure. Chest 82(5), 568–567

Fallat R J 1984 Respiratory monitoring. In: Critical care: A comprehensive approach. Ed. R. C. Bone. Park Ridge, Il: ACCP, 189–205

Farber M O, Bright T P, Strawbridge R A, Robertson G L, Manfredi F 1975 Impaired water handling in chronic obstructive lung disease. J Lab Clin Pred 85: 141–149

Farber M O, Kiblawi S S O, Strawbridge R A, Robertson F L, Weinberger M H, Manfredi E 1977 Studies on plama vasopression and the renin-angiotension-aldosterone system in chronic obstructive lung disease. J Lab Clin Med 90: 373–380

Farber M O, Roberts C R, Weinberger M H, Robertson G L, Feinberg G S, Manfriedi F 1982 Abnormalities of sodium and water handling in chronic obstructive lung disease. Arch Int Med 142: 1326–1330

Farber M O, Weinberg M H, Robertson F L, Fineberg N S, Manfredi F 1984 Hormonal abnormalities affecting sodium and water balance in acute respiratory failure due to chronic obstructive lung disease. Chest 85(1): 49–54

Farkas G A, Roussos C 1982 Adaptability of the hamster diaphragm to exercise and or emphysema. Journal of Applied Physiology, Respiration, Environment, and Physiotherapy 53: 1263–1272

Flemister G, Goldberg N B, Sharp J T 1981 Dirhythmic breathing. Chest 79(1): 33–39

Field S, Kelly S M, Macklem P T 1982 The oxygen cost of breathing in patients with cardiorespiratory disease. Am Rev Resp Dis 126: 9

Fleury B, Murciano D, Talamo C et al 1985a Work of breathing in patients with chronic obstructive pulmonary disease in acute respiratory failure. Am Rev Resp Dis 131: 822

Fleury B, Murciano D, Talamo G, Aubier M, Pariente R, Milic-Emili J 1985b Work of breathing patients with chronic obstructive pulmonary disease in acute respiratory failure. Am Rev Resp Dis 131: 822–827

Flick M R, Block A J 1979 Nocturnal vs. diurnal cardiac arrhythmias in patients with chronic obstructive pulmonary disease. Chest 75: 8–11

Francis P B 1983 Acute respiratory failure in obstructive lung disease. Med Clin North Am 67: 657–668

Freedman S 1970 Sustained maximum voluntary ventilation. Resp Phys 8: 230–244

George R 1985 Long term hospitalization of the ventilator dependent patient. Arch Int Med 145: 2089

Gibney R T N, Wilson R S, Pontoppidan H 1981 Comparison of work of breathing on high gas flow and demand value continuous positive airway pressure system (abstract). Chest 80: 382

Gilbert R, Ashutosh K, Auchincloss J H et al 1975 Asynchronous breathing movements in patients with chronic obstructive pulmonary disease. Chest 67: 553–557

Gilbert R, Ashutosh K, Auchincloss J H et al 1977 Prospective study of controlled oxygen therapy: Poor prognosis of patients with asynchrynous breathing. Chest 71: 456–462

Goldman M D, Grassino A, Mead J, Sears T A 1978 Mechanics of human diaphragm during voluntary contractions: Dynamics. J Appl Phys 44: 840–848

Goldstein R S, Ramcharan V, Bowes G et al 1984 Effects of supplemental nocturnal oxygen on gas exchange in patients with severe obstructive lung disease. N Engl J Med 310(7): 425–429

Gonzales N C, Gerbrandt M, Brown E B 1976 Changes in skeletal muscle cell pH during graded changes in pCO_2. Resp Physio 26: 207–212

Gottlieb L S, Balchum D J 1973 Course of chronic obstructive pulmonary disease following first onset of respiratory failure. Chest 63: 5–8

Grassino A, Macklem P T 1984 Respiratory muscle fatigue and ventilation. Ann Rev Med 35: 625

Grassino A, Goldman M D, Mead J, Sears T A 1978 Mechanics of the human diaphragm during voluntary contractions: Statics. J Appl Phys 44: 829–837

Gross N J, Skorodin M S 1984a Role of the parasympathetic system in airway obstruction due to emphysema. N Engl J Med 311: 421–425

Gross N J, Skorodin M S 1984b Anticholinergic antimuscurinic bronchodilator. Am Rev Resp Dis 129: 856

Gross D, Grassino P, Ross W R D, Macklem P T 1973 Electromyogram pattern of diaphragmatic fatigue. J Appl Phys 46: 1–7

Gross P, Riley E, Ladd A, Macklem P T 1978 Influence of resistive training on respiratory muscle strength and endurance in quadraplegia (abstract). Am Rev Resp Dis 117: S343

Gross D, Ladd H W, Riley E J, Macklem P T, Grassino A 1981 The effect of training on strength and endurance of the diaphragm in quadriplegia. Am J Med 68: 27–34

Guilleminault C, Cummiskey J, Motta J 1980 Chronic obstructive airway disease and sleep study. Am Rev Resp Dis 122: 397

Hendeles L, Weinberger M 1983 Theophylline: A state of the art review. Pharmacotherapy 3: 2–44

Hermansen L 1981 Effect of metabolic changes on force generation in skeletal muscle during maximum exercise. In: Porter R, Whelan J, eds. Human Muscle Fatigue: Physiological mechanism. London Pittman 75–88 (Ciba Foundation Symposium 1982)

Hill N S 1986 Fluid and electrolyte considerations in diuretic therapy for hypertension in patients with chronic obstructive lung disease. Arch Int Med 146: 129–133

Holford F D, Mithoefer J C 1973 Cardiac arrhythmia in hospitalized patients with chronic obstructive pulmonary disease. Am Rev Resp Dis 108(4): 879–885

Holloszy J O, Booth F W 1976 Biochemical adaptions to endurance exercise in muscles. Ann Rev Physio 38: 273–291

Huddy R B, Jones D M, Lee H G 1973 Tetracycline and co-trimoxocole in acute exacerbation of chronic bronchitis. Brit J Dis Chest 67: 212–215

Hudson L D, ed. 1981 Adult respiratory distress syndrome. Seminar in Respiratory Medicine 2: 99–174

Hutchinson D C S, Flenley D C, Donald M W 1964 Controlled oxygen therapy in respiratory failure. Brit Med J 2: 1159–1166

JPPB Trial Group 1983 Intermittent positive pressure breathing therapy of chronic obstructive pulmonary disease. Ann Int Med 99: 612–620

Jenne J W 1984 Pulmonary drugs. In: Critical Care: A Comprehensive approach, R C Bone, ed., Park Ridge, IL: ACCP, pp 223–250

Jenne J W, Slever J R, Druz W S, Solano J V, Cohen S M, Sharp J T 1984 The effect of maintaining theophylline therapy on lung work in severe chronic obstructive pulmonary disease while standing and walking. Am Rev Resp Dis 130(4): 600–605

Juan G, Calverley P, Talamo C, Schrader J, Roussos C 1984 Effect of carbon dioxide on diaphragmatic function in humans. N Engl J Med 310(14): 874–879

Katz A M, Hecht H M 1969 The early 'pump' failure of the ischmic heart. Am J Med 47: 497–502

Kawakami Y, Irie T, Kishi F 1982 Criteria for pulmonary and respiratory failure in chronic obstructive pulmonary disease patients — A theoretical study based on clinical data. Respiration 43: 436–443

Kawakami Y, Kishi F, Yamamoto H, Miyamoto K 1983 Relation of oxygen delivery, mixed venous oxygenation and pulmonary hemodynamics to prognosis in chronic obstructive pulmonary diseaes. N Engl J Med 308: 1045–1049

Keens T G, Krastins I R B, Wannamaker E M, Levinson H, Crozier D N, Bryan A C 1977 Ventilatory muscle endurance training in normal subjects and patients with cystic fibrosis. Am Rev Resp Dis 116: 853–860

Keens T G, Chen V, Patel P, O'Brien P, Levinson H, Ianuzzo D 1978 Cellular adaption of ventilatory muscles to a chronic respiratory load. J Appl Phys 44: 905–908

Kelly S M, Rosa A, Field S et al 1984 Inspiratory muscle strength and body composition in patients receiving total parenteral nutrition therapy. Am Rev Resp Dis 130: 33 37

Khan F, Parekh A, Patel S et al 1981 Result of gastric neutrilization with hourly antacids and cimetidine in 320 intubated patients with respiratory failure. Chest 79(4): 409–412

Kim M J, Druz W S, Danon J, Sharp J T 1979 Force length characteristics of canine diaphragm. American Review of Respiratory Disease 119: supp. 37–39

King T K, Ali N, Briscoe W A 1973 Treatment of hypoxia with 24% oxygen: A new approach to the interpretation of data obtained in a pulmonary intensive care unit. Am Rev Resp Dis 108(1): 19–29

LaForce F M, Eickhoff T C 1986 Pneumococcal vaccine: The evidence mounts. Ann Int Med 104(1): 106–109

Lamont H, Van der Straeten M, Pauwel R et al 1982 The combined effect of theophylline and terbutaline in patients with chronic obstructive airway disease. Eur J Resp Dis 63(1): 13–22

Lee J, Read J 1967 Effects of oxygen breath on distribution of pulmonary blood flow in chronic obstructive lung disease. Am Rev Resp Dis 96: 1173–1180

Leith D E, Bradly M 1976 Ventilatory muscle strength and endurance training. J Apply Phys 41: 508–516

Levine S 1977 Role of tissue hypermetabolism in stimulation of ventilation by dinitrophenol. J Appl Phys 43: 72

Levine S 1979 Ventilatory response to muscle exercise: Observation regarding a humoral pathway. J Appl Phys 47: 126

Lieberman P A, Maxwell C C, Faukner J A 1972 Adaption of guinea pig diaphragm muscle to aging and endurance training. Am J Phys 222: 556–560

Lieberman D A, Faulkner J A, Crais A B T R, Maxwell L L 1973 Performance and histochemical composition of guinea pig and human diaphragm. J Appl Phys 34: 233–237

Lindstrom L, Magnusson R, Peterson I 1970 Muscle fatigue and action potential conduction velocity changes studied with frequency analysis of electromyogram signals. Clin Neurophysiol 10: 341

Lippmann M, Fein A 1981 Pulmonary embolus in the patient with chronic obstructive lung disease: A diagnostic dilemma. Chest 79: 39

Luce J M, Pierson D J, Hudson L D 1981 Intermittent mandatory ventilation. Chest 79: 6

Luft U C, Mustyn E M, Loeppky J A, Venters M D 1981 Contribution of the Haldane effect to the rise of arterial PCO_2 in hypoxic patients breathing oxygen. Crit Care Med 9(1): 32–37

McFadd E R (ed.) 1985 Update on Methylxanthine therapy. Am J Med 79(6A): 1–79

Macklem P T, Permutt S (eds) 1979 The Lung in Transition Between Health and Disease. 1st Ed NY, Marcel Deckker, pp. 389–398

McNicholas W T, Caster J L, Rutherford et al 1982 Beneficial effects of oxygen in 1° alveolar hypoventilation. Am Rev Resp Dis 125: 773

Martin R J, Sanders M H, Gay B A et al 1982a Acute and long-term ventilatory effect of hyperoxia in the adult sleep apnea syndrome. Am Rev Resp Dis 125: 175

Martin T R, Lewis S W, Albert R H 1982 The prognosis of patients with chronic obstructive pulmonary disease after hospitalization for acute respiratory failure. Chest 82(3): 310–314

Mathur P N, Pugsley S O, Powles A L, McEwan M P, Campbell E J 1984 Effect of diuretics on cardiopulmonary performance in severe chronic airflow obstruction. A controlled clinical trial. Arch Int Med 144(11): 2154–2157

Matthay R A, Berger H J, Loke J et al 1978 Effects of Aminophylline upon right and left ventricular performance in chronic obstructive pulmonary disease. Am J Med 65: 903–910

Medical Research Council 1981 Long term domiciliary oxygen in chronic hypoxic cor pulmonale complicating chronic bronchitis and emphysema: Report of the Medical Research Council Working Party. Lancet 1: 681–686

Mitchell R S, Webb W C, Filley G F 1969 Chronic obstructive bronchopulmonary disease. III. Factors influencing prognosis. Am Rev Resp Dis 89: 878

Montserrat J M, Ballester E, Sopeina J J, Picado C 1985 Effect of nadoxone on arterial blood gases in chronically obstructed patients with adult respiratory failure. Eur J Resp Dis 66(1): 77–79

Morganroth M C, Morganroth J L, Nett L M et al 1984 Criteria for weaning from prolonged mechanical ventilation. Arch Int Med 144: 1012

Moser K M, Lachsinger P C, Adamson J S et al 1973 Respiratory stimulation with intravenous doxapram in respiratory failure. N Engl J Med 288: 427–431

Murciano D, Aubier M, Lerocguic Y, Pariente R 1984 Effects of theophyline on diaphragmatic strength and fatigue in patients with chronic obstructive pulmonary disease. N Engl J Med 311(6): 349–353

Murray J F and Division of Lung Disease, National Heart, Lung and Blood Institute 1979 Mechanisms of acute respiratory failure. Am Rev Resp Dis 115: 1071–1078

Nakamaru Y, Schwartz A 1972 The influence of hydrogen ion concentration on calcium binding and release by skeletal muscle sarcoplasmic reticulum. J Gen Physio 59: 22–32

Neff T A, Petty T L 1970 Long-term continuous oxygen therapy in chronic airflow obstruction: Mortality in relationship to corpulmonale, hypoxemia, hypercapnia. Ann Int Med 72: 621–626

Nett L M, Morganroth M L, Petty T L 1985 Weaning from mechanical ventilation. A perspective and review of technique. R C Bone, ed. Crit Care: A Comprehensive Approach, Park Ridge, Ill., ACCP, 171–184

Nicholass J T, Gilbert R, Gabe R, Auchincloss J H 1970 Evaluation of an exercise program for patients with chronic obstructive pulmonary disease. Am Rev Resp Dis 102: 1–9

Nicotra M B, Rivera M, Aure R J 1982 Antibiotics therapy in exacerbation of chronic bronchitis: A controlled clinical trial with tetracycline. Ann Int Med 97: 18

Nocturnal oxygen therapy trial group 1980 Continuous or nocturnal oxygen therapy in hypoxemic chronic obstructive lung disease: A clinical trial. Ann Int Med 93: 391–398

O'Donohue W J, Jr, Baker J P, Bell G M et al 1970 The management of acute respiratory failure in a respiratory intensive care unit. Chest 58: 603–610

Paez P N, Phillipson E A, Masangkay M, Sproule B T 1967 The physiological basis for training patients with emphysema. Am Rev Resp Dis 95: 944–953

Pak C C, Kradjan W A, Lakshminasayan S et al 1982 Inhaled atropine sulfate: dose response characteristics in patients with chronic airway obstruction. Am Rev Resp Dis 25(3): 331–334

Pardee N E, Winterbauer R H, Allen J D 1981 Bedside evaluation of respiratory distress. Chest 85: 203–205

Pardy R L, Rivington R N, Despas P J, Macklem P T 1981 Inspiratory muscle training compared with physiotherapy in patients with chronic airflow obstruction. Am Rev Resp Dis 123: 423–425

Petty et al 1969 A comprehensive care program for chronic airflow obstruction. Ann Int Med 70: 1109–1120

Petty T L, Neff T A, Creagh C F et al 1979 Outpatient oxygen therapy in chronic obstructive pulmonary disease. Arch Int Med 139: 28–32

Pierce A K, Taylor H F, Archer R K, Miller W F 1964 Responses to exercise in patients with emphysema. Arch Int Med 113: 78–86

Pingleton S K, Bone R C, Pingleton W W et al 1981 Prevention of pulmonary embolism in a respiratory intensive care unit: Efficacy of low dose heparin. Chest 79(6): 647–650

Pontoppidan H, Geffin B, Lowastein E 1972 Acute respiratory failure in the adult. New Engl J Med 287: 690–698, 743–752, 799–806

Powell J R, Vozeh S, Hopewell P et al 1978 Theophylline disposition in acutely ill hospitalized patients: The effect of smoking, heart failure, chronic airway obstruction and pneumonia. Am Rev Resp Dis 118(2): 229–238

Priebe H J, Skillman S J, Bushnell L S et al 1980 Antacids vs. cimetidine preventing acute gastrointestinal bleed: A randomized trial in 75 critically ill patients. N Engl J Med 302(8): 426–430

Ramsey A G 1955 Muscle metabolism and the regulation of breathing (abstract). J Phys 127: 30
Ramsey A G 1959 Effects of metabolism and anesthesia on pulmonary ventilation. J Appl Phys 14: 102
Renzetti A D, McClement J N, Litt B D. 1966 The V. A. cooperative study of pulmonary function. III. Mortality in relation to respiratory function in chronic obstructive pulmonary disease. Am J Med 45: 115–129
Robertson C H, Foster G H, Johnson R L 1977 The relationship of respiratory failure to the oxygen consumption of, lactate production by and the distribution of blood flow among respiratory muscles during increasing inspiratory resistance. J Clin Invest 39: 31–42
Robotham J L 1981 Cardiovascular disturbances in chronic respiratory insufficiency. Am J Card 47: 941–949
Rochester D F, Bettini G 1976 Diaphragmatic blood flow and energy expenditure in the diaphragm. J Clin Invest 57: 661–672
Rochester D F, Campbell E J M 1979 The proceeding of the international symposium of the diaphragm. Am Rev Resp Dis 119–181
Rodman T, Fennelly J F, Kraft A J, Close P 1962 Effect of ethamivan on alveolar ventilation in patients with chronic lung disease. N Engl J Med 267: 1279–1282
Rogers R M, Weller C, Ruppenthal B 1972 The impact of the intensive care unit on survival of patients with acute respiratory failure. Chest 62(1): 94–97
Roussos C 1985 Function and fatigue of the respiratory muscles. Chest 88(2): 124S–132S
Roussos C, Macklem P T 1977 Diaphragmatic fatigue in man. J Appl Phys 43: 189–197
Roussos C, Macklem P T 1982 The respiratory mechanism. New Engl J Med 307(13): 786–797
Roussos C, Fixley M, Gross D, Macklem P T 1979 Fatigue of inspiratory muscles and their synergistic behavior. J Appl Phys 46: 897–904
Sackner M A, Gonzalez H, Rodriguez M, Belsito A, Sackner D R, Grenvik S 1984 Assessment of asymetric and paradoxical motion between rib cage and abdomen in normal subjects and in patients with chronic obstructive pulmonary disease. Am Rev Resp Dis 132(4): 588–593
Sahn S A, Lakshminaiayan S 1973 Bedside criteria for discontinuation of mechanical ventilation. Chest 63(6): 1002–1005
Sideris P A, Kutsadoros D P, Valianos G et al 1975 Type of cardiac dysrhythmias in respiratory failure. Am Heart J 89(1): 32–35
Sisk J E, Riegelman R K 1986 Cost effectiveness of vaccination against pneumococcal pneumonia: An update. Ann Int Med 104(1): 79–86
Snider G L 1983 A prospective on emphysema. Clin Chest Med 4(3): 329–396
Somner A R 1972 A comparison of trimethoprim/sulfamethazole vs. tetracycline in exacerbation of chronic bronchitis. Brit J Dis Chest 66: 199–206
Sorli J, Grassino A, Lorange G, Milic-Emili J 1978 Control of breathing in patients with chronic obstructive lung disease. Clin Sci Mol Med 54: 295
Stauffer J C et al 1981 Complication and consequences of endotrachial intubation and tracheostomy. Am J Med 70: 65
Sullivan M, Paliotta J, Saklad M 1976 The endotracheal tube as a factor in the measurement of respiratory mechanics. J Appl Phys 41: 590–592
Sunne C J, Pavis J A 1982 Increased exercise performance in patients with severe chronic obstructive pulmonary disease following inspiratory resistive training. Chest 81: 436
Sutton J R, Viol G W, Gray G W, McFadden M, Keaze P M 1977 Renin, aldosterone, electrolyte, and cortisol response to hypoxic decompensation. J Appl Phys 43: 421–424
Sykes N H, McNicol N W, Campbell E M J 1976 Causes, time course and efforts of respiratory failure. In: Respiratory Failure, 2nd Edition. Oxford: Blackwell Scientific Publication, 95–110
Timms R M, Khaja F U, Williams G W 1985 Hemodynamic response to oxygen therapy in chronic obstructive pulmonary disease. Ann Int Med 102(1): 29–36
Tirlapur Y G, Mir M A 1984 Effects of low caloric intake on abnormal pulmonary physiology in patients with chronic hypercapnic respiratory failure. Am J Med 77(6): 987–994
22nd Aspen Lung Conference 1980 Chronic Obstructive Lung Disease. Chest 77: 2 (supplement 249–330)
Van Dellen R G 1979 Theophylline partial application of new knowledge. Mayo Clin Proc 11: 733–745
Van der Elst A M C, Kreukniet J 1982 Some aspects of oxygen transport in patients with chronic lung disease and respiratory insufficiency. Respiration 43: 336–343
Vires N, Aubier M, Murciano D, Fleury B, Talamo C, Pariente R 1984 Effects of Aminophylline on diaphragm fatigue during acute respiratory failure. Am Rev Resp Dis 129: 396–402
Wagner P D, Dantzker D R, Darik R, Clausen J P, West J B 1977 Ventilator-dependent inequality in chronic obstructive pulmonary disease. J Clin Invest 59: 203–216

Warrell D A, Edwards R H T, Godfrey S, Jones N L 1970 Effect of controlled oxygen therapy on arterial blood gas in acute respiratory failure. Brit Med J 2: 452–455

Weaver I M V, Sahndal K, Downs J B, Klein E F, DeSautels D et al 1973 Intermittent mandatory ventilation: A new approach to weaning patients from mechanical ventilation. Chest 64: 331–335

Weisman I M, Rinaldo J E, Rodgers R M, Sanders M H 1983 Intermittent mandatory ventilation. Am Rev Resp Dis 127: 641–647

Weitzman R E 1979 Factory regulating the secretion and metabolism of arginine vasopressin (ADH). In: Brenner B M, Stein J H, eds. Hormonal Function and the Kidney, NY, Churchill, Livingston, 146–168

West J B 1979 Causes of carbon dioxide retention in lung disease. New Engl J Med 284: 1232–1236

Williams M H 1980 Intermittent mandatory ventilation and weaning. Chest 78: 804

Williams J H, Moser K M 1986 Pneumococcal vaccine and patients with chronic lung disease. Ann Int Med 104(1): 106–109

Zwillich C G, Pierson D J, Creagh A E, Sutton F D, Schatz E, Petty T L 1974 Complication of mechanical assisted ventilation. Am J Med 57: 161–170

4. Life-threatening asthma: Pathophysiology and treatment

Claude Perret

Asthma is a common disease characterised by wide variations over short periods of time in resistance to flow and intrapulmonary airways (Scadding, 1983). The acute episodes of bronchial obstruction are usually relieved by bronchodilators and corticosteroids. Occasionally, the patient fails to respond and progresses towards respiratory failure with severe hypoxaemia and hypercapnia. In these circumstances, endotracheal intubation and mechanical ventilation have proved to be life-saving procedures (Marchand et al, 1966; Sheehy et al, 1972; Scoggin et al, 1977; Hugh-Jones, 1978; Webb et al, 1979; Picado et al, 1983; Darioli & Perret, 1984; Lissac et al, 1985). However, in a number of cases, death occurs outside the hospital before the institution of appropriate treatment (Macdonald et al, 1976; Johnson et al, 1984). It is usually due to non-recognition of the severity of the situation or to an extremely rapid development of bronchial obstruction which kills the patient before the doctor's arrival. This chapter briefly reviews the pathophysiology of severe bronchial obstruction and the different aspects of therapy with special reference to mechanical ventilation as a last resort treatment.

Included under the term status asthmaticus are a number of conditions varying from prolonged wheezing (despite therapy) to life-threatening asphyxia. The American Thoracic Society has defined status asthmaticus as 'an acute asthmatic attack in which the degree of bronchial obstruction is either severe from the beginning or increases in severity and is not relieved by the usual treatment such as epinephrine or aminophylline' (Busey et al, 1968). This definition is clearly too wide, as it includes moribund patients as well as those suffering from a transient aggravation, which will respond to a brief course of corticosteroids. The term status asthmaticus should be reserved for patients who are in imminent danger of developing life-threatening respiratory failure, necessitating immediate admission to an intensive care unit. We therefore propose to define status asthmaticus as a condition of acute ventilatory failure, due to severe bronchial obstruction, which is refractory to the usual treatment and presages impending respiratory failure.

SLOW AND RAPID ONSET ATTACKS

The onset of status asthmaticus usually occurs after a period of slow decompensation progressing over several days. In such circumstances, progressive dyspnoea is associated with increasing fatigue and exhaustion. This morphologically corresponds to over-distended lungs with air-trapping and possibly collapse involving groups of secondary lobules; airways are characteristically occluded by thickened viscid mucous plugs, extending from the trachea to the respiratory bronchioles or even to the alveoli (Hayes, 1976; Dunnill, 1982). The bronchial mucosa is markedly oedematous with swelling of endothelial cells and dilatation of capillary blood vessels.

By contrast, some patients may develop acute asphyxia within a few hours or even a few minutes (Williams & Levin, 1966; Gabay, 1982; Agusti et al, 1983). This pattern is much rarer and may occur without apparent precipitating factors. Sometimes the clinical history may indicate an emotional disturbance, a fit of coughing or an allergen exposure. The relatives report the abrupt onset of cyanosis, profuse sweating and extreme distress. Death may supervene before the doctor's arrival. It is probable that in those circumstances, mucous plugging is not the responsible factor. Bronchial obstruction is probably essentially due to muscle spasm, accounting for the extremely rapid onset and usually prompt response to treatment when it can be provided.

A distinction must be drawn between these two patterns of presentation from a therapeutic point of view. It is useless and indeed, dangerous to expect a *rapid* correction of respiratory failure with mechanical ventilation when most airways are occluded by thickened mucous. Relief of obstruction is necessarily progressive and usually requires several days. On the other hand, when spasm is the main cause of obstruction, correction of extreme hypercapnia is obtained as soon as bronchodilator therapy becomes effective, on occasions within a couple of hours, or even less (Perret & Schaller, 1985).

A survey of the circumstances surrounding the deaths from acute asthma of 90 patients in England and Wales (Johnson et al, 1984), clearly showed that the most frequent cause of death was the severity of the attack, the significance of which was not recognised by the patient or his relatives (77%), by the general practitioner (69%) or the hospital doctor (23%). In 26% of the cases, the attack was fatal within less than 1 hour. This survey proves how important it is to educate asthmatic patients in appreciating by themselves the severity of an attack. If treatment is not effective or if symptoms differ from usual, by their intensity or duration, patients have to be encouraged to go directly to the hospital, as do coronary patients facing a prolonged anginal attack which does not respond to nitrates. Hospital staff should also remain vigilant: they too often tend to underestimate the seriousness of the situation. Ideally, all patients undergoing a severe and acute asthmatic attack should be rapidly admitted in an intensive care unit, the only place where the most efficient monitoring and treatment can be guaranteed.

PHYSIOLOGICAL CONSEQUENCES

Acute severe bronchial obstruction is responsible for widespread and almost complete closure of the airways at normal lung volumes (Permutt, 1973; Stalcup & Mellins, 1977). In order to overcome the increased resistance to flow and in an attempt to achieve airway patency, the patient has to breathe at high lung volumes at the cost of extremely negative pleural pressures (Salmon, 1980; Jardin et al, 1982; Martin et al, 1983). So, the primary physiological response to bronchial obstruction in severe asthma is lung hyperinflation. This leads to marked changes in the distribution of lung volumes. Residual volume (RV) has been shown to increase by two- to four-fold so that it can approximate the normal predictive value for vital capacity (FVC) (McFadden et al, 1973; Freedman et al, 1975; McFadden, 1976). Simultaneously, functional residual capacity (FRC) may double or triple. This is attributed to two different mechanisms (Peress et al, 1976; McFadden, 1976): (i) an increase in inspiratory muscle tone is responsible for a shift upwards and to the left of the chest pressure volume relationship; (ii) the inability to achieve complete expiration in the pause determined by respiratory frequency, results in a shift in the mean expiratory level. A reversible increase in total lung capacity (TLC) is usually observed with changes up to 100% increment over predicted control values. It results from a combination of an increased strength of contraction of the inspiratory muscles, an augmented outward recoil of the chest wall and, possibly, an increased pulmonary distensibility due to a transient and reversible loss of elastic recoil (Peress et al, 1976).

Forced vital capacity during an acute episode of asthma is always decreased (McFadden, 1976). It may ultimately be so restricted that it approaches tidal volume. This reduction is another manifestation of complete airway closure at abnormally high lung volumes. The rise in airways resistance secondary to bronchial obstruction accounts for a reduced peak flow rate (PFR) and one-second forced expiratory volume (FEV_1) (Olive et al, 1972; McFadden et al, 1976). However, there is no strict correlation between FEV_1 and the severity of bronchial obstruction. This is due to the fact that the value of FEV_1 not only depends on the degree of bronchoconstriction but also on the extent of chest distension induced by the inspiratory muscles. Thus, a decrease in bronchial obstruction may be masked by a parallel reduction in lung hyperinflation (Even et al, 1985). The ratio between FEV_1 and FVC is usually decreased in acute crisis but it is not a reliable index of the functional impairment.

In short, the functional response to *severe* bronchial obstruction in asthmatic patients is characterised by lung hyperinflation with increased RV, FRC and TLC. This process enables the patency of some airways to be maintained at the cost of extreme negative pleural pressures. If, as seems likely, mucus plugging and bronchial constriction are not uniformly distributed, the implication is that the few patent airways will have a normal or even a supernormal calibre in response to chest distension. In fact, the asthmatic patient, during a severe crisis, breathes with a small and distended part of his lung.

This situation has to be distinguished from that induced by *moderate* bronchial obstruction without airway closure. In this case, the response to airway narrowing is essentially characterised by a reduction in expiratory flow, attesting to increased airways resistance without marked changes in the distribution of lung volumes (Permutt, 1971; Olive & Hyatt, 1972; Permutt, 1973).

Hyperinflation is a compensatory process, which is achieved at the cost of a series of functional disturbances.

1. Lung hyperinflation requires the generation of highly negative pleural pressures. In the asthmatic, during an acute attack, mean pleural pressure during tidal breathing is lower than in normal subjects (Fig. 4.1). During inspiration, pleural pressure decreases to values less than minus 20 cm H_2O and to approximately −40–50 cm H_2O during forced inspiration. It has been shown that mean pleural pressure is significantly correlated with the measured FVC: the more severe the asthma, the more negative the pleural pressure and the smaller the FVC (Stalcup & Mellins, 1977) (Fig. 4.2). During expiration, pleural pressure approaches zero or becomes slightly positive (Permutt, 1973).

    Generation of such pressures by the respiratory muscles represents a huge increase in the inspiratory work. Breathing at high functional residual capacity

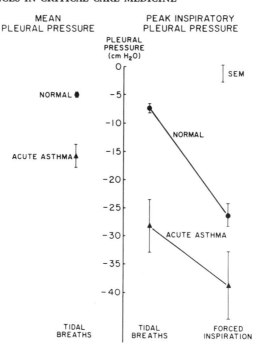

Fig. 4.1   Mean pleural pressure during tidal breathing (left panel) showing pressure to be considerably more negative in eight asthmatic patients than in eight normal children. Right panel demonstrates the peak inspiratory pleural pressures during tidal breathing and forced inspiration in the same groups of children. In asthma, peak inspiratory pleural pressures are more negative because of the need to maintain a high lung volume and because of increased inspiratory air flow resistance. (From Stalcup & Mellins, 1977.)

raises elastic work. With extreme hyperinflation, the cost is even larger due to the decreased slope of the volume/pressure relationship when approaching TLC (Fig. 4.3). The increase in elastic work is associated with a considerable rise in dynamic work developed to overcome the resistances to flow. Such conditions impose an enormous load on the respiratory muscles when their effectiveness is compromised both by the modified geometry of an hyperinflated thorax and by the persistence of some degree of contraction of the inspiratory muscles during expiration (Muller et al, 1980; Martin et al, 1983). The use of accessory muscles cannot prevent progressive fatigue and exhaustion with subsequent inability to maintain hyperinflation. Under such conditions, the decrease in TLC favours the extension of closure to previously patent airways, with further deterioration of gas exchange, alveolar hypoventilation and respiratory acidosis.

2. Variable degrees of bronchial obstruction separate the lung into compartments of different time constants (McFadden, 1976; West, 1976). In some areas, a low ventilation–perfusion ratio leads to hypoxaemia. In others, complete occlusion of bronchi, with maintained perfusion, produces the conditions of a true shunt. Indeed, it is likely that some collateral ventilation is maintained beyond the occluded bronchi, so that the ventilation–perfusion ratio is very low but finite (Wagner et al, 1978). On the other hand, alveolar overdistension in non-obstructed areas impairs capillary perfusion with subsequent increase in dead

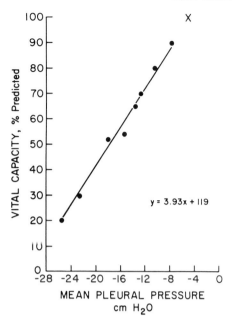

Fig. 4.2   Mean pleural pressure becoming progressively more negative with increasing severity of asthma, indicated by the fall in vital capacity from that predicted by height. ● Denotes individual asthmatic patients, and X mean of eight normal children. (From Stalcup & Mellins, 1977.)

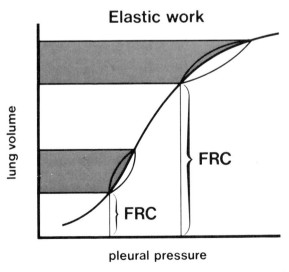

Fig. 4.3   With hyperinflation (increased FRC) secondary to acute bronchial obstruction, the slope of the volume/pressure relationship decreases and the elastic work (grey area) may increase considerably.

space ventilation. In fact, there is little change in VD/VT ratio (Permutt, 1973) suggesting that distribution of perfusion is more homogenous than that of ventilation. At the early stage of an acute attack, ventilatory drive is maintained or even increased, so that $PaCO_2$ remains constant or even decreases in spite of a marked rise in respiratory work (McFadden & Lyons, 1968; Palmer & Flenley, 1976). With progression of obstruction, the patient has to breathe nearer and nearer to TLC, decreasing his tidal volume and increasing the respiratory rate. Alveolar ventilation decreases when, concomitantly, CO_2 production augments in response to the enhanced metabolic requirements of respiratory muscles. Thus the rising PCO_2 in status asthmaticus represents an imbalance between increased metabolic rate and decreased alveolar ventilation.

3. Hyperinflation causes serious circulatory consequences by modifying the extramural pressures surrounding the pulmonary vessels. During inspiration, the large drop of pleural pressure to a markedly negative level is responsible for alveolar overdistension (Permutt, 1971, 1973; Stalcup & Mellins, 1977). Mean alveolar pressure, which is nearly equal to barometric pressure, becomes more positive in relation to pleural pressures and tends to compress the alveolar wall capillaries. Thus, the rise in alveolar volume increases resistance to flow and leads to the derecruitment of micro-vessels (Butler & Paley, 1962). This results in an increased afterload to the right ventricle (Permutt, 1973), with an elevation in end-systolic volume and a decrease in stroke volume (Salmon, 1980; Jardin et al, 1982). Simultaneously, inspiration facilitates venous return to the right chambers, producing right ventricular overdistension with subsequent leftward shift of the intra-ventricular septum. On the left side, stroke volume is reduced. This has two main causes: (i) a decrease in preload, subsequent to diminished venous return and impaired left ventricular distensibility (ventricular interference); (ii) a rise in aortic transmural pressure during inspiration increases the afterload (Jardin et al, 1982).

At the early phase of expiration, pleural pressure becomes suddenly positive and the decrease in alveolar volume reduces micro-vessels' resistances. The drop in afterload in the presence of an overfilled right ventricle provokes first an increase in stroke volume; the septum returns to its normal position and the left ventricle becomes more compliant (Jardin et al, 1982). Subsequently, preload decreases because of the reduced venous return induced by an adverse pressure gradient between the right heart and extrathoracic vessels. Consequently right ventricular volume decreases gradually and systemic pressure progressively declines after an initial increase. These phasic changes in pressures and volumes explain the phenomenon of the pulsus paradoxus, defined as an inspiratory decline of 10 mm Hg or more in the systolic arterial pressure (Rebuck & Pengelly, 1973; Martin et al, 1981; Jardin et al, 1982).

From a haemodynamic point of view, it has been shown that status asthmaticus represents a severe overload for both ventricles. Under normal conditions, mean pleural pressure is nearly equal to barometric pressure and absolute (or intramural) pressures are equivalent to transmural pressures. When pleural pressure is markedly negative, as in an acute attack of asthma, the absolute pressures become much reduced relative to the transmural pressures. Thus, in order to determine the true filling pressures of the ventricles as well as the pulmonary or systemic arterial pressures, it is necessary to measure simultaneously the pleural (or oesophageal) pressure and algebraically subtract it from the absolute values obtained by catheterisation (Permutt, 1973a,b; Freedman et al, 1975; Stalcup et al, 1977). In other words, a moderately increased pulmonary intramural pressure may correspond to a degree of pulmonary hypertension similar to that observed in massive pulmonary embolism. In severe asthma, pulmonary hypertension is mainly due to increase in microvascular resistances secondary to hyperinflation but, the rise in cardiac output and active arteriolar vaso-constriction also contribute. The decreased stroke volume is usually more than compensated for by the increased heart rate.

TREATMENT

Treatment aims at restoring normal gas exchange and adequate circulatory conditions by relieving bronchial obstruction. Usually, this is achieved using simple therapeutic measures, which are now well documented (Rebuck et al, 1971, Derenne et al, 1973, Weiss, 1976; Feldman & McFadden, 1977; Labrousse et al, 1977; Hugh-Jones, 1978; Summer, 1985; Fagon & Aubier, 1985). In some instances, however, the failure of the conservative treatment necessitates recourse to mechanical ventilation (Marchand & Van Hasselt, 1966; Sheehy et al, 1972; Scoggin et al, 1977; Webb et al, 1979; Picado et al, 1983; Darioli & Perret, 1984; Lissac et al, 1985).

Conservative treatment

Oxygen
Hypoxaemia, when severe, may cause pulmonary hypertension, impaired ventricular function and arrhythmias and can even lead to tissue anoxia when cardiac compensation is inadequate. Hence it is important to normalise arterial PO_2 by inhalation of an hyperoxic mixture using a face-mask (Ventimask). The oxygen supply should be adjusted to maintain an arterial PO_2 close to 60 mm Hg, corresponding to a SaO_2 around 90% (Weiss, 1976). A FiO_2 between 28 and 40% is generally sufficient to achieve this objective, except when the mixed venous PO_2 is markedly decreased owing to a drop in cardiac output. In asthmatic patients, contrary to what is usually observed in patients with chronic bronchitis, hyperoxia does not usually induce any substantial reduction in alveolar ventilation, especially when initial arterial PCO_2 is low (Sykes et al, 1976; Summer, 1985). However, some patients, usually with moderate hypercapnia, respond unexpectedly to hyperoxia, with the development of severe respiratory acidosis; hence the necessity for regular blood gas analysis (Sykes et al, 1976).

Hydration and humidification
Most patients reach hospital in a state of advanced dehydration which impairs muco-ciliary action, increases the viscosity and stickiness of the bronchial secretions and favours circulatory instability by reducing ventricular preload. The negative fluid balance is usually explained by increased loss (hyperventilation, fever, sweating) often compounded by reduced fluid intake (Straub et al, 1969). Adequate rehydration is achieved with i.v. administration of 5% dextrose in water or slightly hypotonic saline solution (NaCl 0.5%). The volume infused is adjusted to the patient's requirements

and tolerance—usually about 2 to 4 l for the first 24 hours (Weiss, 1976). Although probably slight, the risk of inducing pulmonary edema by excessive fluid infusion is theoretically more important in severe asthma, as a result of the transfer to the interstitial space of highly negative pleural pressures (Stalcup & Mellins, 1977); hence, the necessity for monitoring plasma and urine osmolarity. Rehydration promotes a better liquefaction of secretions than do conventional humidifiers, whose inadequate droplet size restricts efficiency (Sykes et al, 1976). Ultrasonic nebulisers are more efficient but often badly tolerated by dyspnoeic patients, who react by suffocating when inhaling the dense mist (Weiss, 1976). Humidification units must be correctly set so that the temperature is adequate to prevent bacterial contamination. Aerosol generators are often contaminated by bacterial spores, which can lead to infection.

Of the available mucolytic agents, N-acetylcysteine is the only one capable of reducing significantly the viscosity of the bronchial secretions, which it does by chemical reduction of mucopolysaccharides and mucoproteins. Unfortunately, its use is limited in some patients who develop excessive bronchorrhoea (Weiss, 1976). Special attention must be paid to chest physiotherapy (percussion, vibration of the thorax, suction of secretions) and relaxation of the patient in an effort to achieve optimal cooperation. It is of prime importance that the patient should feel comfortable and secure, thus minimising the possibility of panic reactions due to impending asphyxia. The use of sedatives is proscribed because of the risk of respiratory depression.

Bronchodilators
Theophylline is a methylated xanthine, more soluble when combined with ethylenediamine (aminophylline). Its relaxing action on the bronchial smooth muscle is probably multifactorial (Fagon & Aubier, 1985; Goodman et al, 1985): mechanisms include intracellular calcium translocation; accumulation of cyclic nucleotide, particularly cyclic AMP; blockade of receptors for adenosine. Moreover, it increases diaphragmatic contractility, enhances the sensitivity of the medullary centres to CO_2 and potentiates inhibitors of prostaglandin synthesis.

The intravenous route is the only one to consider when dealing with severe asthma. Several schemes have been proposed, like that of Jusko et al (1977), which suggests a loading dose of 6 mg/kg to be infused within 20–40 min, followed by a maintenance dose of 0.9 mg/kg/h. In the absence of the desired therapeutic response and signs or symptoms of toxicity, an additional 3 mg/kg of aminophylline can be slowly infused. The maintenance dose will be diminished to 0.6 mg/kg/h for elderly patients and to 0.4 mg/kg/h for patients suffering from cardiac failure or liver disease (Weiss, 1976). An increase in the dose may sometimes be required 0.9 mg/kg/h for smokers. In view of the considerable individual variation in pharmacokinetics, it is useful to monitor plasma concentration in order to maintain therapeutic levels (7–15 µg/ml). Signs of intoxication (tachycardia, restlessness, hypotension, chest pain, nausea and vomiting) occur above 20 µg/ml; localised or generalised convulsions usually appear when plasma levels exceed 35 µg/ml.

β_2-adrenergic agents
Drug treatment has been recently improved with the introduction of selective β_2-stimulating agents administered intravenously (McPhillips, 1978). Relaxation of bronchial smooth muscle depends upon a direct action on the β_2-receptors of bronchi

and especially the small airways; the force of contraction of the diaphragm is also stimulated. The drugs generally used are terbutaline and salbutamol (Wolfe et al, 1978; Johnson et al, 1978), with a loading dose of 0.5 mg administered slowly, followed by an infusion of 0.05–0.1 μg/kg/min. It appears that β_2-adrenergic agents potentiate the effects of theophylline and vice versa. These drugs have essentially replaced epinephrine, which is now only rarely used in patients with status asthmaticus complicated by circulatory failure (Lissac et al, 1985) or anaphylaxis. Their main advantage over isoproterenol is their selectivity which makes them easier to use and safer. Nevertheless, in excessive doses, they induce circulatory (tachycardia, hypertension), digestive (nausea, vomiting) and nervous (tremor) disturbances.

Bronchodilators—whatever their mode of action—can paradoxically increase hypoxaemia coincident with the relief of bronchial obstruction. The fall in arterial PO_2 has been related to a further worsening in the distribution of ventilation/perfusion abnormalities throughout the lung, due to reduction of regional vasoconstriction in underventilated areas (Tai & Read, 1967). This phenomenon is somewhat similar to what has already been observed with the use of isoproterenol. It is noteworthy that the vasoconstrictor response to hypoxia may vary widely from patient to patient.

Corticosteroids
Corticosteroid treatment is mandatory in asthma and should be undertaken as soon as possible (Littenberg & Gluck, 1986). The effect of this mode of treatment is dependent upon (Aviado & Carrillo, 1970; Dluhy et al, 1973) its anti-inflammatory action, and upon its ability to relax the bronchial muscles and to produce vasoconstriction and a decrease in permeability of the mucous membrane, resulting in a reduction of oedema. Its action is delayed, starting approximately 2 hours after commencement of intravenous infusion and reaching its peak effect after 6–8 hours. Hydrocortisone hemisuccinate and methylprednisolone succinate are the most frequently used steroids, at a respective dose of 0.5–2 g, and 100–400 mg or more, during the first 24 hours (Rebuck & Read, 1971; Collins et al, 1975; Feldman & McFadden, 1977; Summer, 1985; Littenberg & Gluck, 1986). Treatment is administered by the intravenous route until the bronchial obstruction has subsided. It is then continued orally using decremental doses of prednisone, whilst monitoring the functional improvement—diminishing the dose too rapidly increases the risk of relapse and too slowly, the risk of digestive problems (ulcer, haemorrhage), metabolic alkalosis because of potassium depletion, or even acute psychosis.

Other treatments
Abuse of antibiotics in acute asthma is common, usually on the basis of increased sputum aspect, the presence of a non-specific leucocytosis or simply as a prophylactic measure. Use of these agents should be restricted to patients with bacteriologically proven infection or pulmonary infiltrates on chest X-ray. For such cases, ampicillin, tetracyclines or macrolids are preferred.

Acidosis should be corrected when a disturbance of the metabolic component of acid–base balance is sufficiently severe as to cause a fall in pH to below 7.15 units. Indeed, such a situation rarely occurs apart from very serious attacks for which mechanical ventilation is mandatory. Under these conditions, sodium bicarbonate is administered at a dose which will return pH to around 7.20–7.30; this should be postponed in the presence of hypokalaemia.

Mechanical ventilation

In a few patients, conservative treatment appears to be insufficient and it becomes necessary to proceed to endotracheal intubation with mechanical ventilation. Indications for applying these measures are—apart from apnea and cardiac arrest—exhaustion, rapid rise in arterial PCO_2 during treatment, and severe respiratory acidosis. The presence of hypercapnia upon admission, without significant acidosis (pH > 7.30) is not necessarily an indication for mechanical ventilation. It is often worthwhile waiting for the effects of drug treatment, although one should be ready to proceed immediately to intubation if the situation deteriorates. This requires very careful surveillance and the aim is to avoid unnecessarily invasive measures.

Generally, mechanical ventilation is used to correct alveolar hypoventilation and return arterial PO_2 and PCO_2 to normal (Scoggin et al, 1977). It is a rather simple problem when dealing with non-asthmatic respiratory failure; it can be extremely difficult during acute asthma, since high insufflating pressures have to be used.

In order to analyse the problems of mechanical ventilation in status asthmaticus, one can schematically simplify the lung into three compartments (Fig. 4.4). Airway

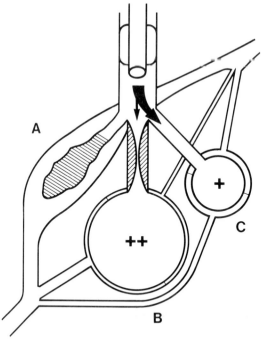

Fig. 4.4   Schematic representation of the lung.

A is perceived to be completely occluded and ventilation is zero. Airway B is obstructed during expiration, but is transiently open during part of the inspiratory phase of ventilation; such a mechanism of inspiratory air-trapping induces intra-alveolar positive pressure with progressive distension and compression of the vessels within the wall. Subsequently most of the ventilation will be distributed to the small non-obstructed compartment C, which is thus overdistended during inspiration. Such conditions favour a derecruitment of alveolar vessels with a shift of perfusion to the areas of lower resistances. In other words, ventilation–perfusion mismatch may even worsen after intubation, increasing the shunt effect and causing more marked hypoxaemia and hypercapnia. Due to high airway resistance and the low compliance of the distended chest, mechanical ventilation requires high insufflation pressures, which increase the hazards of alveolar rupture and barotrauma in the non-obstructed as well as in the air-trapped areas. Furthermore, cardiac output is reduced by two different mechanisms, first the decreased venous return due to an unfavourable abdomino-thoracic gradient and, second, an increased afterload due to the derecruitment of alveolar vessels in hyperinflated areas.

These particular conditions explain the unusually high rate of barotrauma and the relatively high incidence of circulatory failure reported in several series (Scoggin et al, 1977; Webb et al, 1979). A simultaneous decrease in cardiac output and O_2 content dramatically reduces peripheral oxygen delivery, increasing the tendency towards acidosis, arrhythmias and even cardiac arrest. Indeed, excessive airway pressures may be more dangerous than persistent hypercapnia, which mechanical ventilation is intended to correct.

The therapeutic approach favoured by the authors, called controlled hypoventilation, is to use mechanical ventilation as a means of guaranteeing effective oxygen availability without attempting to restore adequate alveolar ventilation (Darioli & Perret, 1984). Correction of hypoxaemia is simply obtained by moderately increasing the oxygen concentration of inspired air. Normalisation of arterial PCO_2 is achieved hours (or even days) later, when the relief of obstruction enables the delivery of adequate volumes with acceptable insufflation pressures. Prolonged hypercapnia has no apparent deleterious effect, provided arterial PCO_2 does not exceed 90 mm Hg.

Technical aspects

Orotracheal intubation is performed after the intravenous administration of diazepam and manual ventilation with hyperoxic mixtures in order to prevent hypoxia during the insertion of the tube. In some cases, administration of pancuronium bromide may be necessary to obtain muscle relaxation and adequate preoxygenation. A large cuffed endotracheal tube is inserted and its position confirmed by X-ray. As soon as the tube has been passed, the patient is again ventilated manually with a hyperoxic mixture. In some cases of extreme obstruction, manual ventilation must be prolonged before the patient can be connected to the ventilator. A nasogastric tube is passed for aspiration of the gastric contents and systematic administration of antacid agents.

The choice of ventilator is important. Only a powerful volume-cycled system will guarantee a steady minute volume against increased airway resistance. The tidal volume should be between 8 and 12 ml/kg with a slow respiratory rate (6–10/min) and an inspiratory–expiratory ratio of 1:2. Maximum insufflation pressures should not exceed 50 cm H_2O. FiO_2 is adjusted to restore a normal arterial PO_2 and saturation. Sedation with diazepam is usually necessary to obtain adequate synchronisation with the ventilator. The use of pancuronium bromide (4 mg/h) is seldom needed.

Continuous positive airway pressure reduces the inspiratory work (Martin et al, 1982) and may improve gas exchange in severe asthma (Tenaillon et al, 1982). Furthermore, ventilation with high level PEEP has also been successfully used in a few patients who could not be adequately ventilated with IPPB, suggesting that an increased mean airway pressure reduces airway closure and resistance (Qvist et al, 1982). These preliminary results have to be confirmed in larger series. Halothane anaesthesia has been reported to be effective in refractory attacks (O'Rourke & Crome, 1982; Rosseel et al, 1985), but its use should be carefully controlled because of the depressant effect on myocardial contractility and arrhythmogenic activity of this agent.

Bronchial lavage has been proposed to facilitate the removal of mucous plugs. The procedure is hazardous and can induce transient deterioration in gas exchange (Sykes et al, 1976). It is probably safer to wait for the benefits of progressive rehydration, which appears to be the best way to liquefy viscid secretions (Weiss, 1976).

Weaning

When clinical signs of obstruction have disappeared and the patient is capable of maintaining a normal arterial PO_2 and PCO_2 under IMV with a FiO_2 of about 30%, extubation can be considered. For this, it is essential to get the patient's active co-operation, hence to alleviate his anxiety. Complete normalisation of arterial PO_2 may take several days. The patient should not be discharged before it is obtained.

Complications

Barotrauma, and especially tension pneumothorax, is a potentially fatal complication. One should keep it in mind and order a chest X-ray whenever an unexplained deterioration occurs.

Development of shock with oliguria and cold extremities is sometimes related to arrhythmias, but more frequently it is associated with hypovolaemia. If not rapidly corrected with volume loading, a haemodynamic investigation including pulmonary artery balloon catheterisation should be performed in order to identify the nature of the disorders.

Transient hypotension when starting artificial ventilation has been frequently described (Riding & Ambiavagar, 1967; Webb et al, 1979; Halttunen et al, 1980). It has been related to a decrease in arterial PCO_2 causing a fall in peripheral resistance and, most likely, to a drop in cardiac output induced by the high insufflation pressure delivered by the ventilator. It is interesting to note that the incidence of barotrauma, hypotension and shock decreased markedly following introduction of the controlled hypoventilation technique, which produces a very slow and progressive correction of hypercapnia, without excessive insufflation pressures.

CONCLUSIONS

Deaths from severe asthma are still too frequent. A better evaluation of the severity of asthma by the physician, the relatives and the patient should result in a decrease in mortality rate outside the hospital. Similarly, in-hospital mortality should be reduced by closer surveillance of the hospitalised patients and adequate use of mechanical ventilation. The latter should be viewed as a safe means of maintaining adequate oxygenation for as long as extensive peripheral bronchial plugging prevents correction of alveolar hypoventilation.

REFERENCES

Agusti A G N, Montserrat J M, Agusti Vidal A 1983 Sudden respiratory arrest from asthma. Chest 83: 933

Aviado D M, Carrillo L R 1970 Antiasthmatic action of corticosteroids: a review of literature on their mechanism of action. Journal of Clinical Pharmacology 10: 3–11

Busey J F, Fenger E P D, Hepper N G et al 1968 Management of status asthmaticus: a statement by the committee on therapy. American Review of Respiratory Disease 97: 735–736

Butler J, Paley H W 1962 Lung volume and pulmonary circulation. The effect of sustained changes in lung volume on pressure-flow relationships in the human pulmonary circulation. Medicina thoracalis 19: 261–267

Collins J V, Clark T J H, Brown D, Townsend J 1975 The use of corticosteroids in the treatment of acute asthma. Quarterly Journal Medicine 174: 259–273

Darioli R, Perret C 1984 Mechanical controlled hypoventilation in status asthmaticus. American Review of Respiratory Disease 129: 385–387

Derenne J P, Canh V N, Pariente R 1973 Traitement de l'état de mal asthmatique. Conception actuelle (à propos de 18 cas). Nouvelle Presse Médicale 2: 1693–1696

Dluhy R G, Lauler D P, Thorn G W 1973 Pharmacology and chemistry of adrenal glucocorticoids. Medical Clinics of North America 57: 1155–1165

Dunnill M S 1982 Asthma. In: Dunnill M S (ed), Pulmonary Pathology, pp 50–66. Churchill Livingstone, Edinburgh, London, Melbourne and New York

Even P, Sors H, Stern M, Bons J, Safran D, Reynaud P, Vivet P 1985 Mécanique respiratoire et circulatoire des asthmes aigus grave (AAG). In: Réanimation et Médecine d'Urgence, pp 338–394. Expansion Scientifique Française, Paris

Fagon J Y, Aubier M 1985 Traitement médicamenteux de l'état de mal asthmatique. In: Réanimation et Médecine d'Urgence, pp 395–406. Expansion Scientifique Française, Paris

Feldman N T, McFadden E R 1977 Asthma. Therapy old and new. Medical Clinics of North America 61: 1239–1250

Freedman S, Tattersfield A E, Pride N D 1975 Changes in lung mechanics during asthma induced by exercise. Journal of Applied Physiology 38, no 6, 974–982

Gabay E L 1982 Sudden respiratory arrest from asthma. Chest 82: 387

Goodman Gilman A, Goodman L S, Rall T W, Murad F (eds) 1985 The pharmacological basis of therapeutics. 7th edition. Macmillan Publishing Company, New York

Hayes J A 1976 The pathology of bronchial asthma. In: Weiss E B, Segal M S (eds) Bronchial Asthma, pp 347–381. Little, Brown and Company, Boston

Halttunen P D, Luomanmäkik K, Takkunen O, Viljanen A A 1980 Management of severe bronchial asthma in an intensive care unit. Annals of Clinical Research 12: 109–111

Hugh-Jones P 1978 Status asthmaticus. Bulletin Européen de Physiopathologie Respiratoire 14: 233–236

Jardin F, Farcot J C, Boisante L, Prost J F, Gueret P, Bourdarias J P 1982 Mechanism of paradoxic pulse in bronchial asthma. Circulation 66: 887–894

Johnson A J, Spiro S G, Pidgeon Bateman S et al 1978 Intravenous infusion of salbutamol in severe acute asthma. British Medical Journal 1: 1013–1015

Johnson A J, Nunn A J, Somner A R, Stableforth D E, Stewart C J 1984 Circumstances of death from asthma. British Medical Journal 288: 1870–1871

Jusko W J, Koup J R, Vance J W, Schentag J J, Kuritzky P 1977 Intravenous theophylline therapy; nomogram guidelines. Annals of Internal Medicine 86: 404–414

Labrousse J, Bousser J P, Tenaillon A, Morgant C, Lissac J 1977 Traitement de l'état de mal asthmatique. Thérapie 32: 49–61

Lissac J, Labrousse J, Tenaillon A, Coulaud J M, Massart J D, Icole B 1985 Traitement instrumental et médications associées dans l'état de mal asthmatique. In: Réanimation et Médecine d'Urgence, pp 407–415. Expansion Scientifique Française, Paris

Littenberg B, Gluck E H 1986 A controlled trial of methylprednisolone in the emergency treatment of acute asthma. New England Journal of Medicine 314: 150–152

Macdonald J B, Seaton A, Williams D A 1976 Asthma deaths in Cardiff 1963–74: 90 deaths outside hospital. British Medical Journal 1493–1495

McFadden E R, Lyons H A 1968 Arterial-blood gas tension in asthma. New England Journal of Medicine 278: 1028–1032

McFadden E R, Kiser R, DeGroot W J 1973 Acute bronchial asthma. Relations between clinical and physiologic manifestations. New England Journal of Medicine 288: 221–225

McFadden E R 1976 Respiratory mechanics in asthma. In: Weiss E B, Segal M S (eds) Bronchial Asthma, pp 259–278. Little Brown, Boston

McFadden E R, Ingram R H 1976 Lung volume and distribution of ventilation in asthma. In Weiss

E B, Segal M S (eds) Bronchial Asthma, pp 279–293. Little Brown, Boston

McPhillips J J 1978 Role of β_2-agents in status asthmaticus. In Weiss E B, Segal M S (eds) Status Asthmaticus, pp 225–233. University Park Press, Baltimore

Marchand P, Van Hasselt H 1966 Last-resort treatment of status asthmaticus. Lancet 1: 227–230

Martin J, Jardin J, Sampson M, Engel L E 1981 Factors influencing pulsus paradoxus in asthma. Chest 80: 543–549

Martin J G, Shore S, Engel L A 1982 Effect of continuous positive airway pressure on respiratory mechanics and pattern of breathing in induced asthma. American Review of Respiratory Disease 126: 812–817

Martin J G, Shore S A, Engel L A 1983 Mechanical load and inspiratory muscle action during induced asthma. American Review of Respiratory Disease 128: 455–460

Muller N L, Bryan A C, Zamel N 1980 Tonic inspiratory muscle activity as a cause of hyperinflation in asthma (abstract). American Review of Respiratory Disease 121, no 4, part 2, 171

Olive J T, Hyatt R E 1972 Maximal expiratory flow and total respiratory resistance during induced bronchoconstriction in asthmatic subjects. American Review of Respiratory Disease 106: 366–376

O'Rourke, P P, Crome R K 1982 Halothane in status asthmaticus. Critical Care Medicine 10: 341–343

Palmer K N V, Flenley D C 1976 Pathophysiology of gas exchange and arterial blood gas and pH in asthma. In Weiss E B, Segal M S (eds) Bronchial Asthma, pp 317–332. Little, Brown and Company, Boston

Peress L, Sybrecht G, Macklem P T 1976 The mechanism of increase in total lung capacity during acute asthma. American Journal of Medicine 61: 165–169

Permutt S 1971 Some physiological aspects of asthma: bronchomuscular contraction and airways calibre. In: Porter R, Birch J (eds) Identification of asthma. CIBA Foundation Study Group no 38, pp 63. Churchill-Livingstone, Londres

Permutt S 1973a Physiologic changes in the acute asthmatic attack. In: Austen F and Lichtenstein L M (eds) Asthma: Physiology, Immunopharmacology, and Treatment, pp 15–27. Academic Press, Inc, New York and London

Permutt S 1973b Relation between pulmonary arterial pressure and pleural pressure during the acute asthmatic attack. Chest 63: 25S–28S

Perret Cl, Schaller M D 1985 Etat de mal asthmatique: définition, signes cliniques et biologiques. In: Réanimation et Médecine d'Urgence, p 324–335. Expansion Scientifique Française, Paris

Picado J M, Montserrat J M, Roca J, et al 1983 Mechanical ventilation in severe exacerbation of asthma. European Journal of Respiratory Disease 64: 102–107

Qvist J, Anderson J B, Pemberton M, Bennike K A 1982 High-level PEEP in severe asthma. New England Journal of Medicine 307: 1347–1348

Rebuck A S, Read J 1971 Assessment and management of severe asthma. American Journal of Medicine 51: 788–798

Rebuck A S, Pengelly L D 1973 Development of pulsus paradoxus in the presence of airways obstruction. New England Journal of Medicine 288: 66–69

Riding W D, Ambiavagar M 1967 Resuscitation of the moribund asthmatic. Postgraduate Medical Journal 43: 234–243

Rosseel P, Lauwers L F, Baute L 1985 Halothane treatment in life-threatening asthma. Critical Care Medicine 11: 241–146

Salmon O 1980 Mécanisme de défaillance cardiaque droite aiguë au cours des crises d'asthme sévère. Thèse médecine (Directeur P Even), no 400, Lyon

Scadding J G 1983 Definition and clinical categories of asthma. In: Clark T J H, Godfrey S (eds) Asthma, 2nd Edition, p 1–11. Chapman and Hall Medical, London

Scoggin C H, Sahn S A, Petty T L 1977 Status Asthmaticus. A nine-year experience. Journal of the American Medical Association 238: 1158–1162

Sheehy A F, DiBenedetto R, Lefrak S, Lyons H A 1972 Treatment of status asthmaticus. A report of 70 episodes. Archives of Internal Medicine 130: 37–42

Stalcup S A, Mellins R B 1977 Mechanical forces producing pulmonary edema in acute asthma. New England Journal of Medicine 297: 592–596

Straub P W, Buhlmann, A A, Rossier P H 1969 Hypovolemia in status asthmaticus. Lancet 2: 923–926

Summer W R 1985 Status Asthmaticus. Chest 87: 1, Suppl 87S–94S

Sykes M K, McNicol W, Campbell E J M 1976 Respiratory failure in patients with acute lung disease. In: Sykes M K, McNicol W, Campbell E J M (eds) Respiratory failure, pp 259–268, 2nd edition. Blackwell Scientific Publications, Oxford

Tai E, Read J 1967 Blood-gas tensions in bronchial asthma. Lancet 1: 644–646

Tenaillon A, Salmona J-P, Burdin M 1982 Continuous positive airway pressure in asthma. American Review of Respiratory Disease 127: 658

Wagner P D, Dantzker D R, Iacovoni V E, Tomlin W C, West J B 1978 Ventilation-perfusion inequality in asymptomatic asthma. American Review of Respiratory Disease 118: 511–524

Webb A K, Bilton A H, Hanson G C 1979 Severe bronchial asthma requiring ventilation. A review of 20 cases and advice on management. Postgraduate Medical Journal 55: 161–170

Weiss E B 1976 Status Asthmaticus. In Weiss E B, Segal M S (eds) Bronchial Asthma, p 875–913. Little, Brown and Company, Boston

West J B 1976 Ventilation-perfusion and diffusion disturbances in asthma. In Weiss E B, Segal M S (eds) Bronchial Asthma, pp 295–316. Little, Brown and Company, Boston

Williams M H, Levin M 1966 Sudden death from bronchial asthma. American Review of Respiratory Disease 94: 608–611

Wolfe J D, Tashkin D P, Calvarese B, Simmons M 1978 Bronchodilator effects of terbutaline and aminophylline alone and in combination in asthmatic patients. New England Journal of Medicine 298: 363–367

5. The changing face of sedative practice

Peter G. M. Wallace   Julian F. Bion   Iain McA. Ledingham

'What distinguishes and worries man is not things as such, but his opinions and fantasies about things'

(Epictetus c. 55–135 A.D.)

INTRODUCTION

The topic of sedation has only recently begun to excite scientific interest amongst intensive care clinicians. While other aspects of treatment have undergone close scrutiny, the provision of sedation has usually been based on the subjective assessment of requirement by attending staff. It has even been suggested that sedative drugs are prescribed to offset the medical staff's own expectations of the Intensive Therapy Unit (ITU) environment (Holland et al, 1973) or to provide convenient nursing conditions, rather than in response to the actual fears or physical needs of patients. Whatever the reason, the use of sedative drugs in the ITU has tended to be empirical and poorly evaluated.

The deficiencies of this uncritical attitude were highlighted during the early part of the present decade when the practice of producing 'long term detachment of the patient from the environment' became popular (Merriman, 1981). While conceived with the best intentions, evidence that this approach benefits patients remains sparse. Indeed, the possibility that such use of sedative agents may be hazardous (Watt & Ledingham, 1984) has provoked considerable concern (Editorial, 1984; Willats, 1985; Dobb & Murphy, 1985; Nightingale & Pleuvry, 1985) and during the last year or two, opinion about the desirable level of sedation for critically ill patients has undergone substantial change. Only a minority of clinicians now favour continuous 'deep' sedation (Bion & Ledingham, 1987) and there is increasing appreciation of the need for objective assessment of all aspects of sedation in the ITU.

PERCEPTIONS AND PROBLEMS OF SEDATION

Discussion of the subject of sedation is complicated by a number of factors, notably, imprecise terminology, variable objectives, the choice, dosage and route of administration of drugs, and possible alternatives to the use of drugs.

Sedation (derived from *sedare*: to soothe or settle) is an ill-defined term which is subject to a variety of interpretations. Some consider the term to imply not only relief of distress but also reduction in level of consciousness. Norris (1969), however, has defined sedation as, 'a state in which pre-existing anxiety is removed or lessened, or in which signs of anxiety do not develop in circumstances in which they would be expected to do so'. Thus sedation need not be viewed as synonymous with altered consciousness.

Contemporary opinion appears to favour attainment of patient comfort without significant depression of consciousness, particularly when sedation is required over a prolonged period. Clearly, certain patients or circumstances may require modification of this approach. For example, regimens involving deeper sedation may be an integral part of the treatment of tetanus (Newton-John, 1984) and head injury (Aitkenhead, 1986). Also manoeuvres such as tracheal intubation or the institution of mechanical ventilation normally require short-term depression of conscious level. Of course, other patients not included in the above categories may at times prove refractory to lighter levels of sedation.

Another problem concerns the choice of available drugs, none of which is ideal. The agents currently available are not selective in their effects and 'most anxiolytics (sedatives) will induce sleep when given in large doses ... and most hypnotics will sedate when given in divided doses' (British National Formulary, 1986). The route and method of administration will also influence response. Continuous intravenous infusion of analgesic drugs may offer certain advantages (Hull, 1985; Stanski, 1987) but in ITU patients this method of administration of sedative drugs may cause unnecessarily prolonged unconsciousness.

Pharmacological methods represent only one component of overall sedative management (Nimmo & MacRae, 1983). Control of the environment and the availability of an adequate number of competent and compassionate attendants are equally if not more important factors.

STRESS: NATURE AND SEVERITY

The reaction of a patient to an illness is determined by the physical effects and perceived outcome of the illness and by the ITU environment (Fig. 5.1). The main psychological aspects of stress in the ITU patient are anxiety, pain and sleeplessness which interrelate with the physiological stress response. Understanding this interrelationship is an important prerequisite to planning appropriate management.

Anxiety

A group of patients will perceive similar situations with different degrees of anxiety, the nature of the individual response being determined by both genetic characteristics and learned behaviour patterns. The level of anxiety may be reduced if the situation is familiar, predictable, understood or can be controlled. Initial admission to an ITU is unlikely to be accompanied by any perception of familiarity or control, and support for patients must be maximised at this time.

Anxiety exceeding the patient's normal emotional defences becomes counterproductive, resulting in psychological disorganisation, manifest as panic, delusions, helplessness or psychosis. These psychiatric aspects of intensive care have been comprehensively reviewed (Baxter, 1974; Strain, 1978; Kornfield, 1980; Bowden, 1983). A patient's coping style in normal life will be reflected in similar reactions to the acute stress of ITU.

Anxiety is particularly liable to occur in patients with excessive neuroticism and in those with high extroversion or affective disorders. By contrast, those with 'psychological hardiness' (Dobson, 1982) are likely to withstand stress to a greater degree. This resilience might lie in basic personality or defensive strategies. Hackett et al

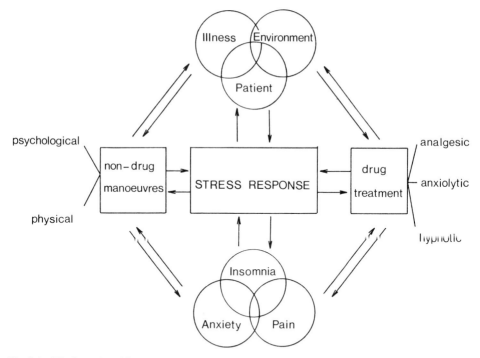

Fig. 5.1 The interplay of factors leading to and resulting from the 'stress response' and the influence of non-drug manoeuvres and drug treatment.

(1968) showed that 'deniers' who tended to minimise or ignore the real significance of serious illness had a lower mortality than patients who were considered to be 'non deniers' and who easily admitted to being frightened. No one however is totally invulnerable and even deniers' defences may be breached if full explanations are attempted (Shipley et al, 1979).

Psychological stress or anxiety appears to produce a neuroendocrine response similar, if somewhat reduced, to that of acute physical stress (Molitch & Hou, 1983). Rapid adaptation and diminution of this response occur with familiarity and/or repeated exposure (Rose, 1985). The earlier a patient can comprehend, evaluate and adapt to the realities of his condition the sooner can the need for sedative supplements be reduced.

Pain

Pain is one of the most frequently noted complaints of ITU patients (Asbury, 1985). Most ITU's generate a large proportion of their admissions from surgical or trauma sources and the presence of acute pain is to be expected. However, continuing distress caused by pain is a measure of inadequate care since the prudent employment of available techniques should achieve acceptable patient comfort (Hug, 1980; Bullingham, 1985).

Numerous reviews (Wallace & Norris, 1975; Utting & Smith, 1979; White, 1982; Dodson, 1985) have commented on the inadequate analgesia often received by hospitalised patients. In ITU the patient's perception of pain is further modulated by the accompanying anxiety and fear of life threatening illness. There is a direct relationship between anxiety and pain, with increased anxiety worsening pain and vice versa (Phillips & Cousins, 1986). The continuation of stress eventually causes a lowering of pain threshold which may be related to alterations in endogenous opioid levels (Madden et al, 1977; Cohen et al, 1982; Szyfelbein et al, 1983).

Insomnia
Circadian rhythmicity, manifest by diurnal variation of physiological function, is a poorly understood phenomenon. The 24-hour cycle is dependent not only on an 'internal clock' of endogenous rhythm but also on external stimuli of 'zeitgebers' such as light, temperature or sound (Moore-Ede et al, 1983a,b). Asynchrony of these internal and external rhythms is well recognised to produce malaise and disorientation in 'jet lagged' travellers or shift workers. The combination of critical illness, treatment and the environment of the ITU is likely to result in similar symptoms and contribute to psychiatric disability (Cousins & Phillips, 1984; Campbell et al, 1986).

The most obvious disturbance of these widely varying inputs is in the sleeping/waking cycles of ITU patients. Sleep deprivation of 4–5 days is recognised to precipitate psychotic symptoms which have been compared to the delirium reported after cardiac surgery (Kornfield et al, 1965). Deterioration of sleep patterns has been recognised following surgery or life threatening illness (Aurell & Elmqvist, 1985). Markedly decreased or absent REM, Stage 3 and Stage 4 sleep has been consistently reported.

The important anabolic contribution of deep levels of sleep to health and tissue restoration after trauma or surgery has been stressed by Adam & Oswald (1984). Growth hormone, for example, is secreted mainly during sleep and protein synthesis and nitrogen balance are adversely affected by sleep deprivation (Adam & Oswald, 1983). Problems arise, however, with attempts to restore sleep: clinically effective doses of hypnotic drugs may further shorten REM and Slow Wave Sleep (Johns, 1975). REM sleep stages have also been associated with bronchospasm in asthmatics (Shapiro et al, 1986) and with sleep apnoea syndromes (Branthwaite, 1986).

The physiological stress response
The significance of the 'stress response' continues to be a source of confusion (Traynor & Hall, 1981; Teich et al, 1985; Kehlet, 1986). The initial sympathoadrenal arousal may cause hypertension and tachycardia and the longer term neuroendocrine effects are known to cause nutritional and immunological disturbance (Blalock et al, 1985; Ganong, 1986). It is accepted, however, that aspects of this stress response have an essential protective function in survival from life threatening illness (Parker et al, 1985; Burke, 1985). The balance required in acute illness is as yet unresolved and it is unclear whether attempts to modify the stress response will prove beneficial (Longnecker, 1984; Editorial, 1985).

This dilemma gave rise to recent controversy with regard to the infusion of etomidate in ITU patients. Most patients suffering a critical illness will respond with higher than normal plasma cortisol levels (Sainsbury et al, 1981; Drucker & Shandling, 1985). In a small number of patients, particularly those with severe sepsis, poor cortisol response is associated with increased mortality (Sibbald et al, 1977). However, Finlay & McKee (1982) in this centre described a much larger group of patients with adrenocorticol suppression who subsequently died; in a later study (McKee & Finlay, 1983), mortality appeared to be reduced by the administration of exogenous steroid. Simultaneously in the same unit, Ledingham & Watt (1983) noted an increase in the mortality rate of trauma patients which they attributed to the use of etomidate by infusion. Subsequent evidence showing that etomidate was a potent inhibitor of adreno-steroidogenesis (Fraser et al, 1984) provided a link between these findings and suggested that failure to mount a cortisol response in acute illness compromised survival. Neumann et al (1986) recently demonstrated in an animal model that survival from septic shock is adversely affected by low cortisol levels secondary to metomidate anaesthesia and is increased by the administration of cortisol. The precise role of cortisol in this regard is unclear (Munck et al, 1984) although the interaction of corticosteroids and catecholamines in vaso-motor control, and the influence of cortisol on plasma volume and intercompartmental fluid shifts, may be important (Burke, 1985).

PATIENTS' OPINIONS OF SEDATION

Bishop's definition of pain (1959) as 'what the patient says hurts' is a wise basis on which to treat acute pain. A similar concept may be used in ITU when assessing requirements for sedation. Although many patients are unable to communicate their immediate feelings and requirements, helpful information may be gleaned from several post-discharge reviews of patients' recollections of intensive therapy (Hewitt, 1970; Jones et al, 1979; Bradburn & Hewitt, 1980; Asbury, 1985; Chew, 1986). These studies surveyed different patient populations and durations of stay in ITU (and few included details of the sedation regimen employed), but there are remarkable similarities in the patients' accounts of their experiences.

Impression of ITU and staff

The hypothesis that intensive therapy is an intolerable ordeal, requiring drugs to obtund consciousness, is not supported by evidence based on patients' recollections. In a group of general ITU patients who had received narcotic and benzodiazepine sedation, to comfort level and not unconsciousness, the opinion of the ITU stay was described as:

Pleasant= 33%
Tolerable= 45%
Unpleasant= 8%
Terrifying= 3%
No opinion= 11%

(Bion et al, 1987).

Jones et al (1979) and Bradburn & Hewitt (1980) showed similar patient acceptance of the ITU environment: 80–90% of patients considered the staff in ITU sympathetic and efficient although 12–20% of patients complained of inadequate explanation from attendant staff.

Memory and orientation

Approximately 25% of patients have no memory of their stay in ITU (Schroeder, 1971; Asbury, 1985). Such memory as is retained is usually associated with the later part of the ITU stay. Patients who have undergone mechanical ventilation have poor recall of this procedure or its duration. This may reflect the seriousness of their illness or the increased drug usage to facilitate mechanical ventilation. Most patients are unable to recall the precise duration of their stay and often complain of marked disorientation in time.

Complaints and worries
Patients most frequently remember the physical aspects of treatment such as physiotherapy and the presence of catheters and intravascular lines (Table 5.1). The physical features most frequently described as unpleasant are thirst and the presence of face mask and nasogastric tube—matters often considered of minor importance by attendant staff. Patients are less likely to recall their subjective feelings than their physical sensations, but when the former are recalled, those invariably described as having caused most distress are anxiety, pain and lack of rest. The occurrence of dreams about ITU which may persist for many months after discharge has also been described as distressing (Asbury, 1985; Schröeder, 1971).

Table 5.1   Patients' recall of ITU (from Bion et al, 1987)

Experience recalled	% of patients recalling experience	% describing experience as moderately or very unpleasant
Physiotherapy	75	33
Urinary catheter	75	17
IV and arterial lines	71	15
Noise	71	4
Thirst	66	60
Face mask	66	52
NG tube	56	47
Anxiety	55	78
Radio	50	33
Lack of rest	45	63
Pain	40	66
ET tube	38	57
Suction	35	24
Dreams	35	—

Of overwhelming importance to individual patients (Henschell, 1977; Donald, 1977; Parker et al, 1984) is human contact and rapport. Nursing staff in particular should provide explanation and support, and demonstrate a caring empathy, not only verbally but visually and by touch (McCorkle, 1974). After 31 days of mechanical ventilation Viner (1985) pleaded for 'a warm smile instead of an air of oblivious indifference' and Kiely (1974) stressed that 'the humanising element of person to person conduct is capable of rapidly desensitising the patient to alarm, fear or bewilderment'. While evidence based on patient information is vital in identifying the precise purpose of sedation there is, however, always the possibility of bias in gratitude for survival.

PSYCHIATRIC STUDIES

There is conflicting evidence concerning the psychiatric sequelae of ITU. Tomlin (1977) claimed that only 0.5% of patients suffer serious psychiatric problems after intensive therapy, whereas Benzer et al (1983) reported that 'after three years of study no single patient was found who had survived the time in ICU without some particular disturbance or handicap'.

Although all forms of disordered thought, mood or behaviour may occur in ITU the most frequently quoted psychiatric complication has been delirium. This psychosis of confusion, disorientation and delusion appears to occur in from 30–70% of patients in ITU, particularly after cardiac surgery (Dubin et al, 1979). Cardiac surgical patients may, however, suffer from organic neurological deficit following cardiopulmonary bypass (Shaw et al, 1985; Bass, 1986; Smith et al, 1986) which will render the diagnosis of psychological impairment alone exceedingly difficult. It is therefore unfortunate that so many ITU studies have used this particular patient model.

Specific settings of intensive therapy have characteristic psychiatric as well as organic causes of mental dysfunction. In the post-surgical ITU, delirium predominates over depression and anxiety, whereas in the Coronary Care Unit and Respiratory Intensive Care Unit, anxiety neurosis and depression feature most frequently (Hackett et al, 1968; Cassem, 1984). Hale et al (1977) observed that 7% of patients in an ITU required psychiatric consultation during a six-month study. Cassem (1984) suggested that there is a fairly predictable time scale in the presentation of these problems with fear and anxiety being exhibited at initial admission, stabilising in about 48 hours. A defensive psychological strategy such as denial is common at this time but at 4–5 days, often after an apparently lucid period, demoralisation presents as personality problems which reflect the patient's previous and lifelong style of coping with stress. This may progress to a passive helplessness described by Tomlin (1977) as apathetic depression, or may be reflected in agitation, belligerent hostility, delirium or other psychosis with a total retreat from reality.

Although patients' recollections may suggest that the psychological effects of intensive care have been exaggerated, the studies discussed above indicate that there is significant incidence of mental disturbance in this population. Indeed, a relationship between psychiatric illness in ICU and increased mortality has been established (Hale et al, 1977; Hackett et al, 1968). Thus if patients can be maintained in a psychologically stable state, both mental and physical benefit will accrue. As yet there is no evidence that different sedation regimens will affect psychiatric outcome. However, identifying those at risk and understanding the precipitating factors at play during the period of critical illness will permit a more logical assessment and effective management.

MANAGEMENT

The previous section has highlighted the important interrelationship between the patient, his environment and those responsible for his care. Management, therefore, is concerned primarily with optimising this relationship, a process involving patient support and encouragement, modification of the environment and the judicious use of drugs.

Non-drug manoeuvres

If admission of an elective surgical patient to ITU can be anticipated, information, orientation and instruction may reduce the incidence of postoperative complications (Egbert et al, 1964; Lazarus & Hagens, 1978). Since most patients admitted to the general ITU are emergencies this will not usually be possible. However, those at most risk of developing acute psychiatric illness, and therefore requiring increased psychological and often drug support, may be identified by their immediate clinical response or by their previous history.

Peck (1986) reviewed the psychological methods which may reduce anxiety and pain. A combination of support, instruction, information and relaxation training have much to offer patients in ITU whether or not they are suffering physical pain. Although many patients will be unable actively to control their physical surroundings, they will undoubtedly be helped by understanding what is happening and knowing what sensations are expected. Even patients undergoing mechanical ventilation who are unable to communicate normally may develop self-coping strategies to divert attention from pain or alter the appraisal of the painful situation. Artificial aids to communication greatly assist these patients (Jones, 1986; MacKereth, 1987). Coping strategies may include imaging pleasant events, disassociating self from pain or concentrating on other sensations.

This support requires sensitive and caring staff in sufficient numbers to permit the development of meaningful communication with each patient (Ashworth, 1980). 'When these precautions are taken a surprising number of patients do accept the reality of the intensive therapy environment quite calmly and do not need sedative drugs' (Schröeder, 1971). The patient's family should also be deeply involved in this psychological support and will themselves require encouragement and reassurance. If staff are insufficient in number or not orientated towards this form of care, it is often easier and more convenient to resort to the use of drug therapy, but this should not be used as a justification for such treatment.

The promotion of appropriate sleep should be a prime objective for all patients (Wilmore et al, 1976). The ITU environment should be structured and ordered to achieve this. The importance of the environment in maintaining a meaningful perception of reality and mental stability has been shown by Keep et al (1980) who found the incidence of delusion to be doubled in an ITU without windows. Daylight and visual distraction should thus be provided if possible (Wilson, 1972; Ulrich, 1984) or at least distinctive day–night lighting patterns. If sedative drugs are given, attempts should be made to fluctuate the level of consciousness in the patient to encourage sleep at night and comprehension during the day. Within the limits of safe practice disturbance of the patient during the night should be minimised, and noise and staff activity controlled. Cues such as calendars, clocks, meals and visitors during waking hours will also help patients to maintain time orientation.

A recent report (Aurell & Elmqvist, 1985) of persistent sleep disturbance after minor surgery (despite efforts to provide a comfortable environment conducive to sleep) suggested that there may be additional, as yet unidentified, endogenous factors which cause disrupted sleep patterns in sick patients. Sedative or hypnotic drug therapy is therefore of major importance in promoting sleep and should be prescribed accordingly but within the limitations described above.

Sedative drug treatment
Although the importance of non-pharmacological manoeuvres in the sedative management of patients in intensive care is not in doubt, it would be unreasonable to suggest that drug treatment has not a central and paramount role in the relief of distress and pain. Nearly all patients will require analgesic, anxiolytic or hypnotic drugs at

some time or other during their stay in ITU. However, there is no evidence that sedative drugs improve outcome and since all have at least some undesirable side effects they should always be prescribed with caution.

Depth and duration of sedation

The increasing popularity of surgery under regional analgesia indicates that if pain relief and reassurance are provided, unconsciousness is not necessary for a large proportion of patients undergoing unpleasant experiences. In the ITU, whilst regional analgesia has its place (see below), systemic agents still predominate. The use of these drugs, particularly by continuous intravenous infusion, make it difficult to achieve sedation without reduction of consciousness. The problem is further complicated by the recent observation that even general anaesthesia may not totally block awareness (Breckenridge & Aitkenhead, 1983). There is increasing evidence that unconscious perception during anaesthesia (Jones & Konieczko, 1986), particularly of auditory input, may influence behaviour at a later date (Bonke et al, 1986). This would suggest that any level of sedation employed in ITU cannot be guaranteed reliably to protect the patient from noxious stimuli.

Prolonged administration of sedative agents creates additional hazards. Immobility may result in negative nitrogen balance (Allison, 1986), an undesirable further insult to an already catabolic ITU patient, and may also contribute to the onset of venous thrombosis or pressure damage to nerves or skin. The immunological status of these patients is compromised by illness or trauma (McIrvine & Mannick, 1983) and possibly by psychological stress or depression (Denman, 1986). Anaesthetic, analgesic and sedative agents may further reduce host defences (Moudgil, 1981) and in the case of morphine an increased incidence of infection has been reported (Tubaro et al, 1983). Attempts to achieve unconsciousness for a prolonged period may thus have significant deleterious results and all options should be fully explored before 'deep sedation' is prescribed.

This is not to suggest that when faced with a confused, agitated, hypoxic patient in respiratory failure the provision of adequate sedation together with mechanical ventilation is inappropriate, but simply that the position should be reviewed at regular intervals. The advantages of a comprehending, co-operative patient are now becoming clear. Not only might physical benefits accrue, but the establishment of human relationships with responding patients improves their dignity and increases rapport both with them and their relatives. The overall effect is to make the ITU a more pleasurable place in which to work and may help to reduce stress amongst staff.

The aims of sedation in ITU, therefore, should be to achieve a pain free, comfortable patient who has periods of sleep but who rouses to a comprehending awareness spontaneously or easily to command. This ideal may not be achievable in every patient all of the time but sedation strategies should be flexible and subject to frequent review. The prospect of one ideal sedative agent (Editorial, 1984) is unrealistic but with careful selection of the agents available and appropriate psychological support the proposed level of sedation should be achievable in the majority of patients for the bulk of their stay in ITU.

Assessment of sedation

Ideally, the patient will be able to communicate feelings of discomfort, pain or anxiety. More often, the subjective feelings of the patient must be interpreted indirectly, either by alteration in physiological variables or by clinical observation.

The most frequently used variable in the assessment of subjective responses has been alteration in cardiovascular function secondary to autonomic arousal (Campbell, 1977). Hypertension and tachycardia can be interpreted as evidence of distress but both are non specific responses to stress. Alterations in forearm blood flow have been shown to relate to levels of analgesia in ITU patients (Campbell, 1970). The psychogalvanic skin response and palmar sweat production have both been used to assess stress (Williams et al, 1975; Grings & Dawson, 1978; Maryniak & Bishop, 1987) but are unreliable in acute illness (Nisbett et al, 1967). The interpretation of hormonal changes, such as catecholamines or cortisol, as a measure of stress has also proved difficult (Utting & Whitford, 1972; Fell et al, 1985). Even with advanced neurophysiological methods, such as the cerebral function analysing monitor and sensory evoked potentials it has proved difficult to assess brain activity under anaesthesia (Editorial, 1986).

Quantitative clinical observation is usually based upon a range of scoring systems (Ramsay et al, 1974) or visual analogue scales. The Glasgow Coma Scale and subsequent derivatives (Shelly et al, 1986) assess conscious level. The quality of sedation such as the presence of agitation, confusion or comprehension are not assessed. Triple analogue scales of consciousness, calmness and comprehension may demonstrate differences between sedative regimens (Fig. 5.2). However, as presently utilised they are unwieldy and too time consuming for use in routine nursing care. There is a need

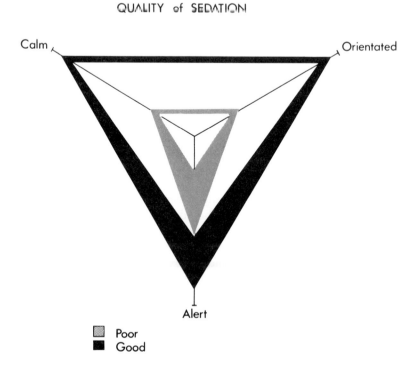

Fig. 5.2   Triple analogue scales of consciousness, calmness and comprehension allowing demonstration of the difference between sedative drug regimens.

for a simple scoring system to assess sedation in ITU which combines subjective observation and objective measurement of response. In the meantime assessment of conscious level including, when appropriate, regular arousal should become a routine component of monitoring and recording the course of a critical illness.

Available drugs
The drugs available for the sedative management of patients in ITU may be conveniently grouped as:

1. Analgesics:
   (a) Systemic.
   (b) Regional.
2. Tranquilisers:
   (a) Benzodiazepines.
   (h) Others
3. Anaesthetic and hypnotic agents:
   (a) Intravenous.
   (b) Inhalational.
4. Miscellaneous:
   (a) Relaxants.
   (b) Antidepressants.
   (c) Others.

Although a wide selection of agents is available, only a small number are currently in regular use in this country (Table 5.2).

Table 5.2 Choice of sedation regimen in UK intensive therapy units (from Bion & Ledingham, 1987)

Preferred choice of sedation regimen	% of ITUs
Opiate alone	37
Opiate plus benzodiazepine	60
Opiate plus other sedative	1
Other drug	2
Preferred opiate	
Papaveretum	33
Phenoperidine	27
Morphine	20
Fentanyl	9
Diamorphine	5
Pethidine	4
Buprenorphine	1
No response	1
Usual mode of administration of drugs	
Infusion plus bolus	55
Mainly infusion	10
Mainly bolus	35

Opiates

Opiates remain the most frequently used drugs for sedation in ITU. The naturally occurring opiates are the most popular of this group despite the development of many synthetic derivatives (Charlton, 1985). The older drugs are familiar, cheap and exhibit more mood elevating effects and psychological 'comfort'.

Morphine

It is widely believed that diamorphine or papaveretum have more pronounced sedative effects than morphine but there is little evidence to support this belief (Kaiko et al, 1981). All three have similar and well recognised side effects (Duthie & Nimmo, 1987).

Particular caution must be observed when morphine is administered by continuous intravenous infusion to patients in renal failure (McQuay & Moore, 1984; Ball et al, 1985; Bion et al, 1986). Difficulties in the assay of morphine have delayed and confused pharmacological interpretation but the prolonged action of morphine in patients with renal failure appears to be due to an accumulation of the active metabolite, morphine-six-glucuronide (Woolner et al, 1986; Osborne et al, 1986), and not to deranged primary metabolism. Although morphine clearance may be impaired by reduced liver blood flow in shock (MacNab et al, 1986), there is also evidence of extra hepatic morphine metabolism (Shelly et al, 1986; Hug et al, 1979).

There is an enormous variation in individual morphine requirement. Dodson (1982) reported a dose requirement between 0.3 and 9.0 mg/h of morphine in a postoperative analgesic study. In the authors' experience infusions varying between 3 and 15 mg/h of morphine resulted in similar sedative effects with widely varying plasma concentrations (Bion et al, 1986). In this study an inverse relationship was noted between sedative requirement and severity of sickness as assessed by the APACHE score (Knaus et al, 1985). In addition, the effect of continuous arterio-venous haemofiltration on drug elimination (Pollock et al, 1986; Bion et al, 1986) may alter requirements.

In a comparative study in this centre, morphine, administered as the only agent, resulted in satisfactory sedation in the great majority of patients without significant adverse effect (Ledingham et al, 1986).

Pethidine

This drug has been the model for much work on individual variation of opiate effect (Mather & Phillips, 1986). Although there may be a relationship between plasma concentration and effect in an individual patient a fourfold variation between patients has been shown (Austin et al, 1980). Pethidine has been infused post-operatively (Church, 1979) and in the ITU (Yate et al, 1986) but its prolonged use has been challenged in view of the possible accumulation of its metabolite, norpethidine, which may cause CNS excitement and convulsions (Inturrisi & Umans, 1983).

Phenoperidine

Although popular in ITU's (Table 5.2) this agent receives little attention in recent texts (Dodson, 1985; Bullingham, 1983). Phenoperidine may result in cardiovascular instability but there is probably little to choose between pethidine and phenoperidine in this respect. Both agents remain useful drugs if histamine release is particularly undesirable e.g. in asthmatics.

Fentanyl

Fentanyl is now probably the most frequently used analgesic in anaesthetic practice (Stanley, 1987) but its use in intensive therapy has been limited. This agent has little effect on the cardiovascular system, does not release histamine and, being lipid soluble, has a rapid onset of action. However, with an elimination half life of 2–5 hours its reputation as a short-acting drug is unjustified, particularly when used in large doses or by infusion.

Alfentanil

With its shorter terminal half-life of approximately 1–2 hours alfentanil may well prove more valuable. Favourable reports of the use of this drug by long-term infusion in critically ill patients may presage its wider acceptance (Yate et al, 1986; Cohen & Kelly, 1987). However, there is evidence that a proportion of patients show a non-uniform metabolism of alfentanil (McDonnell et al, 1984; Shafer et al, 1986). The drug is a most valuable agent when short-term analgesic supplementation is required and may prevent the autonomic responses to short-term painful procedures.

Newer agonist/antagonist analgesics

These agents (Charlton, 1985) have received little attention as ITU sedatives. Their lower addiction potential is probably of little import in acute care (Porter & Jick, 1980). Buprenorphine, perhaps the most widely studied of this group, has not become established as a superior alternative to older analgesics in intensive therapy. However, it has been claimed to have antidepressant properties (Emrich et al, 1982) and its availability as a sublingual preparation is an attractive feature.

Benzodiazepines

In the quarter century since benzodiazepines have been introduced they have become one of the most commonly prescribed of all drugs. They produce anxiolysis, hypnosis, amnesia, muscle relaxation and anticonvulsant effects, a combination suggesting that they might provide the ideal sedative agent for use in ITU. Benzodiazepines reduce the MAC value of halothane during anaesthesia (Melvin et al, 1982) and have been used in the management of postoperative pain (Derrick et al, 1967) but are not normally considered to have significant analgesic properties. They result in a moderate degree of cardiovascular and respiratory depression and some may have a protective function against cerebral ischaemic damage (Reves et al, 1985; Nugent et al, 1982).

Diazepam

The prolonged action of diazepam is now recognised to be due to its elimination half-life of approximately 36 hours and the production of active metabolites. Diazepam continues to be widely used but may result in prolonged recovery times of several days (Kendall & Clark, 1972; Ochs et al, 1982). Care should be taken to limit use of this drug to bolus administration.

Lorazepam

Lorazepam does not have active metabolites and has a slightly shorter elimination half-life of 10–12 hours but potential for inadvertent prolonged depression also exists with this agent. It has been used as a supplementary sedative in intensive therapy with excellent amnesic results (Dundee et al, 1976; Simpson & Eltringham, 1981).

Midazolam

This water-soluble, non-irritant preparation has been widely investigated as an induction and maintenance agent for anaesthesia and as a sedative during local anaesthetic procedures (Dundee et al, 1984; Reves et al, 1985). It has gained popularity for use in the ITU (Gast et al, 1984; Bion & Ledingham, 1987) and its rapid elimination half-life of approximately 2 hours has encouraged its use by continuous infusion. Prolonged recovery of consciousness has been observed in certain patients (Byatt et al, 1984), with accumulation of midazolam and persistently low concentrations of its metabolite 1-hydroxymidazolam (Lloyd-Thomas & Booker, 1986). In the critically ill, impaired metabolism may be associated with poor hepatic perfusion but such impairment has also been demonstrated in some normal volunteers (Dundee et al, 1986).

A number of reports attest to the successful use of midazolam in adults and children undergoing intensive therapy (Shapiro et al, 1986; O'Dea & Hopkinson, 1987; Newman et al, 1987a). The dosage employed has varied from 1 mg to 20 mg/h. Following cardiac surgery in children a dosage of $4 \mu g/kg/min$ was required when midazolam was used alone but if morphine was added the requirement for midazolam was reduced to approximately $3 \mu g/kg/min$ (Booker et al, 1986). Little relationship was observed between plasma levels of midazolam and clinical effect (Lloyd-Thomas & Booker, 1986). Time of awakening was also associated with enormous variation in plasma midazolam levels (78–3315 ng/ml).

Observations in this centre suggests that while midazolam may be an adequate agent in the management of uncomplicated intensive care patients, in others, the drug (even in low doses) may produce an undesirable depression of consciousness. In patients who remain awake, impairment of comprehension and a degree of disorientation is often apparent.

The development of the benzodiazepine antagonist, RO 15/1788, may provide an improved degree of control of benzodiazepine sedation (Ashton, 1985) but as yet this agent is not available in the United Kingdom. The antagonist appears a valuable agent (Alon et al, 1987; Sage et al, 1987) both in the treatment and diagnosis of coma and in the elective reversal of sedation. Careful monitoring is required because of the relatively brief action of the antagonist.

Other systemic agents

Psychotropic drugs other than opioids and benzodiazepines have limited use in ITU practice. However, these drugs may be of value in individual difficult patients.

Barbiturates

The use of barbiturates is now restricted to specific indications, such as status epilepticus or cerebral protection in hypoxic brain damage. In the latter instance these agents reduce intracranial pressure and cerebral oxygen consumption but their influence on long-term prognosis remains controversial (Shapiro, 1985). Thiopentone when infused at approximately 100 mg/h for several days results in awakening time of up to 48 hours (Carlon et al, 1978). The shorter half life of methohexitone (approximately 2 hours) may offer promise but this agent has been reported to cause involuntary movements (MacKenzie & Grant, 1985). All barbiturates may cause hypotension and depress the immune response (Moudgil, 1981; Ward et al, 1985).

Short-acting intravenous agents
Etomidate and althesin, now effectively withdrawn as sedatives, were particularly valuable in neurosurgical practice or when rapid recovery of consciousness was desirable. The new agent, propofol, although not as yet licensed for prolonged sedation appears promising (MacKenzie & Grant, 1987). Preliminary studies (Grounds et al, 1987; Newman et al, 1987b) suggest that this agent, infused at a dose of 1–3 mg/kg/h, is a useful sedative in ITU, the majority of patients being readily maintained in a comfortable yet rousable state. Cardiovascular instability may be a problem in the critically ill patient but no adverse effects on adrenocortical function are apparent.

Inhalational agents
Nitrous oxide 50% in oxygen (Entonox) is a potent and useful short-acting analgesic supplement although its interaction with vitamin B12 and subsequent bone marrow changes (Nunn, 1987) suggest that caution with its use should be exercised. The volatile agents may also be used in low concentrations for analgesia and sedation (McLeod et al, 1985; Parbrook et al, 1987) and may offer particular advantages in the management of severe asthmatics (O'Rourke & Crone, 1982; Bierman et al, 1986).

Ketamine
This agent is also useful as an alternative sedative and analgesic in asthmatic patients (Rock et al, 1986). Infusion of 3 µg/kg/min has been proposed for ITU sedation (Nimmo & McRae, 1983) but has gained little popularity.

Chlormethiazole
This agent has hypnotic and anticonvulsant effects and has found favour in the management of delirium tremens and pre-eclampsia. Although unlikely to cause respiratory or cardiovascular depression in moderate doses (Mather & Cousins, 1980) it requires close supervision and if infused for any substantial period, a slow recovery can be expected (Robson et al, 1984).

Phenothiazines
Of the major tranquillisers, chlorpromazine is the most widely employed and produces sedation, increased duration of sleep and antipsychotic effects. It is limited by its anticholinergic and dyskinetic side-effects, potential hepatic damage and hypotension caused by alpha-adrenergic blockade. When sedation together with vasodilatation is sought, chlorpromazine is useful in small doses provided care is taken to maintain intravascular volume. However, its main indication in the ITU is in the treatment of acute confusional states (Kornfield, 1980).

Butyrophenones
These drugs may be used as alternatives to phenothiazines in treatment of confusion or delirium in ITU (Ayd, 1978). They are also potent antiemetics. Side effects are similar to chlorpromazine but haloperidol in small doses is claimed to exert its antipsychotic effect with less depression of consciousness and hypotension.

Antidepressants
ITU patients who develop symptoms of major depression will often respond to anti-depressants and beneficial results have been reported (Brock-Utne et al, 1976; Bronheim et al, 1985). The tricyclic group have been most commonly used (Dobb & Murphy, 1985), and although the mood elevating effect may take several days to become apparent, in patients with sleep disturbance the use of antidepressants may have a rapid effect in re-establishing improved sleep patterns.

Central nervous stimulants
Although Cassem (1986) has suggested that the amphetamines may have a place in the treatment of depressive states in ITU they cannot be recommended for general use without close psychiatric supervision. They have been reported to augment the analgesia provided by morphine (Forrest et al, 1977).

Adrenergic blocking agents
In some patients whose autonomic responses are difficult to control even with profound sedation, the use of alpha and beta adrenergic blocking agents can be a useful short-term adjuvant if care is taken to prevent hypotension and bronchospasm. The beta blocking agents may indeed have an innate antianxiety effect in their own right (Wheatley, 1981), and may decrease oxygen consumption and the metabolic response to stress (Kehlet & Schulze, 1986).

Muscle Relaxants
Although not sedative agents, muscle relaxants have been used as a component of sedative regimens for many years (Miller-Jones & Williams, 1980). In the past 5 years or so their use has decreased (Merriman, 1981; Gast et al, 1984; Bion & Ledingham, 1987). They may be useful as short-term adjuvants in controlling difficult patients but their long-term use should be deprecated unless clearly indicated and adequate sedative hypnotics have been prescribed simultaneously (Booij, 1986). Although Donald (1977) has claimed 'the inability to struggle lessens the pain' it is generally accepted that to be paralysed and aware is an extremely unpleasant experience (Parker et al, 1984). Specific indications for the use of relaxants other than to facilitate intubation include tetanus, raised intracranial pressure and severe hypoxia with stiff lungs (Willatts, 1985). The new relaxant agents, atracurium and vecuronium (Torda, 1987), may cause less cardiovascular instability than their predecessors and are suitable for continuous infusion (Beemer, 1987).

Regional anaesthetic techniques
The aim of regional anaesthetic techniques is to provide high-quality analgesia without obtunding consciousness. These techniques may be employed to control severe pain in patients breathing spontaneously, to avoid the need for mechanical ventilation, to reduce the requirement for systemic sedation in ventilated patients, or to promote blood flow in ischaemic limbs (Armitage, 1986; Bowler et al, 1986; Morgan, 1987; Cousins & Bridenbaugh, 1986). The environment of the ITU is ideal for the application of these techniques, and yet they are comparatively uncommon in UK practice. This is in part because patients may have pain from more than one site, or may already

be receiving parenteral opiates for mechanical ventilation; but it may also reflect an extension from the operating theatre of a preference for general anaesthesia rather than regional techniques. In addition, these techniques involve certain risks including hypotension (local anaesthetic agents), respiratory depression (opioids), and trauma and infection. Finally, these procedures require specialised expertise and are time consuming.

Epidural analgesia
Epidural catheters allow long-term delivery of analgesic agents. Infusion of local anaes-thetic agents is associated with higher total doses than bolus administration (Li et al, 1985), but is a convenient method of administration and does not produce abrupt changes in sympathetic tone. Low concentrations of bupivacaine (0.125–0.25%) are less likely to cause hypotension, and usually provide adequate analgesia. Epidural opiates are particularly advantageous in the ITU where respiratory depression may be treated rapidly; they provide good analgesia, allow a reduction in parenteral analge-sic and sedative drugs (Rawal & Tandon, 1985), and partially suppress stress responses (Cowen et al, 1982). Diamorphine is less commonly associated with delayed respiratory depression than morphine. It is more lipid-soluble, and passes more rapidly into the spinal cord; it is rapidly converted in neural tissue to the more water-soluble morphine, and rostral spread in the CSF is limited.

The combination of a local anaesthetic agent and an opiate given together, either simultaneously or consecutively, may be advantageous (Rankine & Comber, 1984; Hjortso et al, 1986).

Intrathecal analgesia
The intrathecal route is technically easier for single injections, and diamorphine or morphine in doses of less than 1.0 mg, will provide analgesia for up to 24 hours; higher doses are more likely to produce late respiratory depression (Barron & Strong, 1984). Stress responses are partially suppressed (Child et al, 1985). Indwelling catheters have been used primarily in the treatment of chronic pain (Leavens et al, 1982) and are not normally used in the ITU. Unlikely drugs, such as clonidine and midazolam, possess significant analgesic activity when given by the epidural or intrathecal route (Coombs et al, 1985; Yaksh, 1985; Serrao & Goodchild, 1987) but their role is not yet well defined.

These techniques should be performed with full antiseptic precautions, particularly as the critically ill may be both bacteraemic and immunologically impaired. The spinal route is contraindicated in patients who are receiving anticoagulant drugs or who have coagulation disorders; these may be related to haematological malignancy, mas-sive blood transfusions, sepsis, or liver disease, all common problems in intensive care. Following subarachnoid injection, spinal haematomata have been reported in patients with these predisposing factors, particularly when technical difficulties were encountered (Owens et al, 1986). Epidural injections can produce marked rises in intracranial pressure in the presence of intracranial hypertension (Hilt et al, 1986); and a dural tap may produce fatal coning (Richards & Towu-Aghanste, 1986); the technique is best avoided in such patients.

Brachial plexus block

Brachial plexus block may be an appropriate adjunct in some patients, and is best provided as a continuous infusion using a catheter placed by the axillary (Ang et al, 1984) or interscalene (Kirkpatrick et al, 1985) routes.

Intercostal nerve block

Intercostal nerve blocks are appropriate for the relief of pain from circumscribed sites in the thorax and upper abdomen (Crawford & Thompson, 1986). Single or multiple site injections may be equally effective. Intermittent administration is the normal practice but continuous local infusion is also feasible (Murphy, 1983; Baxter et al, 1987). This procedure should not be performed by inexperienced, unsupervised staff on ventilated patients in view of the danger of pneumothorax.

Sympathetic nerve blockade

Sympathetic nerve block is usually regarded as a side-effect of regional anaesthesia, but may be used specifically to relieve chronic sympathetic-dependent pain (algo-dystrophies), and to improve blood flow to ischaemic tissues. Spinal anaesthesia preserves leg blood flow post-operatively (Foate et al, 1985), and this may diminish the risk of deep venous thrombosis, but it does not appear to reduce the incidence of subsequent amputation in patients presenting for vascular surgery (Cook et al, 1986).

Transcutaneous electrical nerve stimulation (TENS)

TENS is of some value in relieving labour pain, but does not relieve acute post-operative pain (Cushieri et al, 1985); its usefulness in intensive care is likely to be limited.

CONCLUSIONS

The essential ingredient of successful sedation are human contact, relief of pain and anxiety, and adequate sleep. It is no longer deemed appropriate to achieve these in conjunction with prolonged unconsciousness. Depression of conscious level may be necessary at certain circumscribed stages of an illness but in the long term, comprehension and co-operation aid recovery.

The importance of psychological support has been underestimated as, indeed, has the resilience and ability of many patients to adapt to unpleasant circumstances. The patient's innate psychological defences should be reinforced by members of staff, by family and friends, and by the provision of a suitable environment. Simple repeated explanations, reassurance and distraction are required.

Pharmacological agents are of undoubted value in the management of the distressed and exhausted patient but attending staff should have a clear understanding in each case of the desired level of sedation. Drugs should be administered with due care and their effects regularly monitored. The choice of agent varies but the opiates, and morphine in particular, appear to be suitable for the majority of ITU patients. The benzodiazepines are valuable adjuvants if prescribed prudently. Of the newer agents, alfentanil and propofol deserve further investigation as does the more widespread adoption of regional techniques.

To those not directly involved in the practice of intensive therapy, the patient's environment is perceived as one in which emotional needs are neglected in favour of technical expertise (Rawles, 1986). Sedation policies have in the past contributed to the undignified image of a patient appearing like 'an object as impersonal as the machines to which she was connected' (Paton, 1969). The changing face of sedation in recent times has already done much to reduce patient indignity and improve overall care.

REFERENCES

Adam K, Oswald I 1983 Protein synthesis, bodily renewal and the sleep–wake cycle. Clinical Science 65: 561–567

Adam K, Oswald I 1984 Sleep helps healing. British Medical Journal 289: 1400–1401

Aitkenhead A 1986 Cerebral Protection. British Journal of Hospital Medicine 35: 290–298

Allison S P 1986 Some metabolic aspects of injury. In: Little R A, Frayn K N (eds) The Scientific Basis for the Care of the Critically Ill. Manchester University Press, pp 169–183

Alon E, Baitella L, Hossli G 1987 Double-blind study of the reversal of midazolam supplemented general anaesthesia with RO 15-1788. British Journal of Anaesthesia 59: 455–458

Ang E T, Lassale B, Goldfarb G 1984 Continuous axillary brachial plexus block—a clinical and anatomical study. Anesthesia and Analgesia 63: 680–684

Armitage E N 1986 Local anaesthetic techniques for prevention of postoperative pain. British Journal of Anaesthesa 58: 790–800

Asbury A J 1985 Patients' memories and reactions to Intensive Care. Care of the Critically Ill 1: 12–13

Ashton C H 1985 Benzodiazepine overdose: are specific antagonists useful? British Medical Journal 290: 805–806

Ashworth P 1980 Care to communicate. Royal College of Nursing, London

Aurell J, Elmqvist D 1985 Sleep in the surgical intensive care unit. British Medical Journal 290: 1029–1032

Austin K L, Stapleton J V, Mather L E 1980 Relationship between blood meperidine concentrations in analgesic response. Anesthesiology 53: 460–466

Ayd F S 1978 Intravenous haloperidol therapy. International Drug and Therapeutics Newsletter 13: 19–23

Ball M, Moore R A, Fisher A, McQuay H J, Allen M C, Sear J 1985 Renal failure and the dose of morphine in intensive care. Lancet i: 784–786

Barron D W, Strong J E 1984 The safety and efficacy of intrathecal diamorphine. Pain 18: 279–285

Bass C 1986 Psychological problems following coronary artery bypass surgery. British Journal of Hospital Medicine 35: 111–115

Baxter A D, Jennings F O, Harris R S, Flynn J F, Way J 1987 Continuous intercostal blockade after cardiac surgery. British Journal of Anaesthesia 59: 162–166

Baxter S 1974 Psychological problems of intensive care. British Journal of Hospital Medicine 11: 875–885

Beemer G H 1987 Continuous infusions of muscle relaxants—why and how? Anaesthesia and Intensive Care 15: 83–89

Benzer H, Mutz N, Pauser G 1983 Psychosocial sequelae of Intensive Care. International Anesthesiology Clinics 21: 169–180

Bierman M I, Brown M, Muran O, Keenan R L, Glavser F L 1986 Prolonged isoflurane anaesthesia in status asthmaticus. Critical Care Medicine 14: 832–833

Bion J F, Ledingham I McA 1987 Sedation in intensive care: A postal study. Intensive Care Medicine 13: 215–216

Bion J F 1987 Recollections of Critical Illness. Unpublished observations

Bion J F, Logan B K, Newman P M, Brodie M J, Oliver J S, Aitchison T C, Ledingham I M 1986 Sedation in intensive care: morphine and renal failure. Intensive Care Medicine 12: 359–365

Bishop G H 1959 Quoted in Beecher H K: Measurement of subjective responses. P6. Oxford University Press, New York

Blalock J E, Smith E M, Meyer W J 1985 The pituitary–adrenocortical axis and the immune system. Clinics in Endocrinology and Metabolism 14: 1021–1038

Bonke B, Schmitz P I M, Verhage F, Zwaveling A 1986 Clinical study of so called unconscious perception during general anaesthesia. British Journal of Anaesthesia 58: 957–964

Booij L H 1986 Rational use of muscle relaxants during intensive care treatment. In: Vincent J L (ed) Update in Intensive Care and Emergency Medicine. Springer-Verlag, Berlin, pp 509–514

Booker P D, Beechey A, Lloyd-Thomas A R 1986 Sedation in children requiring artificial ventilation using an infusion of midazolam. British Journal of Anaesthesia 58: 1104–1108

Bowden P 1983 Psychiatric aspects of intensive care. In: Tinker J, Rapin M (eds) Care of the Critically
    Ill. Springer-Verlag, Berlin, pp 787–797
Bowler G M R, Wildsmith J A, Scott D B 1986 Epidural administration of local anaesthetics. Clinics
    in Critical Care Medicine 8: 187–235
Bradburn B G, Hewitt P B 1980 The effect of the intensive therapy ward environment on patients
    subjective impressions: A follow-up study. Intensive Care Medicine 7: 15–18
Branthwaite M 1986 Role of sleep and fatigue in Genesis of Respiratory Insufficiency. In: Vincent J L (ed)
    Update in Intensive Care and Emergency Medicine. Springer-Verlag, Berlin, pp 55–56
Breckenridge J L, Aitkenhead A R 1983 Awareness during anaesthesia. A Review. Annals of the Royal
    College of Surgeons (England) 65: 93–96
British National Formulary 1986 Number 12, p 133. British Medical Association, London
Brock-Utne J G, Cheetham R W S, Goodwin N M 1976 Psychiatric problems in intensive care. Anaesthesia
    31: 380–384
Bronheim H E, Iberti T J, Benjamin E, Strain J J 1985 Depression in the intensive care unit. Critical
    Care Medicine 13: 985–988
Bullingham R E S (ed) 1983 Opiate analgesia. Clinics in Anaesthesiology. WB Saunders, London,
    Philadelphia, Vol 1, No 1
Bullingham R E S 1985 Optimum management of post-operative pain. Drugs 29: 376–386
Burke C W 1985 Adrenocortical insufficiency. Clinics in Endocrinology and Metabolism 14: 947–976
Byatt C M, Lewis L D, Dawling S, Cochrane G M 1984 Accumulation of midazolam after repeated
    dosage in patients receiving mechanical ventilation in an intensive care unit. British Medical Journal
    289: 799–800
Campbell D 1970 The management of pain in the Intensive Care Unit. British Journal of Surgery 57: 721–
    722
Campbell D 1977 The management of post-operative pain. In: Harcus A W, Smith R B, Whittle B A (eds)
    Pain—New Perspectives in Measurement and Management. Churchill Livingstone, Edinburgh, pp 103–
    109
Campbell I T, Minors D D S, Waterhouse J M 1986 Are circadian rhythms important in intensive care?
    Intensive Care Nursing 1: 144–150
Carlon G C, Kahn R C, Goldiner P L, Howland W S, Turnbull A 1978 Long term infusion of sodium
    thiopental. Critical Care Medicine 6: 411–416
Cassem N H 1984 Critical care psychiatry. In: Shoemaker W C, Holbrook P R (eds) Textbook of Critical
    Care. WB Saunders, Philadelphia, pp 981–989
Cassem N H 1986 Psychiatric aspects of critical care. In: Vincent J L (ed) Update in Intensive Care and
    Emergency Medicine. Springer-Verlag, Berlin, pp 543–544
Charlton J E 1985 Newer analgesics in the control of post-operative pain. In: Smith J A R, Watkins J (eds)
    Care of the Postoperative Surgical Patient. Butterworths, London, Boston, pp 39–57
Chew S L 1986 Psychological reactions of intensive care patients. Care of the Critically Ill 2: 62–65
Child C S, Kaufman L 1985 Effect of intrathecal diamorphine on the adrenocortical, hyperglycaemic
    and cardiovascular responses to major colonic surgery. British Journal of Anaesthesia 57: 389–393
Church J J 1979 Continuous narcotic infusion for relief of postoperative pain. British Medical Journal
    ii: 977–979
Cohen A T, Kelly D R 1987 Assessment of alfentamil by intravenous infusion as long-term sedation
    in intensive care. Anaesthesia 42: 545–548
Cohen M R, Pickar D, Dubos M 1982 Stress-induced plasma beta endorphin immunoreactivity may
    predict postoperative morphine usage. Psychiatry Research 6: 7–12
Cook P I, Davies M J, Cronin K D, Moran P 1986 A prospective randomised trial comparing spinal
    anaesthesia using hyperbaric cinchocaine with general anaesthesia for lower limb vascular surgery.
    Anaesthesia and Intensive Care 14: 373–380
Coombs D W, Saunders R L, Lachance D, et al 1985 Intrathecal morphine tolerance: use of intrathecal
    clonidine, DADLE, and intraventricular morphine. Anesthesiology 62: 358–363
Cousins M J, Bridenbaugh P O 1986 Spinal opioids and pain relief in acute care. Clinics in Critical
    Care Medicine 8: 151–185
Cousins M J, Phillips G D 1984 'Sleep pain and sedation'. In: Shoemaker W C, Thompson W (eds)
    Textbook of Critical Care. WB Saunders, Philadelphia, pp 981–989
Cowen M J, Bullingham R E S, Paterson G M C, et al 1982 A controlled comparison of the effects
    of extradural diamorphine and bupivacaine on plasma glucose and plasma cortisol in postoperative
    patients. Anesthesia and Analgesia 61: 15–18
Crawford R D, Thompson G E 1986 Intercostal block. In: Cousins M J, Phillips G D (eds) Acute Pain
    Management. Clinics in Critical Care Medicine. Churchill Livingstone, New York, Edinburgh,
    8: pp 237–249

Cushieri R J, Morran C G, McArdle C S 1985 Transcutaneous electrical stimulation for postoperative pain. Annals of the Royal College of Surgeons (England) 67: 127

Denman A M 1986 Immunity and depression. British Medical Journal 293: 464

Derrick W S, Wette R, Hill D B 1967 Librium in the recovery room. Anesthesia and Analgesia 46: 171–175

Dobb G J, Murphy D F 1985 Sedation and analgesia during intensive care. Clinics in Anaesthesiology 3: 1055–1085

Dobson C B 1982 Stress: the hidden adversary. MTP Press, Lancaster

Dodson M E 1985 The Management of Postoperative Pain. Edward Arnold, London

Dodson M E 1982 A review of methods for relief of postoperative pain. Annals of the Royal College of Surgeons (England) 64: 324–327

Donald I 1977 Pain—a patient's view. In: Harcus A W, Smith R, Whittle B (eds) Pain: New perspectives in measurement and management. Churchill Livingstone, Edinburgh, London, pp 1–4

Drucker R, Shandling M 1985 Variable adrenocortical function in acute medical illness. Critical Care Medicine 13: 477–479

Dubin W R, Field H L, Gastfriend D R 1979 Postcardiotomy delirium: a critical review. Journal of Thoracic and Cardiovascular Surgery 77: 586–594

Dundee J W, Collier P S, Carlisle R J T, Harper K W 1986 Prolonged midazolam elimination half life. British Journal of Clinical Pharmacology 21: 425–429

Dundee J W, Halliday N J, Harper K W, Brogden R N 1984 Midazolam: A review of its pharmacological properties and therapeutic use. Drugs 28: 519–554

Dundee J W, Johnston H M L, Gray R C 1976 Lorazepam as a sedative-amnesic in an intensive care unit. Current Medical Research and Opinion 4: 290–295

Duthie D J R, Nimmo W S 1987 Adverse effects of opioid analgesic drugs. British Journal of Anaesthesia 59: 61–77

Editorial 1984 Sedation in the Intensive-care Unit. Lancet i: 1388–1389

Editorial 1985 Analgesia and the metabolic response to surgery. Lancet 1: 1018–1019

Editorial 1986 The depth of anaesthesia. Lancet 2: 553–554

Egbert L D, Battit G E, Weich C E, Bartlett M K 1964 Reduction of postoperative pain by encouragement and instruction of patients. New England Journal of Medicine 270: 825–828

Emrich H M, Vogt P, Herz A, Kissling W 1982 Antidepressant effects of buprenorphine. Lancet ii: 709

Fell D, Derbyshire D R, Maile C J D, Larsson I M, Ellis R, Achola K J, Smith G 1985 Measurement of plasma catecholamine concentrations—an assessment of anxiety. British Journal of Anaesthesia 57: 770–774

Fellows I W, Woolfson A M J 1985 Effects of therapeutic intervention on the metabolic responses to injury. British Medical Bulletin 11: 287–294

Finlay W E I, McKee J F 1982 Serum cortisol levels in severely stressed patients. Lancet i: 1414–1415

Foate J A, Horton H, Davis F M 1985 Lower limb blood flow during transurethral resection of the prostate under spinal or general anaesthesia. Anaesthesia and Intensive Care 13: 383–386

Forrest W H, Brown B W, Brown C R, Defaique R, Gold M, Gordon H E, James K E, Katz J, Mahler D L, Schroff P, Teutsch G 1977 Dextroamphetamine with morphine for the treatment of postoperative pain. New England Journal of Medicine 296: 712–715

Fraser R, Watt I, Gray C E, Ledingham I McA, Lever A F 1984 The effect of etomidate on adrenocortical function in dogs before and during haemorrhagic shock. Endocrinology 115: 2266

Ganong W F 1986 Neuroendocrine response to injury. In: Little R A, Frayn K N (eds) The Scientific Basis for the Care of the Critically Ill. Manchester University Press, pp 61–73

Gast P H, Fisher A, Sear J W 1984 Intensive care sedation now. Lancet 2: 863–864

Gordon H L 1986 Morphine intoxication in renal failure: the role of morphine-6-glucuronide. British Medical Journal 293: 818

Grings W W, Dawson M E 1978 Emotions and bodily responses: A psychophysiological approach. Academic Press, New York

Grounds R M, Lalor J M, Lumley J, Royston D, Morgan M 1987 Propofol infusion for sedation in the intensive care unit. Preliminary report. British Medical Journal 294: 397–400

Hackett T P, Cassem N H, Wishnie H A 1968 The coronary care unit: and appraisal of its psychological hazards. New England Journal of Medicine 25: 1365–1370

Hale M, Koss N, Kerstein M, Camp K, Barash P 1977 Psychiatric complications in a surgical ICU. Critical Care Medicine 5: 199–203

Henschell E O 1977 The Guillain-Barré syndrome; A personal experience. Anaesthesiology 47: 228–231

Hewitt P B 1970 Subjective follow-up of patients from a surgical Intensive Therapy Ward. British Medical Journal 4: 669–673

Hilt H, Gramm H J, Link J 1986 Changes in intracranial pressure associated with extradural anaesthesia. British Journal of Anaesthesia 58: 676–680

Hjortso N C, Lund C, Mogensen T, Bigler D, Kehlet H 1986 Epidural morphine improves pain relief and maintains sensory analgesia during continuous epidural bupivacaine after abdominal surgery. Anesthesia and Analgesia 65: 1033–1036

Holland J, Sgroi S M, Marwit S J, Solkopp N 1973 The ICU syndrome: fact or fancy. Psychiatry Medicine 4: 241

Hug C C 1980 Improving analgesic therapy. Anesthesiology 53: 441–443

Hug C C, Aldrete J A, Sampson J F, Murphy M R 1979 Morphine anesthesia in patients with liver failure. Anesthesiology 51: S30

Hull C J 1985 The case for patient-controlled analgesia. In: Smith J A R, Watkins J (eds) Care of the Postoperative Surgical Patient. Butterworths, London, pp 22–38

Inturrisi C E, Umans J G 1983 Pethidine and 1/3 active metabolite norpethidine. In: Bullingham R E S (ed) Opiate Analgesia Clinics in Anaesthesiology. WB Saunders, London, pp 123–138

Johns M W 1975 Sleep and hypnotic drugs. Drugs 9: 448–478

Jones E 1986 Communication aids for the critically ill. Care of the Critically Ill 2: 117–122

Jones J, Hoggart B, Withey J, Donaghue K, Ellis B W 1979 What the patients say: A study of reactions to an Intensive Care Unit. Intensive Care Medicine 5: 89–92

Jones J G, Konieczko K 1986 Hearing and memory in anaesthetised patients. (Editorial). British Medical Journal 292: 1291–1292

Kaiko R F, Wallenstein S L, Rogers A G, Grabinski P Y, Houde R W 1981 Analgesic and mood effects of heroin and morphine in cancer patients with postoperative pain. New England Journal of Medicine 304: 1501–1505

Keep P, James J, Inman M 1980 Windows in the Intensive Therapy Unit. Anaesthesia 35: 257–262

Kehlet H 1986 Pain relief and modification of the stress response. In: Cousins M J, Phillips G D (eds) Acute Pain Management. Clinics in Critical Care Medicine. Churchill Livingstone, New York, Edinburgh, 8: pp 49–75

Kehlet H, Schulze S 1986 Modification of the injury response. In: Little R A, Frayn K N (eds) The scientific basis for the care of the critically ill. Manchester University Press, pp 153–168

Kendall M J, Clarke S W 1972 Prolonged coma after tetanus. British Medical Journal 2: 354–355

Kiely W F 1974 Psychiatric aspects of critical care. Critical Care Medicine 2: 139–142

Kirkpatrick A F, Bednarczyk L R, Hime G W 1985 Bupivacaine blood levels during continuous interscalene block. Anesthesiology 62: 65–67

Knaus W A, Draper E A, Wagner D P, Zimmerman J E 1985 Apache II: a severity of disease classification system. Critical Care Medicine 13: 818–829

Kornfield D S 1980 The Intensive Care Unit in adults; Coronary Care and general medical/surgical. Advances in Psychosomatic Medicine 10: 1–29

Kornfield D S, Zimberg S, Malm J R 1965 Psychiatric complications of open-heart surgery. New England Journal of Medicine 273: 287–292

Lazarus H, Hagens J 1978 Prevention of psychosis following open heart surgery. American Journal of Psychiatry 124: 1190–1195

Leavens M E, Hill C S, Cech D A, et al 1982 Intrathecal and intraventricular morphine for pain in cancer patients: initial study. Journal of Neurosurgery 56: 241–245

Ledingham I McA, Watt I 1983 Influence of sedation on mortality in critically ill multiple trauma patients. Lancet i: 1270

Ledingham I McA, Bion J, Newman L H, Wallace P G M 1986 Experience of sedation in intensive care with special reference to midazolam. In: Ledingham I McA, Hetzel W (eds) Midazolam and Ro15-1788 in ICU, Hexagon (Roche). Basle, Switzerland, pp 9–15

Li D F, Rees G A D, Rosen M 1985 Continuous extradural infusion of 0.0625% or 0.125% bupivacaine for pain relief in primigravid labour. British Journal of Anaesthesia 57: 264–270

Lloyd-Thomas A R, Booker P D 1986 Infusion of midazolam in paediatric patients after cardiac surgery. British Journal of Anaesthesia 58: 1109–1115

Longnecker D E 1984 Stress free: to be or not to be. Anesthesiology 61: 643–644

McCorkle R 1974 Effects of touch on seriously ill patients. Nursing Research 23: 125–132

McDonnell T E, Bartkowski R R, Kahn C 1984 Evidence for polymorphic oxidation of alfentanil in man. Anesthesiology 61: A284

McIrvine A J, Mannick J A 1983 Lymphocyte function in the critically ill surgical patient. Surgical Clinics of North America 63: 245–261

McKee J I, Finlay W E I 1983 Cortisol replacement in severely stressed patients. Lancet i: 484

MacKenzie N, Grant I S 1985 Comparison of the new emulsion formulation of propofol with methohexitone and thiopentone for induction of anaesthesia in day cases. British Journal of Anaesthesia 57: 1167–1172

MacKenzie N, Grant I S 1987 Propofol for intravenous sedation. Anaesthesia 42: 3–6

MacKereth P A 1987 Communication in critical care areas: competing for attention. Nursing 15: 575–578

McLeod D D, Ramayya G P, Tunstall M E 1985 Self administered isoflurane in labour—A comparative study with entonox. Anaesthesia 40: 424–426

MacNab M S P, MacRae E G, Grant I S, Feely J 1986 Profound reduction in morphine clearance and liver blood flow in shock. Intensive Care Medicine 12: 366–369

McQuay H, Moore A 1984 Be aware of renal function when prescribing morphine. Lancet ii: 284–285

Madden J, Akil H, Patrick R L, Barchas J D 1977 Stress induced parallel changes in central opioid levels and pain responsiveness in the rat. Nature 265: 358–360

Maryniak J K, Bishop V A 1987 Palmar sweat and heart rate changes during stress response attenuation with alfentanil. British Journal of Anaesthesia 59: 133–134

Mather L E, Cousins M J 1980 Low dose chlormethiazole infusion as a supplement to central neural blockade: blood concentrations and clinical effects. Anaesthesia and Intensive Care 8: 421–425

Mather L E, Phillips G D 1986 Opioids and adjuvants: Principles of use. In: Cousins M J, Phillips G D (eds) Acute Pain Management. Churchill Livingstone, New York, Edinburgh, pp 77–103

Melvin M A, Johnson B H, Quasha A L, Eger E L 1982 Induction of anesthesia with midazolam decreases halothane MAC in humans. Anesthesiology 57: 238–241

Merriman H M 1981 The techniques used to sedate ventilated patients. Intensive Care Medicine 7: 217–224

Miller-Jones C M H, Williams J H 1980 Sedation for ventilation. Anaesthesia 35: 1104–1107

Molitch M E, Hou S H 1983 Neuroendocrine alterations in systemic disease. In Scanalon M F (ed) Neuroendocrinology: Clinics in Endocrinology and Metabolism. WB Saunders, Philadelphia, London, 12: no 3, pp 825 851

Moore-Ede M C, Czeisler C A, Richardson G S 1983a Circadian timekeeping in health and disease. Part 1. Basic properties of circadian pacemakers. New England Journal of Medicine 309: 469–476

Moore-Ede M C, Czeisler C A, Richardson G S 1983b Circadian timekeeping in health and disease. Part 2, Clinical implications of circadian rhythmicity. New England Journal of Medicine 309: 530–536

Morgan C J, Branthwaite M A 1986 Severity scoring in intensive care (Editorial). British Medical Journal 292: 1546

Morgan M 1987 Epidural and intrathecal opioids. Anaesthesia and Intensive Care 15: 60–67

Moudgil G C 1981 Effect of premedicants, intravenous anaesthetic agents and local anaesthetics on phagocytosis in vitro. Canadian Anaesthetists' Society Journal 28: 597–601

Munck A, Guyre P M, Holbrook N J 1984 Physiological functions of clucocorticoids in stress and their relation to pharmacological action. Endocrine Reviews 5: 25–43

Murphy D F 1983 Continuous intercostal blockade for pain relief after cholecystectomy. British Journal of Anaesthesia 55: 521–524

Neumann R, Worek F, Gutsch W, Pham L, Zimmermann G, Blumel G, Pfeiffer V 1986 Reconstitution of cortisol prevents circulatory failure in septic pigs anesthetised with metomidate. Intensive Care Medicine 12: 242

Newman L H, McDonald J C, Wallace P G M, Ledingham I McA 1987a Propofol infusion for sedation in the intensive care unit. British Medical Journal 294: 970

Newman L H, McDonald J C, Wallace P G M, Ledingham I McA 1987b Propofol infusion for sedation in intensive care. Anaesthesia 42: 929–937

Newton-John H F 1984 'Tetanus'. Medicine International 2: 80–84

Nightingale P, Pleuvry B J 1985 Analgesia and sedation in intensive care. Intensive Care Nursing 1: 25–37

Nimmo W S, MacRae W A 1983 'Sedation and Analgesia'. In: Ledingham I McA, Hanning C D (eds) Recent Advances in Critical Care Medicine. Churchill Livingstone, Edinburgh, London, pp 29–44

Nisbet H I A, Norris W, Brown J 1967 Objective measurement of sedation: IV: The measurement and interpretation of electrical changes in the skin. British Journal of Anaesthesia 39: 798–805

Norris W 1969 'The quantitative assessment of premedication'. British Journal of Anaesthesia 41: 778–784

Nugent M, Artru A, Michenfelder J D 1982 Cerebral metabolic, vascular and protective effects of midazolam maleate. Comparison to diazepam. Anesthesiology 56: 172–176

Nunn J F 1987 Clinical aspects of the interaction between nitrous oxide and vitamin B12. British Journal of Anaesthesia 59: 3–13

Ochs H R, Greenblatt D J, Lauven P M, Stoeckel H, Rommelsheim K 1982 Kinetics of high dose IV diazepam. British Journal of Anaesthesia 54: 849–852

O'Dea J, Hopkinson R 1987 Alfentamil-midazolam infusion. Care of the Critically Ill 3: 20–21

O'Rourke P P, Crone R K 1982 Halothane in status asthmaticus. Critical Care Medicine 10: 341–343

Osborne R J, Joel S P, Slevin M L 1986 Morphine intoxication in renal failure: the role of morphine-6-glucinoxide. British Medical Journal 292: 1548–1549

Owens E L, Kaster G W, Hessel E A 1986 Spinal subarachnoid hematoma after lumbar puncture and heparinization. Anesthesia and Analgesia 65: 1201–1207

Parbrook G D, James J, Braid D P 1987 Inhalational sedation with isoflurane—an alternative technique of inhalational sedation in dentistry. British Dental Journal 163: 88–92

Parker L N, Levin E R, Lifrak E T 1985 Evidence for adrenocorticol adoption to severe illness. Journal of Clinical Endocrinology and Metabolism 60: 947–952

Parker M M, Schubert W, Shelhamer J H, Parillo J E 1984 Perceptions of a critically ill patient experiencing therapeutic paralysis in an ICU. Critical Care Medicine 12: 69–71

Paton A 1969 Personal View. British Medical Journal 3: 691

Peck C L 1986 Psychological factors in acute pain management. In: Cousin M J, Phillips G D (eds) Acute Pain Management. Churchill Livingstone, New York, pp 251–274

Phillips G D, Cousins M J 1986 Neurological mechanisms of pain and the relationship of pain anxiety and sleep. In: Cousins M J, Phillips G D (eds) Acute Pain Management. Churchill Livingstone, New York, Edinburgh, pp 21–48

Pollock E M M, Dougall J R, Bryce C, McIntosh M, Wallace P G M, Hallworth M 1986 Loss of ranitidine during continuous haemofiltration. British Journal of Anaesthesia 58: 1322

Porter J, Jick H 1980 Addiction rare in patients treated with narcotics. New England Journal of Medicine 302: 123

Ramsay M A E, Savage T M, Simpson B R J, Goodwin A 1974 Controlled sedation with alphaxalone-alphadolone. British Medical Journal ii: 657–659

Rankine A P N, Comber R E H 1984 Management of fifty cases of chest injury with a regimen of epidural bupivicaine and morphine. Anaesthesia and Intensive Care 12: 311–314

Rawal N, Tandon B 1985 Epidural and intrathecal morphine in intensive care units. Intensive Care Medicine 11: 129–133

Rawles J 1986 Personal view. British Medical Journal 293: 1432

Reves J G, Fragen R J, Vinik H R, Greenblatt D J 1985 Midazolam: Pharmacology and uses. Anesthesiology 62: 310–324

Richards P G, Towu-Aghanste E 1986 Dangers of lumbar puncture. British Medical Journal 292: 605–606

Robson D J, Bion C, Gaines P, Flanagan R J, Henry J A 1984 Accumulation of chlormethiazole during intravenous infusion. Intensive Care Medicine 10: 315–316

Rock M J, Rocha S R, L'Hommedieu C S, Truemper E 1986 Use of ketamine in asthmatic children to treat respiratory failure refractory to conventional therapy. Critical Care Medicine 14: 514–516

Rose R M 1985 Psychoendocrinology. In: Wilson J D, Foster D W (eds) Textbook of Endocrinology (7th Edition). WB Saunders, Philadelphia, London, pp 653–681

Sage D J, Close A, Boas R A 1987 Reversal of midazolam sedation with anexate. British Journal of Anaesthesia 59: 459–464

Sainsbury J R C, Stoddart J C, Watson M J 1981 Plasma cortisol levels: a comparison between sick patients and volunteers given intravenous cortisol. Anaesthesia 36: 16–21

Saunders D 1981 Anaesthesia awareness and automation. (Editorial). British Journal of Anaesthesia 53: 1–2

Schroeder H G 1971 Psycho-reactive problems of Intensive Therapy. Anaesthesia 26: 28–35

Serrao J M, Goodchild C S 1987 Intrathecal midazolam in the rat. Evidence for spinally-mediated analgesia. British Journal of Anaesthesia 59: 125

Shafer A, Sung M-L, White P F 1986 Pharmacokinetics and pharmacodynamics of alfentanil infusions during general anesthesia. Anesthesia and Analgesia 65: 1021–1028

Shapiro C M, Catterall J R, Montgomery I, Raab G M, Douglas N J 1986 Do asthmatics suffer broncho-constriction during rapid eye movement sleep. British Medical Journal 292: 1161–1164

Shapiro H M 1985 Barbiturates in brain ischaemia. British Journal of Anaesthesia 57: 82–95

Shapiro J M, Westphal L M, White P F, Sladen R N, Rosenthal M D 1986 Midazolam infusion for sedation in the intensive care unit: effect on adrenal function. Anesthesiology 64: 394–398

Shaw P J, Bates D, Cartlidge N E F, Heaviside D, Julian D G, Shaw D A 1985 Early neurological complications of coronary bypass surgery. British Medical Journal 291: 1384–1387

Shelly M P, Cory E P, Park G R 1986 Pharmacokinetics of morphine in two children before and after liver transplantation. British Journal of Anaesthesia 58: 1218–1223

Shelly M, Dodds P, Park G 1986 Assessing sedation. Care of the Critically Ill 2: 170

Shipley R H, Butt J H, Horwitz E A 1979 Preparation to re-experience a stressful medical examination. Effect of repetitions video tape exposure and coping style. Journal of Constitutional and Clinical Psychology 47: 485–492

Shovelton D S 1979 Relections on an Intensive Therapy Unit. British Medical Journal 1: 737–738

Sibbald W J, Short A, Cohen M, Wilson R F 1977 Variations in adrenocortical responsiveness during severe bacterial infections. Annals of Surgery 186: 29–33

Simpson P J, Eltringham R J 1981 Lorazepam in intensive care. Clinical Therapeutics 4: 150–163

Smith P L C, Treasure T, Newman S P, Joseph P, Ell P J, Schneidav A, Harrison M J G 1986 Cerebral consequences of cardiopulmonary bypass. Lancet 1: 823–825

Stanley T H 1987 Opiate anaesthesia. Anaesthesia and Intensive Care 15: 38–59

Stanski D R 1987 Narcotic pharmacokinetics and dynamics: the basis of infusion applications. Anaesthesia and Intensive Care 15: 23–26

Strain J J 1978 Psychological reactions to acute medical illness and critical care. Critical Care Medicine 6: 39–44

Szyfelbein S K, Osgood P F, Carr D B 1983 Pain assessment and beta-endorphin plasma levels in burned children. Anesthesiology 59: A198

Teich S, Sharpe S, Chernow B 1985 Endocrine function in the critically ill. In: Dobb G (ed) Current Topics in Intensive Care. Clinics in Anaesthesiology. WB Saunders, London, Philadelphia, 3: no 4, pp 999–1026

Tomlin P J 1977 Psychological problems in intensive care. British Medical Journal 2: 441–443

Torda T A 1987 The 'new' relaxants. A review of the clinical pharmacology of atracurium and vecuronium. Anaesthesia and Intensive Care 15: 72–82

Traynor C, Hall G M 1981 Endocrine and metabolic changes during surgery: Anaesthetic implications. British Journal of Anaesthesia 53: 153–160

Tubaro E, Borelli G, Croce C, Cavallo G, Santiangelli C 1983 Effect of morphine on resistance to infection. Journal of Infectious diseases 148: 656–666

Ulrich R S 1984 View through a window may influence recovery from surgery. Science 224: 420–424

Utting J E, Smith J M 1979 Postoperative analgesia. Anaesthesia 34: 320–332

Utting J E, Whitford J H W 1972 Assessment of premedicant drugs using measurements of plasma cortisol. British Journal of Anaesthesia 44: 12–16

Viner E D 1985 Life at the other end of the endotracheal tube: a physician's personal view of critical illness. In: Massion W H (ed) Progress in Critical Care Medicine. Karger, Basel, 2: pp 3–13

Wallace P G M, Norris W 1975 The management of postoperative pain. British Journal of Anaesthesia 47: 113–120

Ward J D, Becker D P, Miller J D, Newlon P 1985 Failure of prophylactic barbiturate coma in the treatment of severe head injury. Journal of Neurosurgery 62: 383–388

Watt I, Ledingham I McA 1984 Mortality amongst multiple trauma patients admitted to an intensive therapy unit. Anaesthesia 39: 973–981

Wheatley D 1981 Beta-Blocking drugs in anxiety. In: Wheatley D (ed) Stress and the Heart. Raven Press, New York, pp 73–89

White D C 1982 The relief of postoperative pain. In: Atkinson R S, Langton Hewer C (eds) Recent Advances in Anaesthesia and Analgesia. Churchill Livingstone, Edinburgh, London, pp 121–139

Willats S M 1985 Intravenous sedation (by infusion) on the Intensive Therapy Unit. British Journal of Parenteral Therapy 1: 13–16

Willats S M 1985 Paralysis for ventilated patients? Yes or No? Intensive Care Medicine 11: 2–4

Williams J G, Jones J R, Workhoven M N, Williams B 1975 The psychological control of preoperative anxiety. Psychophysiology 12: 50–54

Wilmore D W, Long J M, Mason A D, Pruitt B A 1976 Stress in surgical patients as a neurophysiological reflex response. Surgery, Gynecology and Obstetrics 142: 257–269

Wilson L M 1972 Intensive care delirium. The effect of outside deprivation in a windowless unit. Archives of International Medicine 130: 225–226

Woolner D F, Winter D, Frendin T J, Begg E J, Lynn K L, Wright G J 1986 Renal failure does not impair the metabolism of morphine. British Journal of Clinical Pharmacology 22: 55–59

Yaksh T L 1985 Pharmacology of spinal adrenergic systems which modulate spinal nociceptive processing. Pharmacology and Biochemical Behaviour 22: 845–858

Yate P M, Thomas D, Short S M, Sebel P S, Morton J 1986 Comparison of infusions of alfentanil or pethidine for sedation of ventilated patients on the ITU. British Journal of Anaesthesia 58: 1091–1099

6. Diagnosis and management of bleeding disorders in the critically ill

Kaj A. Jørgensen

NORMAL HEMOSTASIS

The blood contains systems which, in conjunction with the vessel wall, keep the vascular bed intact and the blood fluid; thus it fulfils the task of transporting substances to and from organs. Vasoconstricting substances, platelets, and fibrin produced during coagulation endeavour to plug leaks in the vascular bed, while vasodilating substances, platelet function inhibitors, coagulation inhibitors and the fibrinolytic system aim to keep the blood fluid. Thrombosis or bleeding arises when this thrombo-hemorrhagic balance is disrupted (Nilsson, 1974).

Platelets
Vessel injury is immediately followed by platelet adhesion, aggregation and release of vasoconstricting substances at the point of injury. This stops the blood flow (primary hemostasis) and enables the coagulation system to form a firm fibrin clot. Platelets are activated by exposed subendothelial collagen, but they can also be activated by a variety of other substances such as epinephrine, ADP, and thrombin. Upon activation, the phospholipids of the platelets release arachidonic acid which is metabolised to lipoxygenated and cyclooxygenated products. Among the latter is the very potent platelet aggregation stimulator and vasoconstrictor thromboxane A_2 (TXA_2). During aggregation the platelets release a variety of biologically active substances, which are important for the reparative healing process, including a mitogenic factor (Jørgensen, 1982). Leucocytes and erythrocytes also play a role in both acute hemostasis and the subsequent reparative process. PAF (platelet aggregating factor) is a small lipid molecule, which can induce platelet aggregation even if prostaglandin and thromboxane production is inhibited (Cusack, 1980). It is normally found in blood together with its inhibitor PAFI (Lian et al, 1979).

Coagulation (Fig. 6.1)

The intrinsic cascade
The surface activity of subendothelial collagen exposed following disruption of the vessel wall will, in the presence of prekallikrein and high molecular weight kinogen, activate the Hagemann factor (F XII) to a proteolytic enzyme, which activates factor XI (PTA = plasma thromboplastin antecedent or antihemophilia factor C) to a proteolytic enzyme, which again activates factor IX (Christmas factor or antihemofilia factor B) to a proteolytic enzyme. F IXa (activated factor IX) needs Ca^{++} and a phospholipid, usually platelet factor 3 (PF-3) produced by platelets during aggregation, before it

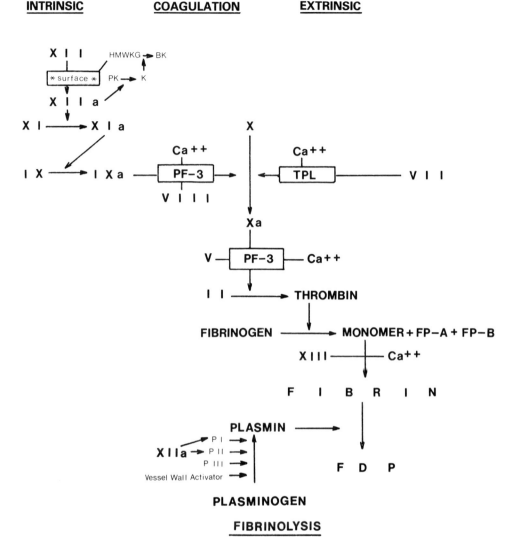

Fig. 6.1 Coagulation and fibrinolysis. The roman numerals depict coagulation factors; 'a' indicates that the factor is activated. HMWKG: High molecular weight kininogen. BK: Bradykinin; K: Kallikrein; PK: Prekallikrein; TPL: Tissue thromboplastin; PF-3: Platelet factor 3 (phospholipid); P-I, P-II, P-III: Circulating plasminogen activators.

can activate factor X (Stuart factor). Factor VIII (antihemophilia factor A) is an accelerator of this process, but parts of the F VIII molecule are of great importance in platelet adhesion (Von Willebrand factor).

The extrinsic cascade
Factor X can also be activated by tissue thromboplastin (a phospholopid present in most tissues) in the presence of Ca^{++} and factor VII (proconvertin). Some of the coagulation factors (F X, F IX, F VII, F II) are only active if they contain a gamma-

carboxyl group, which can bind Ca^{++}. Vitamin K is necessary for the incorporation of this group in the coagulation factor.

The common pathway

F Xa (activated factor X) activates prothrombin (F II) to thrombin in the presence of PF-3 and Ca^{++}, this reaction being accelerated by FVa (activated proaccelerin). Thrombin cleaves fibrinopeptides A and B from fibrinogen (F I) producing the fibrin monomers, which polymerize under the influence of factor XIII (fibrin stabilising factor) and Ca^{++} to form the firm fibrin clot.

The hagemann connection

In a review of this type it is convenient to present a view compartmentalizing physiologic functions, but in fact the systems described are interrelated. The platelets are important for the coagulation system in that they bind some coagulation factors, producing a high concentration of the active factors in the 'platelet atmosphere' and in presenting PF-3 as shown above. On the other hand thrombin is a potent stimulator of platelets and fibrinogen is necessary for normal platelet function. Furthermore there is a connection between the coagulation system, the immunological system, the kinins and the fibrinolytic system (Brozovic, 1977; Murano, 1978; Ogston & Bennet, 1978). The activation of F XII results in the production of kallikrein, which in turn produces bradykinin and other kinins from high molecular kininogen. The system is even linked to the renin-angiotensin system, in that bradykinin is degraded by the converting enzyme. The kinins can produce hypotension, increased vascular permeability, pain, and inflammation. Kallikrein enhances the activation of F XII by a positive feed-back mechanism. F XIIa may also activate the complement system resulting in cytolysis and inflammation. Furthermore F XIIa accelerates the extrinsic coagulation system and it induces fibrinolysis (see below).

Fibrinolysis

There is also both an extrinsic and an intrinsic fibrinolytic system (Müllertz, 1979; Stormorken, 1979). Both systems activate the circulating plasminogen to plasmin, which degrades fibrin to its split products (FDP). Activation of the intrinsic system is initiated by means of circulating activators. Two of these are dependent on the activation of factor XII. An important activation mode is the release of extrinsic activators from the vessel wall by a variety of different stimuli such as ischemia, stasis, and the antidiuretic hormone. Plasminogen can also be activated directly by proteolytic enzymes such as urokinase and streptokinase.

Antithrombins

The coagulation cascades have a great potential for amplification, resulting in many activated coagulation factors. There are many regulatory steps in the cascades with both positive and negative feed-back mechanisms. However, activated factors must be neutralised; if not, all fibrinogen would in the end be converted to fibrin. This inactivation of activated coagulation factors is done by enzyme inhibitor proteins such as antithrombin III, alfa-2-macroglobulin, alfa-1-antitrypsin and C-1-esterase inhibitor. Of these AT-III possesses about 50% of plasma antithrombin activity (Mortensen & Jørgensen 1983).

The factor/antithrombin complexes are removed by the reticuloendothelial system (RES). The protein fibronectin, which is found in cells, in the matrix and also in plasma is of great importance for this RES function (Mosesson & Amrani, 1980; Saba & Jaffe, 1980). It is generally accepted that heparin exerts its anticoagulatant effect by greatly increasing the velocity by which AT-III neutralises coagulation factors, although another heparin cofactor (heparin cofactor II) has been described (Sie et al, 1985).

The vessel wall
The endothelial surface of the vessel wall has the unique property that it does not activate coagulation or platelets, while such an activation immediately occurs if subendothelial collagen becomes exposed. The basis for this property is unknown. The endothelial cells of the capillaries have a receptor called thrombomodulin, which binds and inactivates thrombin. The thrombomodulin/thrombin complex will activate a vitamin K dependent plasma glycoprotein, protein C, which inactivates the regulatory coagulation factors VIII and V (Owen, 1982). The endothelial cells also produce prostaglandins, especially prostacyclin (PGI_2), which is a very potent antiaggregatory and vasodilating substance (Jørgensen 1982). The endothelial cell participates in the production of F VIII/von Willebrand factor. The endothelial cell thus plays an important role in the regulation of platelet aggregation, coagulation and activation of fibrinolysis. The muscle cells of the vessel wall are also of great importance in hemostasis in that they are targets for vasoactive substances from plasma, blood cells, and the endothelial cell.

CAUSES OF BLEEDING IN THE CRITICALLY ILL PATIENT

Patients with acquired or congenital chronic hemorrhagic diathesis may become critically ill, but treatment of these conditions, which is mainly replacement of the absent activity, is beyond the scope of the present communication. In liver disease there is thrombocytopenia and multiple defects in the coagulation and fibrinolytic systems, and the production of AT-III is impaired. In the intensive care unit vitamin K deficiency may be due to parenteral nutrition, if the lipid soluble vitamin K is not substituted. Bleeding in the massive transfusion syndrome is due to loss of activity potential of unstable coagulation factors during storage of blood. It is important to correct Ca^{++} deficit.

CIRCULATING ANTICOAGULANTS

Apart from hemophilia there are also other conditions, such as autoimmune disease and dysproteinemia, where antibodies against coagulation factors appear (Factors II, V, VII, IX, XI, XII, TPL, kallikrein, and probably many other factors), (Green, 1972). They are detected by adding the patient plasma to normal plasma and thereby causing loss of activity. Especially well known is the so called 'lupus anticoagulant' which seems to be directed against the PF-3 part of the prothrombin activator complex (Boxer, 1976). It has been seen in many diseases other than SLE. The treatment of choice involves immunosuppression and substitution of the factor activity even though this regimen gives poor results. Treatment with high concentrations of activated coagulation factors is a difficult procedure. Bleeding in the critically ill patient may, however, be due to disseminated intravascular coagulation (DIC) or occasionally to primary pathological fibrinolysis.

DISSEMINATED INTRAVASCULAR COAGULATION

Schneider introduced the term 'disseminated intravascular coagulation' in 1951 to describe the acute syndrome of defibrination and bleeding associated with late pregnancy. However, Wooldridge had already recognized the coexistence of intravascular coagulation and a hemorrhagic diathesis in 1886. Lasch et al (1961) emphasised the decrease in coagulation factors and termed the condition 'Verbrauchskoagulopathie' ('consumption coagulopathy'). Defibrination syndrome and pathological proteolysis are other names for this syndrome; where activation of the coagulation process is no longer localised and active thrombin can be detected in the circulation.

Experimental animal models (generalised Schwartzman reaction)

DIC can be produced in animal models by endotoxin, bacteria, antigen-antibody complexes, homologous thromboplastin, thrombin, snake venoms, virus, different non biological substances, and shock. The following factors predispose to and stimulate the onset of DIC: Activation of coagulation, reduced fibrinolytic capacity, blocking of RES, vasoactive substances (e.g. epinephrine), cortisone and ACTH, and hyperlipemia. The following factors have an inhibiting effect: Anticoagulation, activation of fibrinolysis, stimulation of RES, blocking of the adrenergic system, prostacyclin and angiotensin II inhibitors (Müller-Berghaus & Lasch, 1975; Watanabe & Tanaka, 1977; Wing et al, 1978; Ståhl et al, 1981; Krausz et al, 1981).

Etiology, pathophysiology and symptoms

DIC is not itself a disease, but an exaggeration of normal defence processes in response to a wide variety of underlying disorders (Bick, 1978; Hamilton et al, 1978; Hewitt & Davies, 1983). The incidence is uncertain. DIC was found in 3% of a large autopsy survey, but only in a small portion of these had the syndrome been clinically suspected (Kim et al, 1976). The key to a high index of suspicion is to note the appropriate symptoms in the appropriate clinical setting. The disease categories in which DIC may be seen are shown in Table 1. The DIC syndrome arises when the mechanism

Table 6.1 Some diseases associated with DIC

Disease category	Example
Injury	Trauma, drowning, heat stroke, burns, envenomation
Infections	Bacterial, viral, rickettsial, protozoal
Immunological	Blood transfusion reactions, autoimmune disease
Circulatory	Shock, pulmonary embolism, dissecting aneurysm
Obstetric	Amniotic embolism, abruptio placentae, retained dead fetus
Neoplastic	Leukaemia, solid tumours
Metabolic/endocrine	Diabetic ketoacidosis, acute fatty liver of pregnancy
Congenital abnormalities	Cavernous hemangioma, hyaline membrane disease

triggering the coagulation is so powerful that it overcomes the systems which normally limit the coagulation locally. This results in diffuse microthrombosis in the capillaries

of the organs resulting in the clinical picture of organ failure. The organs most frequently affected are the kidneys, the liver, the lungs, the heart, and the brain (Siegal
et al, 1978). Signs of microthrombosis may, however, also be seen in the gastrointestinal tract and in the skin. In autopsy series the most frequently affected organ
is the brain followed by the heart, the lungs, the kidneys and the adrenals (Kim
et al, 1976). Very often more than one organ may be affected. The symptoms may
therefore be drowsiness, confusion or coma, increasing problems with oxygenation
of blood, declining renal function or anuria, peripheral cyanosis or gangrene, and
cardiovascular instability. Very often, however, the patients do not present any clinical
symptoms clearly attributable to microthrombosis before the other main symptom
of DIC occurs, namely bleeding.

The mechanism triggering coagulation depends upon the disease which has provoked DIC and many different mechanisms may be active at the same time. The
etiology of DIC may be endotoxin (e.g. in septicemia, chorio-amnionitis, or purpura
fulminans), particulate or colloid substances (e.g. amnion or fat particles), antigen–
antibody complexes and complement activation (e.g. in blood transfusion reactions
or in immune diseases), ischemia, tissue thromboplastin (e.g. in trauma or severe
infections), or the etiology may be proteolytic enzymes in the circulation as seen
in pancreatitis or following snake bites.

The bleeding is due to a decrease in the concentration of coagulation factors, decrease
in the number of platelets, defective polymerization of fibrin monomers to fibrin,
and increased fibrinolysis (Fig. 6.2). The decrease in the number of platelets is due
to platelet plugging in the circulation. The appearance of fibrin/fibrinogen split products in the circulation inhibits platelet aggregation. The typical 'platelet bleeding'
involves petechiae, purpura, and bleeding from the nose and gingiva, but gastrointestinal or genito-urinary bleeding may also be seen. Decrease in the concentration
of coagulation factors occurs when consumption is greater than production. This
will in itself result in decreased fibrin formation and therefore defective plugging
of injured vessels. The characteristic bleeding is therefore characterised by continuous
oozing of blood from intravascular sites, such as intravenous (IV) catheters, needle
punctures for blood sampling and hematomas around injection sites (Spero et al,
1980). The same type of bleeding is due to rapid digestion of fibrin due to increased
fibrinolysis. Increased fibrinolysis will often be triggered together with coagulation,
but it may also be triggered by the resulting ischemia. The increased plasmin activity
will attack fibrinogen as well as fibrin. Some of the resulting split products have
a high affinity for fibrin monomers forming the so-called 'soluble fibrin monomers'
which are formed before the fibrin monomers can polymerize to fibrin. This again
results in the above mentioned type of bleeding.

Besides microthrombosis and bleeding the many interactions between the hemostatic
system and other systems in the blood are important in the pathophysiology of DIC.
The connections through the Hagemann factor have been mentioned. Besides degradation of fibrin, plasmin is also capable of degrading a number of coagulation factors,
ACTH, growth hormone, complement, and insulin. This is why DIC often is termed
'pathological proteolysis' (Bick, 1978). These pathophysiological aspects explain the
variety of symptoms seen in DIC. In some cases the microthrombosis is most prominent, in other cases bleeding may be the most prominent symptom, while both manifestations may appear at the same time.

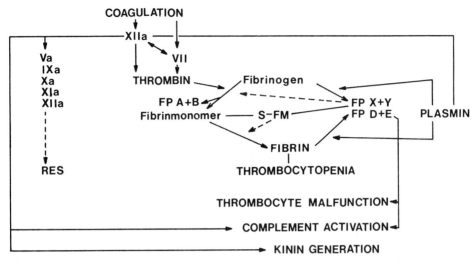

Fig. 6.2   Pathophysiology of DIC. FP: Fibrinopeptide. S-FM: soluble fibrinomonomers. Solid line depicts activation, while an interrupted line depicts inhibition.

Laboratory investigations

Bearing in mind that we are trying to define active coagulation and fibrinolysis in circulating blood, it follows that blood samples must be taken from clean venous punctures discarding the first few ml of blood. Stasis should be minimal to avoid activation of fibrinolysis. If blood samples are taken near a vessel lesion or from a hematoma the tests will naturally reveal active coagulation, but this will be a local phenomenon and not DIC. Abnormal results may also be due to contamination with heparin from a heparinized syringe or from heparin released from a catheter, through which heparin has been given earlier.

Although a wide variety of tests have been used to demonstrate DIC, acute DIC in the critically ill patient requires quick and accurate tests for defining the state and estimating the depletion of platelets and coagulation factors. Defining DIC as active thrombin in the circulation, tests for fibrin monomers or fibrinopeptides A and B would come close to the definition (Figs. 6.1 and 6.2). At present tests for fibrinopeptides A and B are too time-consuming and accurate test for fibrin monomers are still being evaluated for clinical use:

1. *The ethanol or protamine sulfate gelation tests:* These tests utilise the insolubility of the 'soluble fibrin monomers' (see Fig. 6.2) in certain concentrations of ethanol (or protamine sulfate) (Seaman, 1970; Kisker, 1979). Of the quick clinically available tests, they come closest to the definition of DIC and have therefore been widely used in the diagnosis of the syndrome. They are usually positive in DIC, but if the fibrinogen concentration is very low (defibrination syndrome) the test will be negative. This will theoretically also be the case if there is no fibrinolysis, since no 'soluble fibrin monomers' will be produced in these situations. The relatively high frequency of 'false positive tests' are, however, a greater problem. High fibrinogen concentrations give a similar reaction. Positive tests have also been demonstrated in acute myocardial infarction, pulmonary

embolism, extensive deep vein thrombophlebitis, and in contraceptive pill users, without any clinical evidence of DIC. The tests will become negative when the intravascular process has been stopped. They are therefore valuable in the monitoring of the effect of therapy.

2. *Fibrin/Fibrinogen Degradation Products (FDP):* This test is often called fibrin/ fibrinogen related antigens. All fibrinogen is converted to fibrin with thrombin after inhibition of fibrinolysis. The sample is then tested with antibodies against fibrinogen; most commercial kits utilise antibody-coated latex particles (Hedner & Nilsson, 1974). FDP titer will only be elevated if there is increased fibrinolysis. The actual titer may therefore bear little relationship to the clinical course of the intravascular clotting process. A greater problem is that the clearing of FDP is dependent upon renal and RES function. The titer will therefore often be elevated after the intravascular coagulation process has been stopped. Finally circulating proteolytic enzymes may simple degrade fibrin to products that are undetectable by commercial kits.

3. *Antithrombin III:* The invention of chromogenic substrates for determination of coagulation factor activities has resulted in quick, reliable tests for determination of AT-III activity (Abildgaard et al, 1977). The activation of coagulation factors results in a great consumption of AT-III and the activity will be decreased in DIC. AT-III production will very often be decreased in the critically ill patient. Almost any surgical procedure results in a significant decrease in AT-III activity, even though there are no signs of DIC (Jørgensen et al, 1980). A decreased value may therefore have other explanations than DIC. In DIC the A1-III activity is a valuable test in the choice of treatment and evaluation of the progression of the disease (Bick et al, 1977; Blauhut et al, 1980; Laursen et al, 1981a; Jespersen et al, 1982).

4. *Platelet count:* Thrombocytopenia is present in most cases of DIC, indicating consumption of platelets. The platelet count may, however, be within the normal limits. A fall in platelets count is therefore a better diagnostic tool. The condition provoking DIC may in itself cause a decrease or an increase in the number of platelets.

5. *Prothrombin-proconvertin (PP, prothrombin time etc.):* In these tests Ca^{++} is added to citrate plasma after the addition of tissue thromboplastin (often also after addition of fibrinogen and F V in excess). The test therefore in part describes the extrinsic coagulation cascade. The activity is often reduced (time increased) indicating a consumption of these coagulation factors. These tests are more frequently abnormal than tests for the intrinsic cascade.

6. *Activated Partial Thromboplastin Time (APTT):* In this test cephalin (phospholipid) and kaolin (or other substance with great surface activity) is added to citrate plasma before the addition of Ca^{++}. This and other similar tests in part describe the intrinsic coagulation cascade.

7. *The euglobulin clot lysis time:* This test precipitates plasmin in the euglobulin fraction by decreasing pH to 5.5. The plasmin inhibitors are in the supernatant and are discarded. The precipitate is then dissolved and a clot formed by addition of thrombin. The time until this clot is lysed is then determined. This is the most simple and the cheapest test for determination of increased fibrinolytic activity (Boberg & Killander, 1983). If the euglobulin lysis time

is under 60 min in blood sampled without (or with only slight) stasis, the fibrinolytic activity will be increased. It is easy to understand that there must be fibrinogen present in plasma in order to perform the test.

8. *Fibrinogen:* Exact determinations of fibrinogen are too time-consuming for clinical use. The most often used tests determine the time taken to form a clot after addition of excess thrombin. Since FDPs inhibit thrombin, high FDP titers may give misleadingly low values. Fibrinogen is an 'acute phase reactant' and will be increased in almost all conditions provoking DIC. A decrease in the fibrinogen concentration may therefore be of greater diagnostic value than the actual value, as is the case with platelets.

9. *Thrombin time:* This test has its advocates as a valuable diagnostic tool. Depending upon the amount of thrombin used, the time will be dependent on the concentration of fibrinogen and FDP. Abnormal times due to heparin can be corrected by addition of protamine sulfate.

10. *Other tests:* A large battery of other tests including determination of individual coagulation factors, individual fibrinolytic components, substances released by platelets, protein C, and special degradation products have been utilised in DIC, but these tests are still too laborious or expensive to be used in common clinical situations (Ockelford & Carter, 1980; Marlar et al, 1985).

It is essential to understand that none of the above mentioned tests are specific for DIC and that they all have their limitations. It is therefore important, when evaluating the results of the differing tests, to emphasise the clinical situation and to consider the patient's general condition. The importance of correct sampling technique cannot be overemphasised.

Therapy

As previously indicated DIC is not a disease in itself, but an intermediary (or secondary) mechanism of disease occurring within the context of a primary disease process. The most important principle of treatment is adequate management of the underlying disease so that the factors responsible for triggering DIC are rapidly reduced and ideally eliminated (Bick, 1978; Hamilton et al, 1978; Hewitt & Davies, 1983). Acute DIC has a high mortality (some physicians believe DIC stands for Death Is Coming). The reasons for this are several fold. Many disease states associated with DIC are in themselves often fatal. Understanding of the pathophysiology of the syndrome has been poor. The development of effective therapy has been slow. The clinical features often appear after severe organ damage has occurred. Finally, it will sometimes be impossible to remove the triggering process even though its presence may be recognised.

Since the resulting organ damage (ischemia, hypoperfusion, necrosis) can trigger intravascular coagulation, it is obviously important to give the best possible supportive therapy for organ failure. Situations will often arise where the triggering mechanism cannot be removed at once. In these situations, it seems logical to consider therapy aimed at stopping the intravascular coagulation process. The difficulty lies in the fact that this is done utilizing substances which normally enhance bleeding. Many physicians are reluctant to giving anticoagulant therapy if the patient presents a clinical picture of severe bleeding or if the risk of severe life-threatening bleeding is high.

Another problem is that acute DIC is relatively rare and the great variation in the clinical picture and underlying disease makes if difficult to evaluate different therapeutic modalities.

1. *Heparin:* A large number of clinical accounts have been published claiming a beneficial effect of heparin in DIC (Lasch et al, 1961; Kazmier et al, 1974; Astrup & Jespersen, 1984). In larger series there is a trend to a reduced mortality in heparin-treated patients, but the differences are not significant (Spero et al, 1980). Prospective randomised trials are still lacking and will probably never be performed due to the difficulties mentioned above. With this uncertainty about the effect of heparin (Feinstein, 1982) it is not surprising that there is no agreement upon the dose of heparin. If one wants to monitor the anticoagulant effect of heparin with e.g. APTT, it is best to give a bolus dose of about 100 IU/kg and thereafter continuous iv heparin, due to the special kinetics of heparin (Bounameaux et al, 1980; Estes, 1971). Some have claimed low dose heparin (5000 IU 2–3 times daily) to be equally effective (Bick et al, 1980).

2. *Antithrombin III:* There are also many clinical reports of the favourable effect of antithrombin concentrate infusion in DIC (Schipper et al, 1978; Blauhut et al, 1982; Hellgren et al, 1984). In a small randomised study AT-III seemed more effective than heparin alone (Blauhut et al, 1985). The addition of heparin to AT-III seemed to increase the risk of bleeding compared with AT-III or heparin alone, but did not seem to affect the clinical course. There are therefore some indications that AT-III substitution is better and carries a smaller risk than heparin treatment.

3. *Blood component replacement:* Fresh frozen plasma, cryoprecipitate, prothrombin complex concentrates and platelets are all occasionally used in DIC. It is essential when trying to substitute defective coagulative activity that the intravascular clotting has been controlled. The addition of procoagulant activity in the face on continued DIC may 'add fuel to the fire' (Bick et al, 1976; Bick, 1978). In many cases fresh plasma has been used primarily to replace antithrombin and other coagulation inhibiting substances in the absence of AT-III concentrates. This approach is probably acceptable, especially if anticoagulation therapy has been started.

4. *Antifibrinolytic therapy:* This therapy is rarely indicated in DIC. The increased fibrinolysis is almost always secondary to microthrombosis and it is essential for clearing fibrin and restitution of organ function. There are, however, some who believe that a syndrome of primary hyperactivated fibrinolysis exists. This is especially the case in some obstetric situations and following surgery on the prostate. In these cases plasmin activators are released from the tissue and antifibrinolytic therapy is indicated. It must be stressed, however, that laboratory test should confirm this before treatment is started. In DIC, antifibrinolytic therapy may worsen the microthrombosis and thereby increase the chance of irreversible organ failure.

It is very difficult to give general recommendations for treatment of the coagulation abnormalities present in DIC. Anticoagulation with heparin seems logical as does replacement therapy with AT-III, which may carry a smaller risk. The important thing is to evaluate the patient's whole situation including both the clinical and laboratory status. Though seldom published, clinical experience teaches us that it is easy to make errors of judgment in these dramatic situations. A patient with splenic rupture has been treated with heparin because of a fall in platelet count and fibrinogen concentration, and a positive ethanol gelation test, until an experienced doctor examined the patient's abdomen, made the correct diagnosis, and performed the appropriate surgical operation.

SPECIAL SYNDROMES AND DIC

1. *DIC in Obstetrics:* In these conditions heparin is seldom used, because the triggering process can be removed (Talbert & Blatt, 1979). All patients with abruptio placentae should be investigated for DIC and if confirmed, delivery should be immediate. In the case of DIC associated with retained dead fetus there is usually a more gradual depletion of coagulation factors. If DIC is confirmed, delivery should be immediate. Amniotic fluid embolism with DIC should always lead to prompt evacuation of the uterus. In these cases it may be necessary to substitute blood components. In obstetric practice, DIC may also be seen in association with sepsis, hyatidiform mole, eclampsia and acute fatty liver of pregnancy (Liebman et al, 1983; Laursen et al, 1981).

2. *Thrombotic Thrombocytopenic Purpura (TTP-Moschowitz syndrome):* TTP is characterised by thrombosis and fibrinoid degeneration of small vessels. There is microangiopathic hemolytic anemia with schistocytes (fragmented red blood cells), thrombocytopenia and signs of multiple organ involvement. Diagnosis is made by biopsy (Mammen, 1981; Lian & Savaraj, 1981).

3. *Hemolytic uremic syndrome (HUS-Gassers syndrome):* HUS occurs in children, in pregnant women, in women on contraceptive pills and shortly after delivery. It consists of acute hemolytic anemia, thrombocytopenia, and acute renal failure. It is closely related to TTP. Both lack of a plasma factor which stimulates prostacycline production (Remuzzi et al, 1979; Jørgensen & Pedersen, 1981; Deckmyn et al, 1983) and lack of PAFI have been described in this syndrome (Lian et al, 1979; Editorial, 1979; Monnens, 1985). A large number of these cases respond favourably to plasma transfusion or, better, plasma exchange.

4. *Low-Grade DIC:* The DIC described in this chapter is the acute dramatic form causing bleeding in the critically ill patient in the intensive care unit. In some malignancies and hematological disorders active thrombin is sometimes present in the circulation. Often there will be an increased concentration of fibrinogen and coagulation factors. This is due to synthesis exceeding the slow consumption in these cases. The state is characterized by a tendency towards both venous and arterial thrombosis and it can suddenly change to acute DIC.

5. *DIC and Head Injury:* Brain is a rich source of tissue thromboplastin and the frequency of DIC following severe head injury is high. In these circumstances, however, DIC seems very often to be self-limiting. Although heparin has its advocates in this situation, most clinicians consider heparin contraindicated due to the risk of bleeding. It is believed that prompt diagnosis of DIC followed by factor replacement will save some patients from substantial brain trauma. Fresh frozen plasma is the preparation of choice (editorial, 1982).

CONCLUSION

Research in the field of DIC may help us find new ways to deal with this difficult clinical entity. Investigation of the role of increased thromboxane production (Reines et al, 1982) and decrease in protein C (Marlar et al, 1985) is in progress. It is, however, the opinion of the author that a better outcome is more likely to come from improved understanding of the underlying pathophysiology of DIC and from increased awareness of the limitations of the laboratory tests. Anticoagulation is a potentially dangerous approach in many situations and should be used with care. I do not believe, for example, that prophylactic treatment of all multitrauma patients with heparin (Trentz et al, 1979; Bergman et al, 1980) is justified (Sefrin et al, 1982).

REFERENCES

Abildgaard U, Lie M, Ødegaard O R 1977 Antithrombin (heparin co-factor) assay with 'new' chromogenic substrates (S-2238 and chromozym TH). Thrombosis Research 11: 549–553

Astrup T. Jespersen J 1984 Disseminated intravascular coagulation and the balance between blood coagulation and fibrinolysis. Folia Haematologica (Leipzig) 111: 407–415

Bergman H, Blauhut B, Necek S, Kramar H, Vinazzer 1980 Heparinprophylaxe der Verbrauchskoagulopathie bei Schockpatienten. Anaesthesist 29: 623–626

Bick R L 1978 Disseminated intravascular coagulation and related syndromes: Etiology, pathophysiology, diagnosis, and management. American Journal of Hematology 5: 265–282

Bick R L, Schmalhorst W R, Fekete L 1976 Disseminated intravascular coagulation and blood component therapy. Transfusion 16: 361–365

Bick R L, Dukes M L, Wilson W L, Fekete L F 1977 Antithrombin III (AT-III) as a diagnostic aid in disseminated intravascular coagulation. Thrombosis Research 10, 721–729

Bick R L, Bick M. D, Fekete L F 1980 Antithrombin III patterns in disseminated intravascular coagulation. American Journal of Clinical Pathology 73: 377–383

Blauhut B, Necek S, Kramar H, Vinazzer H, Bergman H 1980 Activity of antithrombin III and effect of heparin on coagulation in shock. Thrombosis Research 19: 775–782

Blauhut B, Necek S, Vinazzer H, Bergman H 1982 Substitution therapy with an antithrombin III concentrate in shock and DIC. Thrombosis Research 27: 271–278

Blauhut B, Kramar H, Vinazzer H, Bergman H 1985 Substitution of antithrombin III in shock and DIC: A randomized study. Thrombosis research 39: 81–89

Boberg M, Killander A 1983 Evaluation of euglobulin clot lysis time as a screening method for determination of blood plasma fibrinolytic activity after venous occlusion. Acta Medica Scandinavica 213: 309–311

Bounameaux H, Marbet G A, Lammle B, Eichlisberger R, Duckert F 1980 Monitoring of heparin treatment. American Journal of Clinical Pathology 74, 68–73

Boxer M, Ellman L, Carvalho A 1976 The lupus anticoagulant. Arthritis and Rheumatism 19: 1244–1248

Brozovic M 1977 Physiological mechanisms in coagulation and fibrinolysis. British Medical Journal 33: 231–238

Cusack N J 1980 Platelet-activating factor. Nature 285: 193

Deckmyn H, Proesmans W, Vermylen J 1983 Prostacyclin production by whole blood from children: Impairment in the hemolytic uremic syndrome and excessive formation in chronic renal failure. Thrombosis Research 30: 13–18

Editorial 1979 Plasma exchange in thrombotic thrombocytopenic purpura. Lancet I: 1065–1066

Editorial 1982 Disseminated intravascular coagulation and head injury. Lancet II: 531

Estes J W 1971 The kinectics of heparin. Annuals of the New York Academy of Science 179: 187–204

Feinstein D I 1982 Diagnosis and management of disseminated intravascular coagulation: The role of heparin therapy. Blood 60: 284–287

Green D 1972 Circulating anticoagulants. Medical Clinician of North American 56: 145–151

Hamilton P J, Stalker A L, Douglas A S 1978 Disseminated intravascular coagulation: a review. Journal of Clinical Pathology 31: 609–618

Hedner U, Nilsson I M 1974 Methods. In: Nilsson I M (ed) Haemorrhagic and thrombotic disease. John Wiley, London. 209–235

Hellgren M, Javelin L, Hagnevik K, Blomback M 1984 Antithrombin III concentrate as adjuvant in DIC treatment. A pilot study in 9 severely ill patients. Thrombosis Research 35: 459–466

Hewitt P E, Davies S C 1983 The current state of DIC. Intensive Care Medicine 9: 249–252

Jespersen J, Rasmussen N R, Toftgaard C 1982 Observations during the treatment with antithrombin III concentrate of a case of tampon-related toxic shock syndrome and disseminated intravascular coagulation. Discrepancies between functional and immunologic determinations of antithrombin. Thrombosis Research 26: 457–462

Jørgensen K A 1982 Studies on the biological balance between thromboxanes and prostacyclins in relation to the platelet vessel wall interaction. Danish Medical Bulletin 29: 169–197

Jørgensen K A, Pedersen R S 1981 Familial deficiency of prostacyclin production stimulating factor in the hemolytic uremic syndrome of childhood. Thrombosis Research 21: 311–315

Jørgensen K A, Stoffersen E, Sørensen P J, Ingeberg S, Huttel M, Ahlbom G. 1980 Alterations in plasma antithrombin III following total hip replacement and elective cholecystectomy. Scandinavian Journal of Haematology 24: 101–104

Kazmier F J, Bowie E J W, Hagedorn A B, Owen C A 1974 Treatment of intravascular coagulation fibrinolysis (ICF) syndromes. Mayo Clinic Proceedings 49: 665–672

Kim H-S, Suzuki M, Lie J T, Titus J L 1976 Clinically unsuspected disseminated intravascular coagulation (DIC). American Journal of Clinical Pathology 66: 31–39

Kisker C T 1979 Detection of fibrin monomer. American Journal of Clinical Pathology 72: 405–409

Krausz M, Utsunimoya T, Feuerstein C, Wolfe J H N, Shepero D, Hechtman H B 1981 Prostacyclin reversal of lethal encotoxemia in dogs. Journal of Clinical Investigation 67: 1118–1125

Lasch H G, Krecke H J, Rodriques-Erdmann F, Sessnre H H, Schutterle G 1961 Verbrauchskoagulopathien. Patogenese und Therapie. Folia Haematologica 6: 325–330

Laursen B, Faber V, Brock A, Gormsen J, Sørensen H 1981a Disseminated intravascular coagulation. Antithrombin III, and complement in meningococcal infections. Acta Medica Scandinavica 209: 221–227

Laursen B, Mortensen J Z, Frost L, Hansen K B 1981b Disseminated intravascular coagulation in hepatic failure treated with antithrombin III. Thrombosis Research 701–704

Lian E C-Y, Harkness D R, Byrnes J J, Wallach H, Nuez R 1979 Presence of a platelet aggregating factor in the plasma of patients with thrombotic thrombocytopenic purpura (TTP) and its inhibition by normal plasma. Blood 53: 333–338

Lian C-Y, Savaraj N 1981 Effects of platelet inhibitors on the platelet aggregation induced by plasma from patients with thrombotic thrombocytopenic purpura. Blood 58: 354–359

Liebman H A, McGhee W G, Patch M J, Feinstein D I 1983 Severe depression of antithrombin III associated with disseminated intravascular coagulation in women with fatty liver of pregnancy. Annals of Internal Medicine 98: 330–333

Mammen (ed) 1981 Management of thrombotic thrombocytopenic purpura. Seminars in Thrombosis and Hemostasis. 7: 1–58

Marlar R A, Endres-Brooks J, Miller C 1985 Serial studies of protein C and its plasma inhibitor in patients with disseminated intravascular coagulation. Blood 66: 59–63

Monnens L, van de Meer W, Langenhuysen C, van Munster P, van Oostrom C 1985 Platelet aggregating factor in the epidemic form of hemolytic-urenic syndrome in childhood. 24: 135–137

Mortensen J Z, Jørgensen K A 1983 Antithrombin III: a review. Danish Medical Bulletin 30: 100–105

Mosesson M W, Amrani D L 1980 The structure and biologic activities of plasma fibronectin. Blood 56: 145–158

Murano G 1978 The 'Hagemann' Connection: Interrelationships of blood coagulation, fibrino(geno)lysis, kinin generation, and complement activation. American Journal of Hematology 4: 409–417

Müller-Berghaus G, Lasch H-G 1975 Microcirculatory disturbances induced by generalized intravascular coagulation. In: Born G R V, Eichler O, Farah A, Herken H, Welch A D (eds) Handbook of experimental pharmacology, new series, vol. 16/3. Springer verlag New York.

Müllertz S 1979 The fibrinolytic system. Scandinavian Journal of haematology suppl 34, 15–23

Nilsson Inga Marie (ed) 1974 Haemorrhagic and thrombotic diseases. John Wiley, London

Ockelford P A, Carter C J 1982 Disseminated intravascular coagulation: the application and utility of disgnostic tests. Seminars in Thrombosis and Hemostasis 8: 198–216

Ogston D, Bennet B 1978 Surface-mediated reactions in the formation of thrombin, plasmin and kallikrein. British Medical Bulletin 34: 107–112

Owen W G 1982 The control of hemostasis. Archives Pathology and Laboratory Medicine 106: 209–213

Reines H D, Halushka P V, Cook J A, Wise W C, Rambo W 1982 PLasma thromboxane concentrations are raised in patients dying with septic shock. Lancet 2: 174–175

Remuzzi G, Marchesi D, Misiani R, Mecca G, deGaetano G, Donati M B 1979 Familial deficiency of a plasma factor stimulating vascular prostacyclin activity. Thrombosis research 16: 517–525

Saba T M, Jaffe E 1980 Plasma fibronectin (opsonic glycoprotein): Its synthesis by vascular endothelial cells and role in cardiopulmonary integrity after trauma as related to reticuloendothelial function. The American Journal of Medicine 68: 577–594

Schipper H G, Jenkins C S P, Kahle L H, ten Cate J 1978 Antithrombin-III transfusion in disseminated intravascular coagulation. Lancet I: 854–856

Schneider C L 1951 'Fibrin embolism' (disseminated intravascular coagulation) with defibrination as one of the end results during placenta abruptio. Surgery, Gynecology, and Obstetrics 92: 27–32

Seaman A J 1970 The recognition of intravascular clotting. Archives of Internal Medicine 125: 1016–1021

Sefrin P, Brunswig D, Wenzel M 1982 Fruhzeitige Heparin-Gabe beim traumatisch-haemorrhagischen Schock. Medizinische Welt 33: 638–639

Sie P, Dupouy D, Pichon J, Boneu B 1985 Constitutional heparin co-factor II deficiency associated with recurrent thrombosis. Lancet ii: 414–416

Siegal T, Seligsohn U, Aghai E, Modan M 1978 Clinical and laboratory aspects of disseminated intravascular coagulation (DIC): A study of 118 cases. Thrombosis and Haemostasis 39: 122–134

Spero J A, Lewis J H, Hasiba U 1980 Disseminated intravascular coagulation. Findings in 346 patients. Thrombosis and Haemostasis 43: 28–33

Stormorken H, 1979 Interrelations between the coagulation-, the fibrinolytic and the kallikrein-kinin system. Scandinavian Journal of Hematology suppl. 34: 24–27

Ståhl E, Gerdin B, Rammer L 1981 Protective effect of angiotensin II inhibition on acute renal failure after intravascular coagulation in the rat. Nephron 29: 250–257

Talbert L M, Blatt P M 1979 Disseminated intravascular coagulation in obstetrics. Clinical Obstetrics and Gynecology 22: 889–900

Trentz O, Barthels M, Trentz O A, Oestern H-J, Hempelmann G, Kolbow H 1979 Coagulation and fibrinolysis in multiple trauma after early heparinizing. Advances in Shock Research 2: 103–110

Watanabe T, Tanaka K 1977 Electron microscopic observations of the kidney in the generalized Shwartzman reaction. Virchows Archives A. Pathology, anatomi and histologi 374: 183–196

Wing D A, Yamada T, Hawley H B, Pettit G W 1978 Model for disseminated coagulation: bacterial sepsis in rhesus monkeys. Journal of Laboratory and Clinical Medicine 92: 239–251

Wooldridge L C 1886 Ueber intravaskulare gerinnungen. Archiw Anatomica et Physiologica (Leipzig) 397: 399

7. Right ventricular dysfunction, detection and treatment

John D. Ducas   Richard M. Prewitt

INTRODUCTION

An increase in right ventricular (RV) afterload may decrease CO in several clinical conditions, such as acute pulmonary embolism (Sashara, 1980; Sharma & McIntyre, 1984; Albert et al, 1976) and the Adult Respiratory Distress Syndrome (Zapol & Snider, 1977). This review considers pathophysiology and treatment of decreased cardiac output (CO) complicating increased RV afterload. Recent work investigating pathophysiology and treatment of pulmonary hypertension per se is also reviewed.

TREATMENT OF SHOCK COMPLICATING PULMONARY EMBOLISM

Despite reports that patient mortality may exceed 30% if hypotension develops in the setting of acute pulmonary embolism (Albert et al, 1976; Urokinase Pulmonary Embolism Study Group, 1973) and despite a variety of recommendations, few studies have systematically investigated treatment of acute circulatory instability complicating pulmonary embolism.

A recent canine study investigated treatment of shock in pulmonary embolism (Molloy et al, 1984). Autologous blood clots were injected over approximately 25 minutes, and when mean systemic arterial blood pressure (BP) had fallen to 70 mm Hg (shock), dogs were treated according to prior randomisation. Four groups of six dogs were studied. One group served as controls. Another group was treated with volume expansion, a third with isoproterenol and the final group with norepinephrine (NE).

As per experimental design, blood clot emboli decreased mean BP to 70 mm Hg (mean CO to <0.7 l/min) prior to onset of therapy. In controls and in dogs treated with volume or isoproterenol, hemodynamic state continued to deteriorate, and all dogs died within ten minutes. In contrast, all six dogs treated with NE demonstrated marked hemodynamic improvement and remained stable during one hour of continuous infusion.

Table 7.1 illustrates the hemodynamic effects of pulmonary emboli and NE. Note the marked deterioration in RV function when afterload increased. That is, despite

Table 7.1   Hemodynamic effects of noradrenaline treatment*

	Baseline	Treatment	15 min	60 min
CO (l min^{-1})	3.5 ± 1.5		2.3 ± 0.7	2.3 ± 0.3
BP (mm Hg)	140 ± 22	71 ± 2	112 ± 25	106 ± 16
RVEDP (mm Hg)	0.7 ± 0.8	10 ± 1	5 ± 5	5 ± 3
Mean PAP (mm Hg)	13 ± 3	62 ± 11	55 ± 7	50 ± 6
PVR (mm Hg l^{-1} min)	2.5 ± 0.7		28 ± 8	31 ± 18

* Values are mean ±SD.

an increase in right ventricular end diastolic pressure (RVEDP), CO and BP markedly decreased. NE increased BP, and CO increased from an unmeasurable value to 2.3 l/min. Corresponding to the increase in CO, RVEDP decreased. These changes signal an improvement in RV pump performance, due to a direct inotropic effect and/or increased contractility following increased BP and improved RV perfusion (Vlahakes et al, 1981).

A recent study by Ducas et al (1985) was designed to determine which of the above mechanisms best explained the improvement in RV performance. In an attempt to separate direct inotropic effects from indirect effects due to increased BP and improved RV perfusion, acute hemodynamic effects on NE and methoxamine were compared in the same dogs. RV afterload was increased over approximately two hours via injection of small (80–120 μm) glass beads to decrease BP to approximately 65 mm Hg. In this model of glass bead embolisation, this was the lowest BP at which hemodynamic stability was maintained. Mean results are illustrated in Table 7.2.

Table 7.2   Hemodynamic effects of embolisation, noradrenaline and methoxamine

	Baseline	Embolisation	Noradrenaline	Time control	Methoxamine
CO (l min)	4.8 ± 1.4	$1.0 \pm 0.3^{\dagger}$	$2.0 \pm 0.5\ddagger$	1.2 ± 0.4	1.1 ± 0.3
BP (mm Hg)	144 ± 10	$64 \pm 13\ddagger$	$122 \pm 5\ddagger$	68 ± 18	$121 \pm 10\ddagger$
Mean PAP (mm Hg)	16.2 ± 1.6	$47.8 \pm 16.5^{\dagger}$	52.1 ± 16.6	38.3 ± 9.1	37.9 ± 10.4
RVEDP (mm Hg)	4.4 ± 2.0	$10.7 \pm 4.3^{\star}$	8.0 ± 3.1	8.4 ± 3.2	12.8 ± 4.0
PVR (mm Hg l^{-1} min)	1.5 ± 0.6	$44 \pm 17\dagger$	$24 \pm 12\dagger$	28 ± 11	28 ± 15
RVCPP (mm Hg)	132 ± 10	$35 \pm 11\ddagger$	$93 \pm 10\ddagger$	48 ± 17	$94 \pm 7\dagger$

$\star$ p < 0.05 *vs* previous baseline.
$\dagger$ p < 0.01 *vs* previous baseline.
$\ddagger$ p < 0.001 *vs* previous baseline.
RVCPP = Right ventricular coronary perfusion pressure.

Note that embolisation dramatically decreased CO, BP and RV coronary perfusion pressure. NE doubled BP and CO and almost tripled RV coronary perfusion pressure. Note that PVR, calculated as PVR = PAP − LVEDP/CO decreased with NE. In contrast, despite a similar improvement in BP and RV coronary perfusion pressure, CO did not change with methoxamine. The calculation of PVR assumes that in Zone III the LVEDP is the effective pulmonary vascular outflow pressure. However, in certain conditions, this assumption may be incorrect. This is discussed in detail later (see section on flow resistive characteristics of the pulmonary vasculature).

The above results suggest that norepinephrine improved RV pump performance primarily via a direct inotropic effect. While it is possible that the failure of RV function to improve with methoxamine was due to an increase in coronary vascular resistance, offsetting the increase in coronary perfusion pressure, previous work does not support this possibility (West & Aviado, 1956).

The results of this study complement those of Vlahakes et al (1981). In the latter study, RV function in the setting of marked systemic hypotension was improved by infusion of an α agonist (phenylephrine). The authors attributed the increased RV function to the improvement in BP and RV coronary perfusion pressure reversing RV ischemia. However, in that study, BP was lower during RV failure (48 mm Hg) than in the study of Ducas et al in which an α agonist had no effect on RV function. Accordingly, the more pronounced level of hypotension prior to treatment probably explains the increase in CO which occurred with phenylephrine, whereas direct inotropic effects were necessary to improve CO and RV function without profound shock.

While isoproterenol was ineffective in the treatment of shock due to acute pulmonary emboli (Molloy et al, 1984), can isoproterenol improve RV performance in the setting of pulmonary hypertension without frank circulation instability?

To test this hypothesis, a recent study compared the acute cardiopulmonary effects of NE and isoproterenol in a canine model of increased RV afterload and decreased CO (Molloy et al, 1985). In six anesthetised dogs, autologous blood clots were injected over approximately two hours to increase RV afterload and decrease CO 40%. Mean results are illustrated in Table 7.3. Note that while both drugs increased SV, only

Table 7.3 Hemodynamic effects of inotropic agents in pulmonary hypertension

	CO l/min	SV ml/beats	PAP mm Hg	RVEDP mm Hg	BP mm Hg	PVR mm Hg l^{-1} min
Control 1	1.3 ± 0.3	8 ± 2	44 ± 5	9 ± 4	93 ± 16	34 ± 10
Isoproterenol	$3.0 \pm 0.8^{\star}$	$15 \pm 4^{\star}$	$49 \pm 9\ddagger$	5 ± 3	$71 \pm 11^{\star}$	$16 \pm 4^{\star}$
Control 2	1.2 ± 0.4	7.5 ± 3.5	40 ± 6	9 ± 4	84 ± 18	33 ± 10
Noradrenaline	1.4 ± 0.5	$12 \pm 5^{\star}$	45 ± 11	8 ± 5	$117 \pm 20^{\star}$	32 ± 14
Control 4	1.2 ± 0.4	7.4 ± 2.5	42 ± 5	9 ± 4	90 ± 18	34 ± 12

$\star$ = $p < 0.01$, $\dagger$ = $p < 0.025$, $\ddagger$ = $p < 0.05$.
Comparing control 1 to isoproterenol.
Comparing control 2 to noradrenaline.

isoproterenol increased CO. Corresponding to the increase in flow, RV filling pressure and PVR decreased with isoproterenol.

McDonald et al (1968) gave isoproterenol to patients with pulmonary embolism. Intravenous isoproterenol increased CO, did not effect PAP and decreased PVR.

ADULT RESPIRATORY DISTRESS SYNDROME

Zapol & Snider (1977) reported beneficial hemodynamic effects of isoproterenol in patients with ARDS and pulmonary hypertension. In another study, Snider et al (1980) investigated effects of isoproterenol in patients with ARDS and mild pulmonary hypertension. Isoproterenol increased CO and caused a small decrease in PVR.

Accordingly, when a moderate decrease in CO complicates an increase in RV afterload, isoproterenol may be an excellent drug to increase CO and improve RV function.

In a variety of conditions vasodilators are used to decrease systemic and pulmonary vascular resistances and increase CO. For example, nitroprusside reduces LV filling pressure and increases CO in patients with congestive heart failure (Pierpont et al, 1980). Similar hemodynamic effects are reported in patients with ARDS (Snider et al, 1980; Wood & Prewitt, 1981; Zapol & Falke, 1985). A recent clinical study investigated acute hemodynamic effects of nitroprusside in patients with ARDS (Zapol & Falke, 1985). Nitroprusside reduced PCWP, PAP and PVR (from 2.2 to 1.5 mm Hg l^{-1} min) and increased CO. Associated with the increase in flow, there was a decrease in mean BP, from 89 to 70 mm Hg, and PaO_2 decreased from 105 to 74 mm Hg. In these studies PVR was normal or only slightly increased. In the setting of marked pulmonary hypertension, a fall in BP could significantly reduce the driving pressure for RV perfusion and thus impair ventricular performance. Also, it is conceivable that in certain conditions such as acute pulmonary embolism, nitroprusside may not significantly affect RV afterload.

Hydralazine is commonly used to decrease LV afterload and improve cardiac performance in patients with congestive heart failure (Chatterjee et al, 1976). In patients with LV failure, PaO_2 remains constant with hydralazine and BP may not decrease (Pierpont et al, 1980).

Hydralazine has been reported to decrease PVR and to improve ventricular performance in patients with primary pulmonary hypertension and in patients with pulmonary hypertension secondary to chronic lung diseases (Rubin & Peter, 1980, 1981). For example, Rubin et al (1982) studied effects of oral hydralazine in patients with chronic pulmonary hypertension and RV failure. Despite unchanged PAP and decreased RVEDP, CO and SV markedly increased with hydralazine. The authors attributed the improvement in RV function to a decrease in PVR. In contrast, results from another study demonstrated that while CO increased, PVR did not change when hydralazine was given to five patients with primary pulmonary hypertension (Rounds et al, 1983). Furthermore, in that study PVR did not decrease and CO did not increase with nitroprusside.

Despite their potential importance, few studies have systematically investigated the cardiovascular effects of vasodilators in conditions where RV afterload is acutely increased.

A recent study compared the acute cardiopulmonary effects of nitroprusside and hydralazine in a canine model of pulmonary hypertension and decreased CO (Lee et al, 1983). Autologous clot injection increased RV afterload and decreased CO. Mean results are illustrated in Table 7.4. Note that while both drugs decreased ventricular filling pressures and systemic vascular resistance, only hydralazine increased CO.

Table 7.4   Hemodynamic effects of increased PVR and vasoactive drugs

	CO l/min	PAP mm Hg	RVEDP mm Hg	BP mm Hg	SVR mm Hg l^{-1} min	PVR mm Hg l^{-1} min
Baseline	3.0 ± 1.3	14 ± 2	3 ± 2	139 ± 21	53 ± 20	3 ± 3
Control 1	1.6 ± 0.7^B	47 ± 5^B	6 ± 3^A	144 ± 32	93 ± 26^B	31 ± 17^B
Nitroprusside	1.8 ± 2.2	44 ± 5	$4 \pm 2^{A,D}$	97 ± 18^B	$63 \pm 25^{B,C}$	30 ± 30
Control 2	1.5 ± 0.6	43 ± 5	5 ± 3	134 ± 26	94 ± 8	29 ± 15
Hydralazine	2.7 ± 1.5^A	42 ± 6	$4 \pm 3^{A,D}$	133 ± 31	$55 \pm 19^{B,C}$	18 ± 12^B

Statistical comparisons: [A] $p < 0.05$ parameters *vs* control; [B] $p < 0.01$ parameters *vs* control; [C] $p < 0.05$ comparing differences from control; [D] not significant, comparing differences from control.

The failure for CO to increase with nitroprusside is explained by the lack of change in RV afterload.

Similar findings with nitroprusside and hydralazine have been reported by Ghignone et al (1985) in a canine model of pulmonary hypertension where PVR was increased with injection of glassbeads. In both these studies (Lee et al, 1983; Ghignone et al, 1985), hydralazine produced a large decrease in PVR so that CO and SV doubled despite a decrease in RVEDP. Note that the PAP and BP did not change with hydralazine, and that while the mean value for arterial O_2 tension decreased with nitroprusside, it increased with hydralazine. Similar results are reported when hydralazine is given to patients with primary and secondary pulmonary hypertension (Rubin & Peter,

1980, 1981; Rubin et al, 1982). Also, one case report describes improved cardiovascular function when oral hydralazine was given for acute pulmonary embolism and a low output state (Bates, 1981).

While several studies indicate that hydralazine may be useful in treatment of a decreased CO complicating increased RV afterload, deleterious effects have been reported. One study of thirteen patients with primary and secondary pulmonary hypertension failed to document significant hemodynamic improvement with oral hydralazine (Packer et al, 1982). Four patients became symptomatically hypotensive, two requiring vasopressors to maintain BP. One death occurred and was attributed to excessive systemic hypotension complicating hydralazine therapy.

Accordingly, while hydralazine may be useful to decrease RV afterload and increase CO when a low output state complicates an acute increase in RV afterload, extreme care should be taken to ensure that excessive falls in BP and RV perfusion do not occur. Conceivably, pressor agents such as NE, which probably do not increase PVR (see section on the flow resistive characteristics of the pulmonary vasculature), could be used in conjunction with a vasodilator if the latter is felt to be indicated. For example, a recent clinical study of patients with pulmonary hypertension and circulatory failure complicating mitral valve replacement reported marked improvement in hemodynamic parameters with NE and PgE_1 (D'Ambra et al, 1985). PgE_1 decreased PVR but caused an excessive decrease in systemic BP; therefore, NE was used to maintain BP and RV perfusion pressure.

The rationale for combined thereapy in conditions of marked pulmonary hypertension and systemic hypotension should be based on the supposition that the increase in systemic BP, via inotropic and/or direct pressor effects, will not be associated with a significant, corresponding increase in pulmonary vascular tone. Clearly, this approach, while theoretically sound, requires systematic investigation.

FIBRINOLYTIC THERAPY

Many investigators and clinicians feel that fibrinolytic agents are indicated in the treatment of life-threatening pulmonary emboli. The phase I multicenter Urokinase Pulmonary Embolism Trial compared the effects of 12 hours of urokinase therapy followed by herarin therapy with the effects of heparin alone. The Phase II Urokinase-Streptokinase Pulmonary Embolism Trial compared the efficacy of 12- and 24-hour urokinase therapy with 24-hour streptokinase therapy (Phase II Results. A Cooperative Study, 1974; Urokinase Pulmonary Embolism Trial (UPET), 1973). Resolution of pulmonary thromboemboli during the first 24 hours of therapy, as assessed by graphic studies (angiography and perfusion lung scan) and hemodynamic measurement, was greater in patients treated with fibrinolytic therapy and heparin than in those treated with heparin alone. Effects were most pronounced in patients with massive emboli. For example, in the Phase I trial the mean values for RVEDP and RVSP decreased from 11 to 7 mm Hg and from 49 to 36 mm Hg respectively with urokinase. There were less obvious changes in the corresponding pressures in patients treated with heparin. There was a higher incidence of early (first 24 hours), severe bleeding complications associated with thrombolytic therapy.

In a more recent study, Petitpretz et al investigated effects of a single bolus of urokinase, 15 000 IU/kg followed by heparin, in treatment of fourteen patients with life-threatening pulmonary emboli (Petitpretz et al, 1984). Two patients did not improve. However, twelve demonstrated rapid and significant hemodynamic and clinical improvement. Sequential hemodynamic measurements, obtained in seven patients demonstrated that the greatest percentage of hemodynamic improvement occurred within three hours of bolus administration of urokinase. In contrast to continuous infusion thrombolytic therapy, no significant complications were reported with the bolus technique. The investigators favorably compared their results with other studies where thrombolytic agents were given as smaller initial dose followed by continuous infusion. They concluded that because of the rapid efficacy and low cost, the bolus technique was probably useful in treatment of patients with acute, life-threatening emboli.

THE FLOW RESISTIVE CHARACTERISTICS OF THE PULMONARY VASCULATURE

Thus far, this review has focused on the pathophysiology and treatment of RV dysfunction complicating acute changes in afterload. The genesis of RV dysfunction in this setting arises from alterations in the pulmonary vascular bed. The physiological mechanisms responsible for the alterations in pulmonary hemodynamics have only recently been investigated.

Conventionally, PVR, calculated as PAP-LV filling pressure ÷ CO, is assumed to reflect the flow resistive properties of the pulmonary vasculature and changes in PVR are felt to reflect changes in effective vascular caliber. This calculation implies that the PAP-CO (P-Q) relationship of the lung is linear and that the effective pulmonary vascular outflow pressure in Zone III of West is the LV filling pressure (Graham et al, 1983; Mitzner, 1983).

Several recent studies have used the pulmonary vascular P-Q relationship to investigate physiology and pathophysiology of the pulmonary circulation (Graham et al, 1982, 1983; Mitzner, 1983; Ducas et al, 1986; Mitzner & Sylvester, 1981; Shoukas, 1975). Using this analysis, two parameters describe hemodynamics: 1. The slope of this relationship, consistently reported as linear over physiological flow rates, defines the incremental vascular resistance (pressure change per unit change in flow); 2. The mean effective vascular outflow pressure is defined by linear extrapolation of the P-Q relationship to zero flow (Graham et al, 1982, 1983; Mitzner, 1983; Ducas et al, 1986; Mitzner & Sylvester, 1981). The effective outflow pressure may be influenced by vascular closing pressure (Graham et al, 1983; Mitzner, 1983; Ducas et al, 1986), left atrial pressure (Shoukas, 1975) and/or by alveolar pressure (Graham et al, 1982). Several studies have confirmed that under certain conditions, the effective outflow pressure may exceed LV filling pressure in Zone III (Ducas et al, 1986) and alveolar pressure in Zone II (Graham et al, 1982, 1983).

Accordingly, in pulmonary hypertension, the elevation in PAP may be related to an increase in effective outflow pressure, an increase in incremental resistance or a combination of these two factors. Similarly, vasoactive compounds may produce alterations in pulmonary hemodynamics, by altering these factors either separately or in combination.

A recent canine study investigated the pulmonary vascular effects of pulmonary emboli and hydralazine (Ducas et al, 1986). To define the vascular P-Q relationship, multiple PAP-Q coordinates were obtained by opening systemic A-V fistulae fitted with variable resistors.

As in previous studies by Rubin & Peter (1980, 1981), Rubin et al (1982), Rounds et al (1983), Lee et al (1983), hydralazine markedly increased CO, decreased calculated PVR and did not affect PAP. In the three experimental circumstances, before and after emboli and after hydralazine, the P-Q relationship was well described by linear regression analysis, mean r value 0.94. Effects of pulmonary emboli and hydralazine on pulmonary P-Q characteristics in four representative dogs are illustrated in Fig. 7.1 (left side). Note that while emboli increased incremental resistance, the predominant emplanation for the increase in PAP was the large increase in effective outflow pressure. Further, note that the predominant effect of hydralazine was not to alter incremental resistance, but to decrease effective outflow pressure (mean change, 24%). To test the hypothesis that the extrapolated pressure intercept reflects the effective downstream or outflow pressure, in four dogs, left atrial pressure was progressively raised by inflating a left atrial balloon at constant CO (see Fig. 7.1, right side). Before embolisation, increases in left atrial (LA) pressure over a given range (approximately 8 to 18 mm Hg) caused similar changes in PAP, indicating LA pressure approximated the effective outflow pressure. In contrast, after embolisation, changes in LA pressure over the same range had absent to trivial effects on PAP. Accordingly, as signalled by the change in extrapolated pressure intercept, embolisation resulted in a marked increase in the effective outflow pressure.

Another recent canine study investigated the effects of pulmonary emboli and NE on P-Q characteristics (Duval et al, 1984). P-Q characteristics were defined as described above (Ducas et al, 1986). Emboli increased mean incremental resistance from 1.9 to 5.5 mm Hg/l/min and caused a marked upward shift in the extrapolated pressure intercept, from 8.1 to 28.3 mm Hg. Both before and after emboli NE produced significant increases in CO and BP. Also, as seen in the studies of Molloy et al (1984) and Ducas et al 1985, NE decreased traditionally calculated PVR. However, as illustrated in Fig. 7.2, NE did not alter incremental resistance or outflow pressure.

These findings further emphasise the utility of NE for treatment of low output states due to increased RV afterload. That is the beneficial inotropic and pressor effects which improve RV function, CO and BP are not associated with increased pulmonary vascular tone so that the increase in PAP with NE is due to the corresponding change in flow.

SUMMARY

When shock complicates an acute increase in RV afterload, initial therapy should be directed toward restoration of an adequate BP (RV coronary perfusion pressure) and CO. Current results indicate that NE may be an excellent agent for acute resuscitation and short-term maintenance of hemodynamic stability.

In the absence of shock, when a moderate decrease in CO complicates pulmonary embolism, isoproterenol, hydralazine or other vasodilators, may be employed to improve flow. However, these agents may decrease BP so careful monitoring is required.

Recent canine studies indicate that an increase in effective outflow pressure is the predominant mechanism explaining the increase in PAP and apparent increase in

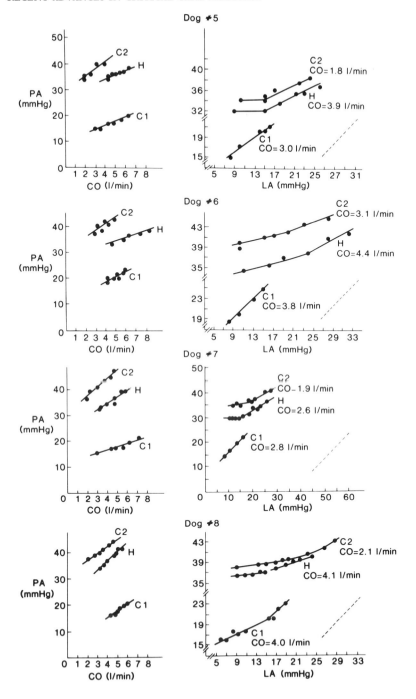

Fig. 7.1 On the left, the coordinates for PA and CO have been plotted for four dogs. The lines drawn are from linear regression. On the right, for each dog, the relationship between PA pressure and LA pressure at constant cardiac output are plotted. The lines drawn are from a visual best fit. The dashed line indicates the slope of the line of identity. See text for further discussion. H = after hydrallazine. C1 = control. C2 = after emboli.

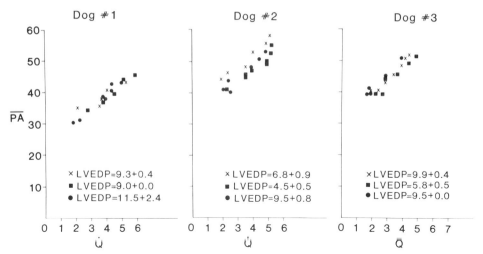

Fig. 7.2   The PA-CO coordinates for three dogs post emboli are plotted prior to noradrenaline (NE) (x) during NE (●), and time control-TC after NE infusion (■). For each dog, analysis of covariance revealed no differences in slope or intercept.

PVR complicating pulmonary embolism. Accordingly, in addition to decreasing vascular resistance, therapy could be directed toward decreasing outflow pressure.

REFERENCES

Albert J S, Smith R, Carlson J, Oskene I S, Dexter L, Salen J E 1976 Mortality in patients treated for pulmonary embolism. Journal American Medical Association 236: 1477–1480

Bates E R, Crevey B J, Sprague F R, Bertram P 1981 Oral hydralazine therapy for acute pulmonary embolism and low output state. Archives Internal Medicine 141: 1537–1538

Chatterjee K, Parmley W W, Massie B, Greenberg B, Werner J, Klausner S, Norman A 1976 Oral hydralazine therapy for chronic refractory heart failure. Circulation 54(6): 879–883

D'Ambra M N, LaRaia P J, Philbin D M, Watkins W D, Hilgenberg A D, Buckley M J 1985 Prostaglandin E_1: A new therapy for refractory right heart failure and pulmonary hypertension after mitral valve replacement. Journal Thoracic Cardiovascular Surgery 89: 567–572

Ducas J, Deutscher R, Prewitt R M 1985 Inotropic vs vasopressor agents in acute right ventricular failure. American Review Respiratory Disease (suppl) 131(4): A149

Ducas J, Girling L, Schich U, Prewitt R M 1986 Pulmonary vascular effects of hydralazine in a canine model of pulmonary thromboembolism. Circulation, 73(5): 1050–1057

Duval D, Ducas J, Molloy W D, Girling L, Prewitt R M 1984 Effects of pulmonary (P) emboli (E) and noradrenaline (NE) on pulmonary pressure-flow relationships. American Review Respiratory Disease 129(4): A63

Ghignone M, Girling L, Prewitt R M, 1985 Effects of vasodilators on canine cardiopulmonary function when a decrease in cardiac output complicates an increase in right ventricular afterload. American Review Respiratory Disease 131: 527–530

Graham R, Skoog C, Macedo W, Carter J, Oppenheimer L, Rabson J, Goldberg H S 1983 Dopamine, dobutamine, and phentolamine effects on pulmonary vascular mechanics. Journal Applied Physiology 54(5): 1277

Graham R, Skoog C, Oppenheimer L, Rabson J, Goldberg H S 1982 Critical closure in the canine pulmonary vasculature. Circulation Respiratory 50: 566

Lee K Y, Molloy W D, Slykerman L, Prewitt R M 1983 Effects of hydralazine and nitroprusside on cardiopulmonary function when a decrease in cardiac output complicates a short-term increase in pulmonary vascular resistance. Circulation 68(6): 1299–1303

McDonald I G, Hirsh J, Hale G S, Cade J F, McCarthy R A 1968 Isoproterenol in massive pulmonary embolism: haemodynamic and clinical effects. Medical Journal Australia (suppl) 201–205

Mitzner W 1983 Resistance of the pulmonary circulation. Clinics Chest Medicine 4(2): 127

Mitzner W, Sylvester J T 1981 Hypoxic vasoconstriction and fluid filtration in pig lungs. Journal Applied Physiology 51(5): 1065

Molloy D W, Lee K Y, Girling L, Schick U, Prewitt R M 1984 Treatment of shock in a canine model of pulmonary embolism. American Review Respiratory Disease 130: 870–874

Molloy W D, Lee K Y, Jones D, Penner B, Prewitt R M 1985 Effects of noradrenaline and isoproterenol on cardiopulmonary function in a canine model of acute pulmonary hypertension. Chest 88: 432–435

Packer M, Greenberg B, Massie B, Dash H 1982 Deleterious effects of hydralazine in patients with pulmonary hypertension. New England Journal Medicine 306: 1326–1331

Petitpretz P, Simmoneay G, Cerrina J, Musset D, Dreyfus M, Vandenbroek M, Duroux P 1984 Effects of a single bolus of urokinase in patients with life-threatening pulmonary emboli: a descriptive trial. Circulation 70(5): 861–866

Phase II results. A cooperative study 1974 Journal American Medical Association 229: 1606

Pierpont G, Hale K A, Franciosa J A et al 1980 Effects of vasodilators on pulmonary hemodynamics and gas exchange in left ventricular failure. American Heart Journal 99: 208

Rounds S, Kellet M, Jacobs A, Ryan T 1983 Failure of vasodilator responses in primary pulmonary hypertension. American Review Respiratory Disease 127(4) Part 2: Abstract 82

Rubin L J, Handel F, Peter R H 1982 The effects of oral hydralazine on right ventricular end-diastolic pressure in patients with right ventricular failure. Circulation 65(7): 1369–1373

Rubin L J, Peter R H 1980 Oral hydralazine therapy for primary pulmonary hypertension. New England Journal Medicine 302: 69

Rubin L J, Peter R H 1981 Hemodynamics at rest and during exercise after oral hydralazine in patients with cor pulmonale. Americn Journal Cardiology 47: 116

Sashara A A 1980 Controversy: the vase of fibrinolytic therapy. Journal Cardiovascular Medicine 5: 793–814

Sharma G V R K, McIntyre K M 1984 Pulmonary embolism. Cardiology Clinics 2(2): 269–274

Shoukas A A 1975 Pressure-flow and pressure–volume relations in the entire pulmonary vascular bed of the dog determined by two-port analysis. Circulation Respiratory 37: 809

Snider M T, Rie M A, Lauer J et al 1980 Normoxic pulmonary vasoconstriction in ARDS: Detection by sodium nitroprusside (N) and isoproterenol (I) infusions Massachsetts General Hospital, Boston, Massachusetts. American Review Respiratory Disease (suppl) 121: 191

Urokinase Pulmonary Embolism Trial (UPET) 1973 Circulation 47 (suppl II): II-I

Urokinase Pulmonary Embolism Study Group 1973 Urokinase pulmonary embolism trial. Circulation 47: 66–73

Vlahakes G J, Turlcy K, Hoffman J I E 1981 The pathophysiology of failure in acute right ventricular hypertension: hemodynamic and biochemical correlations. Circulation 63: 87–95

West J W, Aviado D M 1956 Cardiac output of methoxamine with special reference to intracoronary injection. American Journal Medical Science 231: 599–600

Wood L D H, Prewitt R M 1981 Cardiovascular management in acute hypoxemic respiratory failure. American Journal Cardiology 47: 963

Zapol W M, Falke K J 1985 Acute respiratory failure. Marcel Dekker 7: 241–272

Zapol W M, Snider M T 1977 Pulmonary hypertension in severe acute respiratory failure. New England Journal Medicine 296: 476–480

8. Sepsis, hypermetabolism and organ failure

Frank B. Cerra

Sepsis, hypermetabolism and organ failure continue to account for most surgical intensive care unit admissions staying over five days, and is the cause of death in over 90% of surgical intensive care unit patients (Carrico et al, 1986; Cerra, 1987a). The mean length of stay is 21 days and the mean cost is around $84,000 (Madoff et al, 1985). In those that survive, rehabilitation is mainly a process of rebuilding the skeletal muscle mass that was lost during the SICU phase with a cost twice that of the intensive care unit cost. There has been a progressive reduction in mortality risk from approximately 90% several years ago to the current level of 35–40% (Madoff et al, 1985).

BASIC HYPOTHESIS

The most common setting for the complex has traditionally been infection (Carrico et al, 1986; Cerra, 1987a; Madoff et al, 1985; Cerra et al, 1979a; Border et al, 1976). The systemic response was observed to be independent of the type of invading microorganism, be it virus, bacteria, or fungus (Wiley et al, 1980; Deutschman et al, 1987). Observations made in settings of severe perfusion injury and severe soft tissue damage or retroperitoneal inflammation, such conditions as ruptured aneurysms, soft tissue trauma, and pancreatitis failed to statistically differentiate the systemic manifestations (Tilney et al, 1973). Hence, the concept evolved that the systemic inflammatory response was being manifested in all these settings. One form of this response came from invading microorganisms and that form continues to be called sepsis or the systemic septic response.

A number of predisposing clinical settings have been identified (Carrico et al, 1986; Cerra, 1987a; Cerra et al, 1979a; Cuthbertson & Tilstone, 1977; Wilmore & Orlick, 1980; Cerra et al, 1980; Shoemaker, 1985). These include: a persistent undrained or uncontrolled source of infection; a severe perfusion deficit followed by infection; a severe perfusion deficit alone; a persistent inflammatory focus; or the continued presence of the hypermetabolic state.

The basic hypothesis evolved that the clinical, physiologic, and metabolic responses represent the systemic expression of mediator systems that have been activated by a number of clinical-pathologic settings. These clinical settings that are capable of activating this response include: dead tissue, injured tissue, perfusion deficits, and invading microorganisms. The mediator systems involved include the central nervous system, the classic macroendocrine system, and the cell-cell microendocrine system that includes such agents as the interleukins, various peptides, prostaglandins, leukotrienes, and various components of the coagulation system (Fig. 8.1) (Pomanda, 1980; Heideman & Hugli, 1984; Alberti et al, 1980; Bessey et al, 1984; Clowes et al, 1983; Lefer, 1985; Barracos et al, 1983).

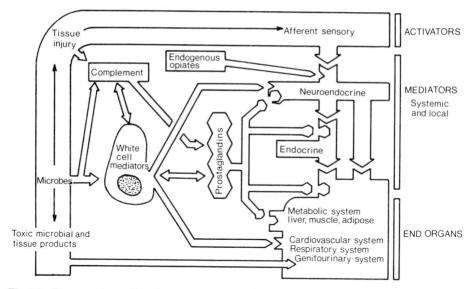

Fig. 8.1 The systemic manifestations are expressions of mediator systems that modulate the end-organs to produce the clinical, physiologic and metabolic manifestations that are present at the bedside (Cerra, 1987a).

THE CLINICAL SYNDROME

In the presence of a septic focus, the metabolic response follows a general pattern. There is an ebb phase that generally coincides with the shock phase of an injury and is characterised by vasoactive phenomena and the output of acute hormones such as cortisol and catecholamines, and high levels of sympathetic and parasympathetic tone (Cuthbertson & Tilstone, 1977). Following this the flow phase occurs during which the metabolic response to injury increases (Cuthbertson & Tilstone, 1977). It usually reaches a peak in 48–72 hours and then begins to spontaneously abate and is usually gone in 7–10 days.

The response is not necessarily temporal and its manifestation depends in large part on the severity of the stimulus and when the practitioner first observes the patient (Fig. 8.2). Thus, it may proceed directly towards death. In other cases the reactivation phase is entered, usually heralding the onset of a new stress stimulus, such as an infectious complication in the surgical patient. If the source is controlled, the recovery phase is again entered. If the source is not controlled, the hypermetabolism continues until such time as the source is controlled or the organ failure stage is entered. In the early organ failure phase, if the source could be controlled, recovery is still possible. This is not true of the later phases of organ failure, however, where the probability of recovery significantly declines.

The typical clinical course then is one of an episode of sepsis with a perfusion deficit that is resuscitated, and appropriately managed medically and surgically. The next day the patient looks quite well. Several days later there is a change in mentation, some tachycardia and sympathomimetic findings, and an increase in respiratory rate. Bilateral pulmonary interstitial infiltrates begin to appear together with hypocapnia and hypoxemia and the progressive need for mechanical ventilation. At this point an effort is made to find a treatable cause and either control it, as with antibiotics,

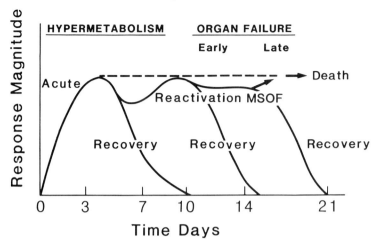

Fig. 8.2 Sepsis proceeds through a sequence of hypermetabolism. With continued injury, infection or perfusion failure, the transition to the organ failure syndrome is made with an associated rise in mortality risk (Cerra, 1987a).

or excise it, as with abscess or the presence of dead or injured tissue. Encephalopathy worsens and the bilirubin begins to rise. Usually ileus is present and a consumptive coagulopathy begins to appear. After several more days the creatinine begins to rise and the renal failure phase of the organ system dysfunction begins. Gastrointestinal bleeding becomes a prominent feature, even in the presence of efforts to control stress ulcers in the stomach. Sites of bleeding further down the intestinal tract are common. Bacteremias and fungal and viral infections become significant features of the process.

PHYSIOLOGIC CHARACTERISTICS

With the onset of sepsis the primary physiological change appears to be an increase in oxygen consumption demand (Fig. 8.3). This increase in demand needs to be met by an increase in supply. Hence, there is a corresponding increase in cardiac output (Shoemaker, 1985). The calculated variable, systemic vascular resistance, falls (Cerra, 1987b). Sequential studies would indicate that the increase in cardiac output is responding to the rise in oxygen consumption demand by a fall in systemic vascular resistance. In the early phases, the arterial venous oxygen content difference (DVO_2) is quite normal (Cerra et al, 1979a, 1980).

As the process progresses and the transition into organ failure begins, the oxygen consumption demand tends to increase. This is associated with an increase in cardiac output and a different relationship of the systemic vascular resistance and DVO_2 to the cardiac output. The systemic vascular resistance falls and, the DVO_2 is narrower than it should be for the existing level of cardiac output, the narrowness in DVO_2 deriving from a failure of venous desaturation (Cerra et al, 1979a, 1980; Shoemaker, 1985).

The precise origin of these latter events is unclear. There is adequate oxygen content and a seemingly adequate oxygen delivery to the periphery. The problem appears to reside in an extraction failure at the periphery. This process was initially felt to be physiologic shunting. However, the metabolic data do not strongly support this

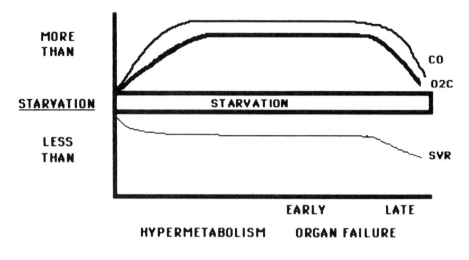

CO = CARDIAC OUTPUT
O2C = OXYGEN CONSUMPTION
SVR = SYSTEMIC VASCULAR RESISTENCE

Fig. 8.3   The horizontal bar represents the spectrum of response in standard starvation. The response in sepsis is characterised by a fall in systemic resistance with an increase on oxygen demand. If the cardiac output can be increased to meet the demand, survival potential is improved (Cerra, 1987b).

hypothesis. The observations that there is not excess lactate production, that there is a reduced oxidation of pyruvate with increased recycling of lactate, that there is a significant increase in alanine production with the nitrogen component originating from the oxidation of amino acids in the Krebs cycle, all serve to indicate that the oxidative mode at this time is one of aerobic metabolism and not one of anaerobic metabolism.

As the organ failure progresses, these physiologic changes worsen. The systemic vascular resistance becomes very low and cardiac output begins to fall, a reflection of left ventricular and frequently biventricular cardiac failure.

CARBOHYDRATE METABOLISM

The mediator systems modulate carbohydrate metabolism in a way that is much different from that of standard starvation (Fig. 8.4). The ratio of carbon dioxide production to oxygen consumption (R/Q) reflects the combustion of substrate that is ongoing for the production of energy (R/Q). In the hypermetabolic septic state this R/Q spontaneously approaches the 0.8–0.85, level, reflecting the oxidation of mixed substrate (Giovannini et al, 1983), carbohydrate, fat, and amino acids. When the organ failure state is entered, this R/Q begins to rise until in late organ failure it approaches and eventually exceeds 1, representing a transition into net lipogenesis.

From the point of view of carbohydrate metabolism, this R/Q indicates that there is a reduction in the fractional energy expenditure that is being derived from the oxidation of glucose. The regulation appears to originate from the reduced function of pyruvate dehydrogenase and therefore the reduced use of pyruvate as an oxidation fuel substrate in the Krebs cycle (Cerra et al, 1979b, 1980; Clowes et al, 1976).

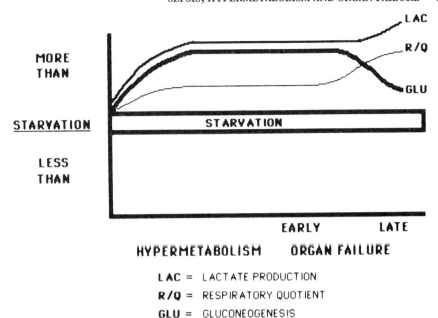

LAC = LACTATE PRODUCTION
R/Q = RESPIRATORY QUOTIENT
GLU = GLUCONEOGENESIS

Fig. 8.4   The format is the same as in Fig. 8.3. The R/Q is 0.8 to 0.85; gluconeogenesis is increased; pyruvate oxidation is reduced (Cerra, 1987b).

In the absence of a perfusion deficit, the lactate and pyruvate output remain proportionately increased without excess lactate production. This lactate appears to serve as an energy substrate in other tissues such as heart which has the capacity to oxidise lactate by direct entry into the mitochondria through the malate shuttle. The liver appears to use lactate as a substrate for gluconeogenesis.

Gluconeogenesis is significantly increased (Elwyn et al, 1979; Long et al, 1976), presumably reflecting the existing mediator milieu and the increased substrate base that is being derived from the carbon skeletons of lactate, alanine, and the large load of amino acids that the liver is being presented with from the periphery. This gluconeogenesis is much less responsive to exogenous glucose administration. Whereas in starvation the administration of exogenous glucose can shut down the production of glucose, this is less easily done in septic hypermetabolism and organ failure (Long et al, 1976).

With the entrance into organ failures, the carbohydrate metabolism continues to change. As the late phase of the organ failures are entered, the R/Q begins to exceed one, lactate and pyruvate production markedly increase but still without excess lactate production until the cardiac output falls. Ultimately gluconeogenesis fails and hypoglycemia becomes a clinical manifestation.

FAT METABOLISM

The most well-described difference between starvation and hypermetabolism occurs with ketone body production by the liver (Fig. 8.5). Ketosis is markedly suppressed in the presence of septic hypermetabolism (Rich & Wright, 1979; Birkham et al, 1981; Watters et al, 1984). This occurs in the presence of reduced lipogenesis, an

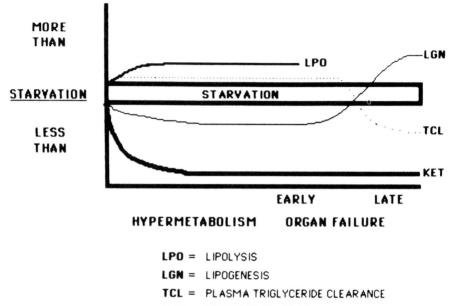

Fig. 8.5   The format is the same as in Fig. 8.3. Ketosis is reduced; fat provides an important source of calories. Eventually triglyceride clearance decrease and net lipogenesis is present, particularly in liver (Cerra, 1987b).

increase in lipolysis and a marked increase in the turnover rate and oxidation of fatty acids of both medium chain and long chain variety. There is likewise an associated increase in triglyceride clearance relative to starvation. The precise origin for the reduction in ketosis is not entirely clear but again is felt to reflect at least in part the high insulin levels that are present in the hypermetabolic state with the selective inhibition of hormone sensitive lipase.

As the organ failure progresses, there is an increase in net lipogenesis that correlates with the progressive rise in R/Q. The site of this lipogenesis appears to be primarily hepatic. The precise reason for this is not clear, with such hypothesis as a failure of hepatic protein synthesis, or primary enzyme dysfunction being proposed. Triglyceride clearance also becomes reduced and spontaneous lipemia or hypertriglyceridimia becomes a prominent feature (Cerra et al, 1980; Lindholm & Rossner, 1983; Cerra et al, 1979c). It in part seems to reflect the reduction in lipoprotein lipase activity, at least in skeletal muscle and adipose tissue (Robin et al, 1981). This observation in a patient carries a high mortality risk.

PROTEIN METABOLISM

With the onset of sepsis, total body protein synthesis is decreased (Fig. 8.6). This is associated with a primary increase in catabolism of the protein stores, particularly in skeletal muscle, loose connective tissue, and intestinal viscera (Cerra et al, 1979a, 1980; Cuthbertson & Tilstone, 1977; Clowes et al, 1976; Birkhan et al, 1980; Long et al, 1981). This catabolism has been coined 'autocannibalism' (Cerra et al, 1980). The clinical correlate is the rapid marked reduction in skeletal muscle mass that

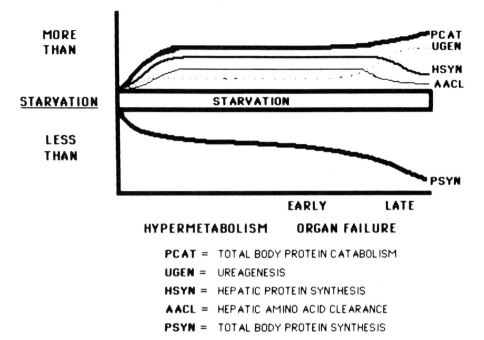

MORE
THAN
                                                                    PCAT
                                                                    UGEN

                                                                    HSYN
                                                                    AACL

STARVATION   STARVATION

LESS
THAN

                                                                    PSYN

                              EARLY   LATE
        HYPERMETABOLISM   ORGAN FAILURE

        PCAT = TOTAL BODY PROTEIN CATABOLISM
        UGEN = UREAGENESIS
        HSYN = HEPATIC PROTEIN SYNTHESIS
        AACL = HEPATIC AMINO ACID CLEARANCE
        PSYN = TOTAL BODY PROTEIN SYNTHESIS

Fig. 8.6   The format is the same as in Fig. 8.3. Protein synthesis is reduced and catabolism is increased, except in liver where protein synthesis is increased. When hepatic protein synthesis fails, hepatic failure is present and the organ failure syndrome has become manifest (Cerra, 1987b).

exceeds that predicted from bed rest alone. This amino acid efflux from the peripheral tissues is not the same for all amino acids. For the branched chain amino acids leucine, isoleucine, and valine, the efflux seems to be less, with an increase in the peripheral oxidation of the branched chain amino acids for energy production (Cerra et al, 1980; Birkhan et al, 1980). This is paralleled by an increase in the total body oxidation of amino acids as energy sources (Long et al, 1981; Powell-Tuck et al, 1984; Long et al, 1977).

In contrast to these observations, hepatic protein synthesis is significantly increased. This is paralleled by an increase in amino acid clearance. The increase in net ureagenesis reflects this balance of catabolism, utilisation of amino acids as gluconeogenic substrate, and net hepatic protein synthesis. When the organ failure phase is entered, total body protein synthesis decreases more. Ureagenesis increases more reflecting the increase in catabolic rate and efflux of amino acids from the peripheral tissue. Hepatic protein synthesis begins to fail, reflected in the reduction in amino acid clearance. There is a continued increase in catabolism and a reduction in total body protein synthesis. The result at this point is a spontaneous increase in ureagenesis with a corresponding increase in the prerenal azotemia that is present throughout the hypermetabolism organ failure complex irrespective of whether exogenous amino acid support is given or not.

This mobilisation of amino acids seems to be regulated by different processes than those that regulate protein synthesis. Exogenous amino acids and/or calories do not effectively control it. Current hypotheses implicate the peptide mediators produced by white cells, particularly macrophages. The loss of this mobile amino acid pool, as in skeletal muscle, serves to meet demands for protein synthesis and energy production and redistribution of protein to the organs 'doing the work', e.g. heart and liver.

ENERGY EXPENDITURE

The increase in energy expenditure is reflected in the oxygen consumption demand and in the observed cardiac output. The substrate base for this increased energy production must come from the oxidation of carbon sources in the Krebs cycle. These carbon sources must come from either carbohydrate, fat, or amino acids.

Relative to standard starvation where in the early phases the primary carbon source for oxidation is glucose and then switches over mostly to fat in the form of fatty acids and ketones, in hypermetabolism and organ failure there is a mixed substrate oxidation (Fig. 8.7). The fraction of the total energy expenditure that is derived

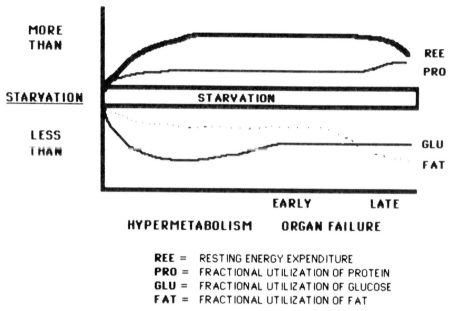

REE = RESTING ENERGY EXPENDITURE
PRO = FRACTIONAL UTILIZATION OF PROTEIN
GLU = FRACTIONAL UTILIZATION OF GLUCOSE
FAT = FRACTIONAL UTILIZATION OF FAT

Fig. 8.7   The format is the same as in Fig. 8.3. REE is increased. The *fractional* amount of energy derived from amino acids is increased, whereas that from glucose and fat is reduced (Cerra, 1987b).

from glucose is significantly reduced, while that derived from the direct oxidation of amino acids in the Krebs cycle is significantly increased, and accounts for much of the nitrogen that appears in alanine and glutamine. The remainder of the energy expenditure is derived from the direct oxidation of fat, presumably of the medium and long chain variety (Cerra et al, 1980; Birkhan et al, 1980; Long et al, 1977, 1981).

As the organ failure phase is entered, this fuel mix continues to change. More is derived from amino acids, and eventually there appears to be a further reduction in the fractional energy expenditure derived from glucose and then from fat. Thus in the later stages of organ failure the predominant oxidative fuel appears to be amino acids, reflected in the unrestricted ureagenesis and marked increase in catabolism that was previously discussed. The mobile amino acid pool conceptually seems to represent the 'gasoline tank'. Its rapid rate of use results in the accelerated appearance of clinical malnutrition.

The link between these initiating factors of dead tissue, injured tissue, perfusion deficits and invading micro-organisms and the observed responses appears to reside in the mediator systems (Powanda, 1980; Heideman & Hugli, 1984; Alberti et al, 1980; Bessey et al, 1984; Meakins, 1985; Clowes et al, 1983; Lefer, 1985; Barracos et al, 1983). Three general classes of mediators are recognised: the central nervous system, the macroendrocrine, and the microendocrine (cell to cell) mediator systems.

It has been known for some time that the metabolic response to injury is associated with release of hormones from the hypothalamic-pituitary axis as well as an increased outflow from the sympathetic-parasympathetic nervous system. Stimulation of hypo-thalamic nuclei can mimic a number of the metabolic responses; hyperglycemia and triglyceride mobilization are examples. Autonomic tone can mobilise glycogen, stimu-late glucose production and insulin output. Adrenocortical hormones are known to cause salt and water retention, proteolysis and lipolysis; growth hormone-somatomedin output is reduced and associated with reduced protein systhesis. Glucagon and insulin levels are increased with an increased glucagon/insulin ratio and are associated with increased gluconeaogenesis and lactate formation. Catecholamine infusions have been shown to induce glucose intolerance and insulin resistance, and presumably the reduced activity of pyruvate dehydrogenase (Alberti et al, 1980; Bessey et al, 1984).

The interleukin group of mediators are all metabolically active and have the capacity to act directly at the cell level, or indirectly through central nervous system stimulation (Powanda, 1980). They can produce many of the observed responses, such as increased gluconeogenesis and proteolysis. Peptide mediators are being increasingly identified, such as those implicated to cause proteolysis in skeletal muscle (Clowes et al, 1983). A number of the prostanoids have been shown to modulate intracellular biochemical pathways (Lefer, 1985). PgE2 is an example in its ability to modulate protein synthesis (Barracos, 1983).

Other mediator substances seem to be byproducts of the metabolism itself. An example is octopamine. This compound is a product of the nonoxidative metabolism of phenylalanine and can produce many of the altered physiologic changes that are observed: reduced systemic vascular resistance, high cardiac output.

The trade-off for this type of regulatory system is a progressive insensitivity to exogenous intervention. Thus the liver does not have large increases in ketone output; yet the muscle maintains the capacity to metabolise the ketones. The administration of glucose does not reduce the rate of lipolysis or gluconeogenesis. Betahydroxybuty-rate does not modulate lipolysis. The counterregulatory hormones override the insulin effects on hormones sensitive lipase in adipose tissue, but not the effects on fatty acid esterases and ketosis. Indeed, the administration of glucose is associated with an increased activation of the mediator systems, as evidenced by the marked increase in norepinephrine output (Nordenstrom et al, 1981).

The etiology of the hypermetabolism and organ failure is not clear: hypotheses seem to fall into three general categories: a failure to down-regulate, toxic mediation, and malnutrition.

The failure to down-regulate hypothesis purports that we are not programmed to servoregulate these prolonged response states that now occur in the modern SICU. On the other hand, when a local response becomes acutely systemic, the system may have discharged and be unable to further respond. This mode of action seems characteristic of several of the macrophage and white cell responses to stimuli.

The malnutrition hypothesis stems from the marked clinical manifestations of malnutrition that become evident in prolonged hypermetabolism and organ failure. Thus, substrate-limited metabolism could occur with the loss of organ structure and function and a failure of energy production. Muscle biopsies demonstrating reduced ATP and increased ADP and AMP in these clinical settings were consistent with this hypothesis (Fath et al, 1985; Fry et al, 1981).

Toxic mediation encompasses a group of hypotheses. Toxic substances can act directly on cells or indirectly through another regulatory cell. The gut-mediated hypothesis is an example. Bacteria and/or their products are hypothesised to translocate across the bowel and become absorbed into the portal and/or systemic circulation. They can directly injure such cells as hepatocytes or can activate regulatory cells such as Kupffer cells that then injure the hepatocytes.

Another model is exemplified in paired-cell systems, such as the Kupffer cell-hepatocyte system. Data from coculture systems would indicate that regulation of hepatocyte function is mediated by the Kupffer cell. Peptide mediators seem to be involved. Of particular interest is the observation that hypoxia presensitises the Kupffer cell so that when endotoxin is then added, a particularly devastating reduction in hepatic protein synthesis is observed (West et al, 1985; Keller et al, 1985). Recent data indicating macrophage modulation of muscle ATP production under conditions of inflammation is another example of cell-cell mediated metabolism (Morris et al, 1985).

THE EFFECTS OF EXOGENOUS SUBSTRATE ON THE METABOLIC RESPONSE TO SEPSIS

Tables 8.1 and 8.2 summarise the current understanding of septic metabolism relative to starvation and the alterations in fuel requirements that seem to result from that metabolic response.

Table 8.1 Comparison of starvation and sepsis

	Starvation	Sepsis
Energy expenditure	↓	++
Mediator activation	+	+++
R/Q	0.7	0.8–0.85
Fuel	Glucose/fat	Mixed
Gluconeogenesis	+	+++
Protein synthesis	↓	↓↓
Catabolism	---	+++
AA oxidation	±	+++
Ureagenesis	±	++
Ketosis	+++	+
Responsiveness	+++	+
Rate of malnutrition development	+	+++

Table 8.2   Fuel utilisation in sepsis

	Starvation			Organ failure	
	Early	Adapted	Septic	Early	Late
REE	↓	↓ ↓	+ +	+ +	+ +
Glucose	+ + +	+	+	+	+
Fat	+	+ + +	+	+	±
Amino acid	+ +	+	+ +	+ +	+ + +

With the application of standard hyperalimentation and caloric loads exceeding 50 kcal/kg, a number of organ failures appeared. Carbon dioxide production was increased, minute ventilation rose, ventilatory failure occurred; hepatic steatosis was a common finding; nitrogen retention was suboptimal; hyperglycemia with hyperosmolar complications were common; energy expenditure increased (Nordenstrom et al, 1981, 1983; Askanazi et al, 1900a, b, Kirkpatrick et al, 1981, Barke et al, 1976). When the total caloric load was reduced and the glucose load was reduced, the problems were greatly reduced. 35–40 nonprotein calories/kg/day without exceeding 5 mg/kg-min of glucose accomplished the goals.

With the advent of intravenous fat as long chain fatty acid triglyceride emulsion, it became possible to better mimic the 'natural' caloric mix, substitute fat calories for glucose calories, and reduce the problems of excess glucose administration (Nordenstrom et al, 1983; Kirkpatrick et al, 1981; Barke et al, 1976). In addition, it was observed that fat mobilisation and utilisation, although increased early in the process, was not nearly as increased as a comparable stage of nonstressed starvation. If the fat was not administered, the changes of long chain fat deficiency appeared within 5–7 days.

Starvation doses of amino acids (1.0 g/kg/day) were found to not induce reasonable nitrogen retention or balance, or to inhibit the redistribution of the lean body mass. Contrary to starvation, it was observed that the nitrogen retention was proportional to the amino acid load (Cerra et al, 1983). Nitrogen equilibrium also related to the degree of metabolic stress that was present. At moderate to high levels of stress, 2.0–3.0 g/kg/day were necessary to achieve nitrogen equilibrium or 3–4 g/day of positive nitrogen balance (Birkhan et al, 1980; Long et al, 1977, 1981; Cerra et al, 1983, 1984; Bower et al, 1986; Clowes et al, 1980). With the calorie loads as discussed above, this resulted in a nonprotein calorie to nitrogen ratio of 100 : 1; and was consistent with the metabolic observations that had been made.

With these support principles most of the major complications were no longer significant clinical problems. Patients who responded to the support by increasing both the production of acute phase proteins and nutritional proteins had an increased likelihood of survival (Moyer et al, 1981). Total body protein synthesis was increased, but there was no demonstrable reduction in catabolism. Patients who reversed their skin test anergy in response to the substrate support also had an increased likelihood of survival (Meakins et al, 1977). Although the redistribution of nitrogen was not altered, the visceral protein mass and function was better supported.

In an effort to achieve better organ support, the amino acid composition was altered to increase those amino acids where there was an increase in demand, reduce those where there was a reduction in demand or associated hepatotoxic effect and those whose primary function was glucose production. These solutions at best induced better nitrogen retention per gram administered protein nitrogen and more hepatic protein synthesis. A reduction in catabolic rate or an effect on the redistribution of the body nitrogen were not established, although the rate of ureagenesis was less than that for standard formulas. The dose-dependency of the response indicated that amino acids were acting like drugs in the setting of hypermetabolism and organ failure. No demonstrable effect on hypermetabolism was shown although it seemed the patients could be supported longer so that more could recover (cure themselves) without suc-cumbing to malnutrition (Cerra et al, 1982, 1984; Bower et al, 1986).

The phenomenon of flow-dependent oxygen consumption was observed, even in settings where it was felt oxygen consumption was restored by clinical criteria. When applied prospectively as a resuscitation criterion with subsequent maintenance of the high flow state, reduction in organ failures, infectious complications, and mortality was observed (Shoemaker, 1985).

The route of administration has received renewed attention with the demonstration that the small bowel will still function when gastric and colonic atony are present. Early enteral feeding has been associated with improved survival in animal burn models (Alverdy et al, 1985). Gut secretory IgA production was better maintained by enteral nutrition (Saito et al, 1985). In human studies, effective stress ulcer prevention has been achieved with enteral feeding alone (Pingleton & Hadgima, 1983). Enteral modi-fied amino acids have been associated with improved hepatic function and regeneration; the cholestasis and sludging of the biliary tree seems to respond well to enteral feedings (Cerra et al, 1985). A number of randomised, prospective studies are now in progress to evaluate the efficacy of enteral feeding in preventing or treating the organ failure syndrome.

SUMMARY AND CONCLUSIONS

Sepsis, hypermetabolism with organ failure remains a major clinical problem. The pathogenesis seems to reside in the mediated metabolic response to injury; the etiology of the organ failure transition remains elusive. The best treatment remains prevention. When the organ failures occur, even antibiotics and surgical control of the source may not stop the process. No one supportive treatment seems to cure the disease; there seem to be no 'magic bullets'. Rather, the supportive care such as fluids, ventila-tion, antibiotics, buy time for the process to 'cure itself'.

Control of the source and the restoration of oxygen transport remain the mainstays of therapy. Metabolic support has emerged as a clinical tool. It represents a departure from the principles of classic nutrition to those of the support of the structural and functional integrity of organs and organ-systems. It emphasises support of the meta-bolic pathways without forcing them in abnormal and detrimental directions. The criteria of efficacy become those of the evaluation of organ structure and function.

The principles of metabolic support derive from an understanding of the metabolic response to injury and of working within the limits set by the regulatory systems. The complication rate of the support tool has been greatly reduced; efficacy can be demonstrated in several areas. When applied in a setting of knowledgable practice, good surgery, and basic principles of physiology, there has been a progressive reduction in mortality in this class of patients.

The frontiers lie in understanding the mediator systems. It seems unlikely a single 'magic bullet' will emerge for therapy. More likely, combinations of appropriately timed therapy will become useful as support tools or perhaps as means of controlling the metabolic response when it has become a detriment to survival.

REFERENCES

Alberti K G, Batstone G F, Foster K et al 1980 Relative role of various hormones in mediating the matabolic response to injury. JPEN 4: 141

Alverdy J C, Chi H S, Selivanov 1985 The effect of route of nutrient administration on the secretory immune system. ASPEN Clinical Congress

Askanazi J, Rosenbaums H, Hyman A, Elwyn D, Kinney J 1980a Respiratory changes induced by high glucose loads of total parenteral nutrition. Journal of The American Medical Association 243: 1444–1447

Askanazi J, Carpentier Y, Elwyn D, Kenney J 1980b Influence of total parenteral nutrition on fuel utilization in injury and sepsis. Annals of Surgery 191: 40–46

Barke S, Holm I, Hakansson et al 1976 Nitrogen-sparing effect of fat emulsion compared with glucose in the postoperative period. Acta Chirurgica Scandinavica 142: 423–427

Barracos V, Rodemann H P, Dienarello C 1983 Stimulation of muscle protein degradation of PgE$_2$ release by leukocyte pyrogen. New England Journal of Medicine 308: 553–558

Bessey P, Waters J, Soki T, Wilmore D 1984 Combined hormone infusion stimulates the metabolic response to injury. Annals of Surgery 200: 264–281

Birkhan R, Long C, Fitkin D, Geiger J, Blakemore W 1980 Effects of major skeletal trauma on whole body protein turnover in man measured by 1, 14C leucine. Surgery 88: 294–297

Birkhan R, Long C, Fitkin D L, Geiger J, Blakemore W 1981 A comparison of the effects of skeletal trauma and surgery on the ketosis of starvation in man. Journal of Trauma 21: 513–519

Border J H, Chenier R, McMenamy R H 1976 Multiple systems organ failure: muscle fuel deficit with visceral protein malnutrition. Surgical Clinics of North America 56: 1147–1150

Bower R H, Muggin-Sullam M, Vallgren S, Fischer J 1986 Branched chain amino acid-enriched solutions in the septic patient: a randomized, prospective trail. Annals of Surgery 203: 13–21

Carrico C J, Meakins J, Marshall J, Fry D, Maier R 1986 Multiple organ failure syndrome. Archives of Surgery 121: 196–208

Cerra F B 1987a Hypermetabolism, organ failure and metabolic support. Surgery (in press)

Cerra F B 1987b The hypermetabolism-organ failure complex. World Journal of Surgery (in press)

Cerra F B, Siegel J H, Border J, Coleman B 1979a Correlations between metabolic and cardiopulmonary measurement in patients after trauma, general surgery and sepsis. Journal of Trauma 19: 621–628

Cerra F B, Caprioli J, Siegel J, Border J 1979b Proline metabolism in sepsis, cirrhosis and general surgery: the peripheral energy deficit. Annals of Surgery 190: 577–586

Cerra F B, Siegel J H, Border J, Coleman B 1979c The hepatic failure of sepsis: cellular vs substrate. Surgery 86: 409–422

Cerra F B, Siegel J H, Colman B, Border J, McMenamy R H 1980 Autocannibalism, a failure of exogenous nutritional support. Annals of Surgery 192: 570–574

Cerra F B, Upson D, Angelico R, Wiles III C, Lyons J, Paysinger J 1982 Branched chains support postoperative protein synthesis. Surgery 92: 192–199

Cerra F B, Mazuski J, Teasley K, Nuwer N, Lysne J, Shronts E, Konstantinides F 1983 Nitrogen retention in critically ill patients is proportional to the branched chain amino acid load. Critical Care Medicine 11: 775–778

Cerra F B, Mazuski J, Chute E, Teasley K, Konstantinides N 1984 Branched chain metabolic support. Annals of Surgery 199: 286–291

Cerra F B, Shronts E P, Konstantinides N, Thoele S, Konstantinides F, Teasley K, Lysne J 1985 Enteral feeding in sepsis: a prospective, randomized, double-blind trial. Surgery 98: 632–638

Clowes G, George B, Villes 1983 Muscle proteolysis induced by a circulating peptide in patients with sepsis and trauma. New England Journal of Medicine 308: 545–552

Clowes G H A, O'Donnell T F, Blackburn G 1976 Energy metabolism and proteolysis in traumatized and septic man. Surgical Clinics of North America 56: 1169–1172

Clowes G H A, Heidman M, Lindberg B 1980 Effects of parenteral alimentation on amino acid metabolism in septic patients. Surgery 8: 532–535

Cuthbertson D, Tilstone W 1977 Metabolism during the post-injury period. Advances in Clinical Chemistry 12: 1–55

Deutschman C, Simmons R L, Cerra F B The systemic response to cytomegalovirus: further evidence for a host dependent response. Archives of Surgery (in press)

Elwyn D H, Kinney J M, Juvanandum M 1979 Influence of increasing carbohydrate intake on glucose kinetics in injured patients. Annals of Surgery 190: 117–127

Fath J J, St Cyr J A, Cerra F B et al 1985 Alterations in amino acid clearance during ischemia predict hepatocellular ATP changes. Surgery 98: 396–404

Fry D E, Kaelin C R, Giammara B L, Rink R 1981 Alterations of oxygen metabolism in experimental bacteremia. Advances in Shock Research 6: 45–54

Giovannini I, Boldrini G, Castagnato M, Namio G, Pittiniti, Castiolini G 1983 Respiratory quotient and patterns of substrate utilization in human sepsis and trauma. JPEN 7: 226–230

Heideman M, Hugli T E 1984 Anaphylatoxin generation in multisystem organ failure. Journal of Trauma 24: 1038–1043

Keller G, Barke R, Harty J, Humphrey E, Simmons R 1985 Decreased hepatic glutathione levels in septic shock; predisposition of hepatocytes to oxidative stress. Archives of Surgery 120: 941–945

Kirkpatrick J, Dann M, Haynes M 1981 The therapeutic advantages of a balanced nutrition support system. Surgery 89: 370–374

Lefer A 1985 Eicosanoids as mediators of ischemia and shock. Federal Proceedings 14: 275–280

Lindholm M, Rossner S 1983 Rate of elimination of the intralipid fat emulsion from the circulation in ICU patients. Critical Care Medicine 10: 740–746

Long C, Kinney J, Geiger J 1976 Nonsuppressability of gluconeogenesis by in septic patients. Metabolism 25: 193

Long C L, Jeevanaudan M, Kinney J M 1977 Whole body protein synthesis and catabolism in septic man. American Journal of Clinical Nutrition 30: 1340–1345

Long C, Birkhan R, Geiger J 1981 Contribution of skeletal muscle protein in elevated rates of whole-body protein catabolism in trauma patients. American Journal of Clinical Nutrition 34: 1087

Madoff R D, Sharpe S M, Fath J J, Simmons R L, Cerra F B 1985 Prolonged surgical intensive care. Archives of Surgery 120: 698–702

Meakins J 1985 Host defense response to sepsis and septic shock. (In) *Prospective in Sepsis and Septic Shock*, Sibbald W, Sprung C (ed). SCCM Fullerton, Ca

Meakins J L, Pietsch J, Bubenich O 1977 Delayed hypersensitively; indicator of acquired failure of host defenses in sepsis and trauma. Annals of Surgery 186: 241–250

Morris A, Henry W, Shearer J, Caldwell M 1985 Macrophage interaction with skeletal muscle: a potential role of macrophages in determining the energy state of healing wounds 25: 746–751

Moyer F, Border J R, McMenamy R, Cerra F 1981 Multiple systems organ failure V: alterations in plasma protein profile in septic-trauma-effect of intravenous amino acids. Journal of Trauma 21: 645–649

Nordenstrom J, Jeevanandam M, Elwyn D, Kinney J 1981 Increasing glucose intake during total parenteral nutrition increases norepinephrine excretion in trauma and sepsis. Clinical Physiology 1: 525–534

Nordenstrom J, Askanazi J, Elwyn D H, Kenney J 1983 Nitrogen balance during total parenteral nutrition: glucose *vs* fat. Annals of Surgery 197: 27–33

Pingleton S K, Hadgima S K 1983 Enteral alimentation and gastrointestinal bleeding in mechanically ventilated patients. Critical Care Medicine 11: 13–16

Powanda M 1980 Host metabolic alterations during inflammatory stress as related to nutritional states. American Journal of Veterinary Medicine 41: 1905–1911

Powell-Tuck J, Fern E, Garlich P, Waterlow J 1984 The effect of surgical trauma and insulin on whole body protein turnover in parenterally-fed undernourished patients. Human Nutrition and Clinical Nutrition 38: 11–22

Rich A J, Wright P D 1979 Ketosis and nitrogen excretion in undernourished surgical patients. JPEN 3: 350–354

Robin A P, Askanayi J, Greenwood M, Elwyn D, Kenney J 1981 Lipoproteinlipase activity in surgical patients: effects of trauma and sepsis. Surgery 90: 401–405

Saito H, Trocki O, Alexander J 1985 Comparison of immediate postburn enteral *vs* parenteral nutrition. ASPEN Clinical Congress

Shoemaker W 1985 Hemodynamic and oxygen transport patterns in septic shock: physiologic mechanisms and therapeutic implications. (In) *Prospectives in Sepsis and Septic Shock*, Sibbald W, Sprung C (ed), SCCM, Fullerton Ca

Tilney N, Bailey G, Morgan A 1973 Sequential system failure after rupture of abdominal aortic aneurysms. Annals of Surgery 118: 117–122

Watters J, Bessey P, Wilmore D 1984 Catabolic hormones suppress adaptation to starvation. Surgical Forum 35: 82–85

West M A, Keller G, Hyland B, Cerra F, Simmons R 1985 Hepatocyte function in sepsis: Kupffer cells mediate a biphasic protein synthesis response in hepatocytes after endotoxin and killed *E. coli*. Surgery 98: 388–395

Wiles J B, Cerra F B, Siegel J H, Border J R 1980 The systemic septic response: does the organism matter? Critical Care Medicine 8: 55–60

Wilmore D W, Orlick L 1980 Systemic responses to injury and the healing wound. JPEN 4: 147

9. The control of Gram-negative bacterial infection in the ICU

D. Reis Miranda   Dieter Langrehr

INTRODUCTION

It is estimated that hospital acquired infections (HAI) affect 5% of inpatients (Allen et al, 1981; Bennet, 1978; Brachman et al, 1980; Eickhoff et al, 1969; Haley et al, 1981; Haley et al, 1985; Meers et al, 1981; Thoburn et al, 1968). As pointed out by Brachman et al (1980) the incidence of HAI may vary according to the category of hospital studied. Quoting the National Nosocomial Infection Study (NNIS) municipal hospitals have the highest incidence (7%) and community hospitals the lowest (4.3%), suggesting that organisational and functional factors other than illness and treatment may also be of significance in the incidence of HAI. However, the accuracy of the observed incidence is dependent on the effectiveness of the surveillance programes. Eickhoff et al (1969) in a pilot study conducted in six community hospitals estimated that the surveillance programs for determining HAI had an effectiveness of only 40%.

Hospital acquired infection, also known as nosocomial infection, is an infection presenting for the first time more than 48 hrs after admission. This definition separates HAI from infections outside the acquired hospital environment (Community Acquired Infections).

The study of HAI is frequently based upon epidemic outbreaks. The impact of epidemic outbreaks upon hospital policies makes it likely that these are completely studied and evaluated, in contrast with most of the endemic infections. However, the conclusions that can be drawn from epidemic studies are often not of much help in elucidating the mechanism of HAI. In order to characterise hospital-based epidemics Stamm et al (1981) studied 265 consecutive outbreaks occurring between 1956 and 1979. The frequency of pathogenic micro-organisms involved was *Staph. aureus* 19%, *Klebsiella* sp. 14%, *Salmonella* 13%, *Hepatitis B virus* 8%, *E. coli* 5%, *Pseudomonas* sp 4% and Group A *Streptococcus* 4%. The sites of infection were—wounds and skin 29%, gastrointestinal 21%, blood 12%, respiratory tract 11%, liver 10%, urinary tract 7%, meninges 5%, other 5%.

Allen et al (1981), referring to the NNIS covering each year about 1.16 million admissions to US hospitals, gave the frequency of pathogenic microorganisms involved in HAI as follows: *E. coli* 19%, *Staph. aureus*, *D streptococcus* and *Pseudomonas* 9% to 10% each, *Klebsiella pneumonia* and *Proteus* 8%, *Anaerobes* 3.6%. Quoting the same study Brachman et al (1980) gave the following frequency of infected sites in HAI: urinary tract 39%, wounds and skin 32%, respiratory tract 16%, blood 4%, other 5%. These figures are not different from those reported by Eickhoff et al (1969).

Studying the incidence of HAI in the different hospital departments Brachman

(1980) reported 4–6% in surgical wards, 2–6% in obstetric units, and 2–4% in medical wards. Haley et al (1981) studying 169 526 patients admitted to 338 hospitals noted an infection rate of 5.23% and an incidence of 1.3 episodes of infection per patient. 71% of all nosocomial infections occurred in the 42% of admissions who underwent surgical procedures. In view of the fact that 40–65% of all hospital admissions occur in surgical departments (Altemeier et al, 1975) the importance that these wards have in influencing infection control policies is easy to understand. The estimated overall mortality in relation to HAI is 7.4% (Bennett, 1978).

The ICU is generally accepted to be the hospital facility with the highest incidence of HAI. The overall infection rate is reported to lie between 12% and 25% depending upon the type of the unit and the severity of illness amongst the patients admitted (Altemeier et al, 1975; Daschner et al, 1982). The rates of infection increase sharply with the duration of stay in the unit. French & Homi (1979), Northey et al (1974), Stoutenbeek et al (1983) and Thorp et al (1979) have shown infection rates above 50% after the fifth day and above 90% after the tenth day in the ICU.

Depending on several factors to be discussed later, the frequency of infected sites in ICU patients is rather different from that observed in other hospital locations. Thorp et al (1979) report the following frequency: respiratory tract 89%, urinary tract 20%, intra-abdominal 15%, wounds 13% and blood 9%. The incidence observed in this study is similar to that referred by others (Casewell & Philips, 1978a; Daschner et al, 1981; Stoutenbeek et al, 1983).

The mortality rate in relation to infection is very high in the ICU. Depending on several factors such as age, duration of hospitalisation, previous nosocomial or community acquired infection, underlying disease, iatrogenic factors, etc, and on the source of infection, mortality rate varies from 20% up to 100% (Bryan & Reynolds, 1984; Fischer & Polk, 1975; La Force, 1981; Milligan et al, 1978; Molnar & Burke, 1983; Thorp et al, 1979; Watt & Ledingham, 1984). Multiorgan failure is the commonest cause of ICU mortality, almost invariably includes one or more sources of infection and the whole process often starts with a HAI (Clarke, 1985; Meakins et al, 1980; Rapin & George, 1983; Watt & Ledingham, 1984; Zimmerman, 1971).

The observed tendency towards a predominance of Gram-negative bacteria (GNB) in HAI is most obvious in the ICU environment. Between 50% and 80% of ICU infections are caused by GNB (Brachman, 1980; Krieger et al, 1983; Sanford & Pierce, 1979; Stoddart, 1983; Stoutenbeek et al, 1983; Thorp et al, 1979; Watt & Ledingham, 1984). Gram-positive infection is not only less frequent (20% to 40%) but also appears less lethal. The increasing role that GNB play in ICU infection contrasts with their lesser occurrence in community acquired infection. This might not be valid for every site of infection. Mulholland & Bruun (1973) reported a similar incidence of GNB in HAI and community acquired infections of the urinary tract. Petras & Bognar (1981) suggest that the increasing incidence of GNB in HAI was also noted in infections arising outside the hospital.

HAI is a major priority in hospital health care not only because of the associated increase in morbidity and mortality but also because of the increasing costs involved in infection prevention programs. The total annual cost of HAI in the USA was estimated at $1222 million in 1976, or $600 average direct cost per case (Bennett, 1978). This average has a very large standard deviation. Examples of extra cost of hospitalisation relating to HAI are $560 for urinary tract infection (Givens & Wenzel,

1980), $1100 for wound infection (Bennett, 1978) or $4400 for bacteremia (Maki, 1981). An important part of these extra costs corresponds to an average of 3.6 extra days of hospitalisation per case (Haley et al, 1985). In the ICU, because of the severity of infection and consequently longer hospitalisation, these costs can be much higher. Green et al (1982) in a prospective study of HAI in surgical and orthopedic departments concluded that urinary tract infection produced 4.5 extra hospitalisation days, wound infection 11.9 days and both infections together 25 days.

It is understandable why investment in infection prevention programs is substantial. In 1976 the USA spent $216 million in programs to prevent HAI (Bennett, 1978). The effectiveness of these programs in lowering morbidity and mortality did not exceed 25%. And as Bennett noted, the effectiveness of these programs is certainly very low when compared with the effectiveness achieved by other prevention programs, such as for prevention of botulism (95% effective).

The most important reason for the low effectiveness and low rentability per diem expended might be the fact that prevention programs essentially are not directed to the object of prevention (the patient) but to his environment. As we will discuss below, the failure of preventative methods aimed directly at the patient (antibiotics, etc.) led, not surprisingly, to the increased use of indirect methods—isolation of patients, treatment of his environment, isolation of attendants and visitors, etc. and, not least, to major concern about invasive monitoring and therapy.

PATHOGENESIS

The normal flora
Microbial flora exist normally in healthy humans. Table 9.1 shows the predominant microflora as presented by several authors (Bartlett et al, 1977; Finegold et al, 1983; Hill et al, 1985; Mackowiak, 1982; Noble, 1983; Van Saene, 1983). From this table some comments deserve to be made:

1. The digestive tract (DT) is a heavily colonised organ, especially near its orifices—oropharynx and large intestine.
2. Anaerobic micro-organisms are overwhelmingly represented (98%).
3. Amongst those organs in continuity with the outside environment (other than the DT) the lungs are sterile as is the genito-urinary system with the exception of the vagina, which is normally colonised with anaerobic flora and facultative anaerobes.
4. Other than E. coli all other GNB are absent under normal circumstances.

Microbial colonisation begins immediately after birth, depending mostly upon the flora existing in the environment. Within a few weeks colonisation of the neonate becomes qualitatively and quantitatively remarkably similar to that observed in adults (Mackowiak, 1982). Although there might be differences in the representation of microbiological species between individuals the pattern will remain almost constant for any single individual. Holdeman et al (1976) studying the fecal flora of astronauts has shown that there were only small daily variations in the flora of each of them, even when submitted to different diets or environments. In a literature review Van der Waaij (1984) advanced evidence that immunological factors select individual microflora, particularly the anaerobes.

Table 9.1 Normal flora

	Growth density per ml	Incidence (%)
Skin:		
Anaerobes	10^{1-4}	100
Aerobes (mainly Staphylococci)	10^{2-4}	100
Digestive tract:		
Oropharynx		
anaerobes	10^7	100
aerobes: Strep. viridans	10^{5-7}	100
Staph. aureus		
Strep. pneumonia	10^3	<40
Hemoph. influenza		
Gram-negative bacteria	$0-10^3$	<1
Candida albicans	10^3	<40
Stomach:		
anaerobes		
aerobes: Strep. hemolytic		
Staph. epidermidis	$<10^3$	<100*
Candida albicans		
Upper small intestine	0	0†
Lower small intestine and large bowel		
anaerobes	10^{7-11}	100
aerobes: Strep. fecalis	10^{5-7}	100
Staphylococci	10^{5-7}	<30
E. coli	10^{5-7}	100
Other enterobacteriaceae	$<10^3$	<20
Pseudomonadaceae	$<10^3$	<1
Candida albicans	10^3	<40
Vagina.		
Anaerobes	10^9	100
Aerobes (mainly Lactobacilli)	10^8	100

* These counts tend to decrease to zero after meals.
† Lactobacilli $(0-10^4)$ is frequently found.

Before a severe infection arises one or more of the following events tend to occur:

1. Overgrowth of one micro-organism, upsetting the previous equilibrium with other micro-organisms in the local flora.
2. The appearance and growth of micro-organisms normally not present in the normal flora.
3. The penetration and growth of microorganisms into sites normally sterile.

Colonisation

When a potentially pathogenic microorganism (PPM), normally not present in the microflora of an individual, penetrates and grows either among the existing flora or in a normally sterile site, without signs of infections, this new situation is called colonisation. As we will see below, many microorganisms penetrate several body sites during the daily contact with the environment. However, defence mechanisms will prevent them from setting up residence at those sites; colonisation will not take place and the PPMs will not remain for more than a few hours. It is then possible to culture PPMs in occasional samples taken from a given site. Therefore, colonisation with PPMs will only be considered to occur when the same microorganism is isolated from at least two consecutive samples from that site taken over a two day interval.

In the ICU, colonisation with PPMs occurs quickly and after a few hours or days the majority of ICU patients are heavily colonised, particularly in the DT (French & Homi, 1979; La Force, 1977; Mackowiak, 1982; Northey et al, 1974; Stoddart, 1983; Watt & Ledingham, 1984). The individual rapidly loses his capacity to resist colonisation. Sanford (1974) described it as a loss of colonisation immunity. Johanson et al (1972) related the colonisation of the oropharynx with GNB to the general state of health of patients.

Du Moulin et al (1982) established a sequence of transmission of pneumonia due to GNB in 17 of 60 consecutive ICU admissions treated with antacids. The microorganisms responsible for the clinical picture previously had been isolated from the oropharynx and the stomach of these patients. Rosendorf et al (1974) observed after open heart surgery that most patients became colonised with GNB and that the source of colonisation was other heavily colonised, and often infected, long-stay patients. Stoddart (1983) also demonstrated the importance of colonisation and emphasised that the patient is almost invariably the source of his own infection. The microbiologic equilibrium between the individual and his environment is such that colonisation with PPMs normally does not occur in healthy humans; however, in patients it may occur and commonly precedes infection.

Risk factors

In Table 9.2 are listed the commonly accepted risk factors contributing to colonisation/infection with PPMs. The majority are only relevant when associated with other factors. This is certainly true in the case of the environmental factors. With some differences in the relative percent of PPMs, contamination of the environment is not different inside and outside the hospital (Miranda et al, 1983). However, many studies dealing with infection prevention, point to the environment (food, people and equipment) as forming an important source of infection in the critically ill patient. In fact, the environment, by itself, may be the risk factor of least importance if other factors are not present. The second most frequently incriminated group of risk factors is invasive monitoring and therapy. However, too much emphasis is sometimes placed upon these risk factors, which may lead to delayed institution of appropriate monitoring or therapy. The emergence of exacerbation of some of the other listed risk factors is the obvious consequence of such policies.

Concerning ICU patients we consider organ failure and metabolic state as the two most important groups of risk factors contributing to colonisation/infection with PPMs. After all, these are the common reasons for ICU treatment. Wagner (1985) studying the productivity of several ICUs in the USA concluded that aggressive initial therapy aimed at achieving physiologic homeostasis was one of the most important single variables influencing outcome. Without neglecting any of the listed factors we stress that adequate and timely support of threatened or already disturbed organ or system function is more effective in preventing infection than restrictive measures concerning the environment and the clinical management of critically ill patients.

Source of infection. Endogenous vs Exogenous

The classification of infection as 'endogenous' and 'exogenous' is usually utilised to attribute the influence of the environment on infection rate: the term 'endogenous' is used when an infection is caused by PPMs existing in the host's flora and 'exogenous'

Table 9.2   Risk factors contributing to colonisation/infection

---

 I Organ failure:
   Digestive tract (1)
   Respiratory (2)
   Cardiovascular (3)
   Renal (4)
 II Metabolic state:
   Catabolism (anergy, urea, etc.) (5)
   Surgery/trauma (6)
   Anaesthesia (7)
   Acidosis (8)
   Stress (9)
 III Medication:
   Antibiotics (10)
   Corticosteroids (11)
   Immunosuppression (12)
   Antacids (13)
 IV Invasive therapy and monitoring:
   Endotracheal intubation (14)
   Indwelling urinary catheter (15)
   Intravascular catheters (16)
 V Environment:
   Food/beverages (17)
   Equipment (18)
   Other people (19)

References: (1) Buisson & Meakins 1983, Hilman et al 1982. (2) Knighton et al 1984, Altlan 1982. (3) Gould et al 1985. (4) Goldstein & Green 1966, Miller 1984. (5) Meakins et al 1980, Damas 1983, Pietsch & Meakins 1979. (6) Hooton et al 1981, Morris & Bullock 1919, Krivit et al 1979, Saba 1975, Glover & Jolly 1971. (7) Johanson & Sanford 1968, Scott 1982. (8) Goldstein et al 1970. (9) Hodlam et al 1976, Jemmott et al 1983. (10) Slack 1983, Price & Ghonheim 1978, van Saene et al 1983. (11 and 12) Freeman & McGowan 1978. (13) Du Moulin et al 1982. (14) Freeman & McGowan 1978, Boysen et al 1979, French & Homi 1979. (15) Hooton et al 1981, Kunin 1982. (16) Meakins et al 1980. (17) Stoddart 1983, Casewell & Phillips 1978, Mackowiak 1982. (18) Cross & Roup 1981, Stoddart 1983. (19) Smith et al 1984, Freeman & Gowan 1978, Holzman & Scott 1981, Casewell & Phillips 1977, Bixton et al 1978, Meakins et al 1980.

when an infection is caused by PPMs existing in the environment and later observed at the site of infection. A lack of precision in these concepts makes them difficult to understand and not very useful in analysing infection prevention.

Two examples will illustrate common utilisation of these concepts:

Example 1—The clinical diagnosis of lobar pneumonia with *Strep. pneumoniae* is made in a patient. The same microorganism is found in his oropharynx. This is an endogenous infection. This patient has also a urinary tract infection caused by *Kl. pneumoniae* which was also found in his rectum. This is again by definition an endogenous infection.

Example 2—A polytrauma patient, who is intubated and ventilated, presents a severe wound infection complicating a femoral fracture. *Proteus vulgaris* is found in the wound, and the same strain is not cultured anywhere else on the patient or in the unit at that moment. This is an exogenous infection due to wound contamination (? at the scene of accident). The patient also has pneumonia caused by *Ps. aeruginosa*, and the same strain has been isolated at several other sites in the same patient (rectum, urine, etc.) and also in the sputum of another patient occupying the same room as well as on the hands of two nurses who treated the patient. This is usually defined as an exogenous infection. The source is originally the other patient, and the hands of the nurses the factor leading to cross-infection.

The pneumonia in patient 1 was almost certainly an endogenous infection. *Strep. pneumoniae* exists frequently in the microflora of the oropharynx and was known to be present in this patient. The wound infection in patient 2 was quite probably an exogenous infection. But there are no obvious reasons to consider the urinary tract infection in patient 1 endogenous and the pneumonia in patient 2 exogenous. We would prefer to consider both endogenous. In both situations the responsible PPM had the opportunity to grow in other body sites before causing the infection. It is known that ICU patients become colonised during their stay in the unit. As Meakins et al (1980) point out 'the normal flora does change in the hospital and autochthonous organisms are replaced by hospital flora, making infections caused by endogenous bacteria more difficult to treat'. The DT is frequently accepted as the 'natural habitat' of all GNB (Stoddart, 1983). Nothing is more doubtful. The danger of this misconception is that the appropriate importance will not be given to colonisation of the DT. Nonetheless, the direct correlation between colonisation and infection is today fully accepted.

As shown in Table 9.1 *E. coli* is the only GNB usually found in the normal host's flora. All the others are absent or seldom cultured. This is the normal situation and efficient infection prevention should aim at avoiding abnormal colonisation.

We classified the endogenous infections in two groups (Stoutenbeek et al, 1984):

1. Primary endogenous infections caused by PPMs present in the normal residential flora (Table 9.1).
2. Secondary endogenous infections caused by acquired PPMs that have previously colonised the DT.

Exogenous infections are those caused by PPMs which did not colonise the patient previously. The advantage of this modified classification is that it transfers efforts aimed at prevention of infection from manipulating the environment to developing techniques which will prevent colonisation of the DT. Using the proposed classification, Stoutenbeek et al (1984) have shown that in a group of 48 polytrauma and infected patients 86% of the isolated PPMs were of endogenous origin (70% of which were secondary endogenous). In this study it was also demonstrated, in a comparable group of patients, that infection rate was drastically reduced if colonisation of the DT was prevented.

Defence mechanisms

In the pathogenesis of an endogenous infection three steps are distinguished:

1. Colonisation of the skin, DT and or vagina with PPMs. Considering only infections caused by aerobic GNB, the digestive tract is the most important site of colonisation. Once the new bacteria achieve colonisation they will tend to increase progressively in concentration at the colonised site. A new dynamic equilibrium will be established between the physiologic mechanisms of the host against bacterial colonisation, the normal microflora of the colonised site, and the newly introduced PPMs. When the new equilibrium favours the host the invader will be eliminated or its increase kept under control. This explains why

it is possible to find abnormal GNB colonisation of the DT without any evidence of associated illness. However, apart from the risk that it represents to the host, this new situation adds the host to the pool of colonised patients, which is the most significant reservoir of GNB in the ICU.

2. When the new equilibrium favours the invader, the latter will extend out of the colonised site and colonise major organ systems (respiratory tract, urinary tract, blood) and wounds. At this stage of bacterial invasion a compromise between host and invader may be reached in a number of ways without serious prejudice to the host. The host has then to mobilise his defence capacity and thereby eliminate the invader.

3. When the above mechanisms fail and elimination is unsuccessful, infection will occur.

Local Host defence

Table 9.3 presents the commonly accepted factors contributing to local host defence (Buisson & Meakins, 1983; Freter, 1974; La Force & Eickhoff, 1977; Meakins et al, 1980). It is important to note that all these factors are able to exert their effect upon the bacterial content of body cavities (except the skin). Another aspect of great relevance is the importance of motility in evacuating local contents, and the undirectional character of these mechanisms. In the critically ill patient motility is often impaired or absent, facilitating not only local bacterial growth but also its multidirectional extension. Especially in surgical patients the impaired motility is frequently associated with alterations of the normal anatomy with two other important consequences: neutralisation and/or diversion of relevant resistance factors (gastric content, bile, etc.); creation of recesses or blind loops which increase local stasis (duodenal stump, choledocostomy, colostomy, etc.).

Table 9.3   Local host resistance

Site*	Mechanical/chemical	Immunologic
Skin	pH, fatty acids	IgA = Prevents adherence of bacteria
Oropharynx	Chewing, swallowing	= Activates complement cascade
Stomach	Peristalsis, pH	= Bactericidal activity in presence of lysozyme
Upper small intestine	Peristalsis, pH, bile salts	
Lower small intestine and large bowel	Peristalsis, defecation	IgG, IgM = Direct bactericidal effect after passing to the surface of the mucosa
Vagina	pH, menses	
Respiratory tract	Mucous barrier, mucociliary action, coughing	Macrophage mucosal defence network
Urinary tract	Voiding, dilution, pH, osmolarity	

* Common to all sites is integrity of mechanical barriers, cell desquamation, presence of a mucopolysaccharidase (lysozyme) except in the urine, presence of mucin except in the skin.

Integrity of natural mechanical barriers is violated by almost all ICU techniques which involve monitoring and/or artificial support of physiological functions. Particularly threatened by these techniques are the respiratory tract, the urinary tract, the skin and finally the blood. It is of interest that the organs responsible for colonisation, and in particular the DT, are not involved in the undesirable side effects of these life-saving techniques. This suggests that if the patient had a normally functioning digestive tract, i.e. without abnormal colonisation with GNB, secondary endogenous infection with GNB would be impossible even if the integrity of the natural mechanical barriers were violated. The efficacy of local host defences will not only be dependent on the competence of the defence mechanisms, but also on the colonisation pressure exerted by the environment. A more heavily contaminated environment (food, equipment, attendants and other patients) will represent an increased challenge to the local host defences. A more heavily colonised patient will increase the potential environment contamination.

Systemic host defence
When bacterial invasion reaches the third step (infection) systemic defence mechanisms become actively involved in the process. These mechanisms are cell-mediated (T-lymphocyte), humoral (B-lymphocyte) and phagocytic (granulocyte and monocyte macrophages). This topic will not be discussed in detail; the interested reader is referred to the work of Buisson & Meakins (1983) and Roitt (1977).

Different forms of stress (malnutrition, catabolism, shock, hypoxia, etc.) will depress these mechanisms. Extensive colonisation with GNB even without infection, and transient subclinical endotoxemia will tend to exhaust these mechanisms. In such circumstances, systemic resistance is compromised and the host is prone to severe infections should local host resistance for any reason be overcome by bacterial invasion. One study of Meakins et al (1980) illustrates the importance of systemic host defence. In 115 ICU patients after operation or trauma, skin testing with five recall antigens was performed in order to assess responsiveness by cell-mediated immunity. The response of each patient was correlated with outcome. 96 patients (83.5%) presented complete or relative anergy, and 19 (16.5%) had a normal response. In the first group, 59 (61.5%) became septic and 30 (31.3%) died whereas in the second group with normal response to skin testing, 5 (26.3%) became septic and 1 (5.3%) died.

THERAPEUTIC APPROACHES

Systemic Antibiotics. 40 years experience
In the last two decades much effort has been invested in the development of new protocols for the administration of antibiotic drugs aimed at prophylaxis of HAI.

Shapiro et al (1979) studied the use of prophylactic antibiotics (PAB), reviewing 5288 clinical records from twenty general hospitals in Pennsylvania. 10% of all admissions (surgical and medical) received PAB. Total PAB amounted to one third of all antibiotics used during the study period. Surgical patients received 60% of the total of antibiotic drugs, half of which were given as PAB. The majority of PAB (80%) were given for periods exceeding 48 hours. The drugs most frequently used were in the following order of preference—cephalosporins, benzylpenicillins, ampicillins and tetracyclines. There was no obvious correlation between duration of prophylaxis and duration of hospitalisation.

Crossly & Gardner (1981) reviewed the use of PAB in 1021 records of surgical patients admitted to 27 different hospitals. Patients undergoing 'clean surgery' received more than 50% of total antibiotics. The mean duration of PAB exceeded 72 hours (3.4 days) and cephalosporins accounted for more than 50% of all administered antibiotics.

The clinical experience with PAB is not satisfactory. Not only does the infection rate remain high, but the remaining infections are more difficult to treat. Goodman et al (1968), studying prospectively 72 patients undergoing cardiovascular surgery and receiving PAB, observed 20 post-operative infections (28%). The infection rate was not different amongst patients receiving penicillin and streptomycin or oxacillin as compared with the placebo group. It was observed that the infection rate in operations involving bypass was high (17/41) as compared with the infection rate in those operations where bypass was not utilised (3/31). The reduction in host defence caused by the extracorporeal circulation was suggested as a major factor to explain hese observations.

Peterdorf et al (1957) studied the effect of PAB in 72 coma patients. They utilised penicillin and streptomycin, tetracycline, or sulphomanide and nitrofurantoin. 30 patients did not receive PAB. 45% of treated patients had pneumonia in comparison with only 15% of the control group. Seven patients in the treated group had skin infections with *Staph. aureus*, and a further two died with sepsis caused by GNB. No such complications were observed in the control group.

The administration of PAB leads normally to a change in the individual normal flora as again recently demonstrated by Bennett et al (1982). They compared 14 neonates who received ampicillin and gentamicin systemically with 8 comparable neonates who received no antibiotics. After two weeks of age, the control group showed abundant fecal flora growth of aerobes and anaerobes. The treated group presented lower counts particularly of anaerobic bacteria (10/16 cultures had no anaerobic flora). *E. coli* predominated in the fecal flora of the untreated group, whereas *Klebsiella pneumonia* was dominant in the treated group.

The utilisation of systemic antibiotics not only does not achieve the expected reduction in infection rate, but also involves the large-scale use of antimicrobial drugs which is responsible for the emergence of bacterial strains resistant to the antibiotics utilised and for the emergence of superinfections often caused by multi resistant bacteria (Levy, 1982).

The local application of PAB may also have undesirable results as demonstrated by Feeley et al (1975) who instilled polymyxin B in the upper airways of a group of 292 patients, aiming to prevent pneumonia with *Ps. aeruginosa*. They observed an unusual pneumonia rate by polymyxin-resistant organisms, and an unexpectedly high mortality rate.

The unsuccessful outcome of PAB has caused many authors, including Fry et al (1981), to reevaluate and restrict their use in clinical practice.

Alternative modes of therapy to antibiotics, such as the administration of J5 serum as proposed by Ziegler et al (1979, 1982), may be promising as therapeutic adjuvants but have not yet been shown to meet clinical needs. Utilising antiserum from 103 patients with proven GNB sepsis the American group observed a mortality of 23% as compared with 39% in 109 untreated, comparable patients. Glinz et al (1985) in a prospective, randomised and double-blind study in 150 patients comparing the prophylactic effects of immunoglobulins administered intravenously, observed a 37% incidence of pneumonia in the treated group as compared with 58% in the placebo group. In this study the administration of immunoglobulins did not change significantly the occurrence of sepsis and/or other infections; mortality was similar in both groups.

The role of the digestive tract
As described above the DT plays a prominent role in the emergence of infection. The predilection of the DT for this role derives from its functional characteristics—it is in direct contact with the environment, contains nutritional material in the process of decomposition, and its milieu is warm and moist. Eickhoff (1979) reviewed the sources of nosocomial respiratory tract infections and considered the DT as a probable reservoir. The same conclusion was drawn by Schimpff (1979) when reviewing infection in immunocompromised hosts. Montgomerie (1979) has demonstrated the importance of the DT in the 'acquisition–colonisation' mechanism before an individual becomes a reservoir of *Klebsiella* sp. Stoutenbeek et al (1984), studying 122 polytrauma ICU patients, identified 105 infections, isolating 187 PPMs. 84% of these had been isolated from the DT before being identified at the site where infection occurred. Accepting this role of the DT in the pathogenesis of infection we will now discuss possible defence mechanisms responsible for the maintenance of the microflora of the DT within normal patterns.

The concept of colonisation resistance
The normal microflora are usually not responsible for host infections (see Table 9.1). When foreign bacteria invade the DT, such as in food or beverage, elimination is usually effected within 24 hours (Van der Waaij, 1984). This means that such bacteria will be only transiently isolated from the feces of the host (Van Saene et al, 1983b). The persistence of the invading microorganism in the DT depends upon its concentration (number of microorganisms per ingested ml) and the state of health of the host. Van der Waaij & Berghuis (1974) contaminated mice orally with *E. coli* and observed a direct correlation between dose and fecal concentration. When *E. coli* were given in a dose of 10^9–10^{11} the organism would be found in feces the following day in a concentration of about 10^6/g and would still be present after 14 days in a concentration of 10^3/g feces. When the consumption dose was reduced to 10^5–10^7 the concentration in feces would be 10^2/g after one day and only 10^1/g on the 14th day. Reducing the administered does to 10^3 resulted in a concentration of 10^1 in feces the next day and elimination by the 4th day. This experiment showed that administered doses of above 10^7 are likely to become established in, i.e. to colonise, the DT.

The higher the number of ingested *Enterobactereaceae* and the higher the concentration in the DT, the greater the probability of infection and death caused by the contaminant strain in immunocompromised mice. These were the observations of Van der Waaij et al (1978) after contaminating total body irradiated mice with increasing doses of *Enterobacteraeceae* and examining the concentration of these in feces, regional lymph nodes, spleen and blood.

In summary, these studies demonstrate that

1. The normally functioning DT is usually capable of eliminating invading GNB when the colonisation pressure is not high.
2. If elimination does not succeed and colonisation occurs, the colonising bacteria will tend to damage and/or impair the mucosal barrier and invade other organ systems.

Colonisation Resistance (CR) to foreign bacteria was defined by Van der Waaij et al (1978) as the logarithm of an oral dose of the given strain that colonised the DT

in 50% of the animals for more than two weeks. They determined that the CR for
E. coli was 7 and above 9 for *Klebsiella* sp. and *Pseudomonas*. This difference in
CR may explain why *E. coli* is found in almost 100% of healthy humans.

The anaerobic flora have been shown to have an intimate involvement with the
process of colonisation of the DT. Van der Waaij et al (1971) observed a sudden
increase in colonisation and translocation (invasion) by resistant *Enterobactereaceae*
in mice in which the intestinal flora were previously and totally eliminated by the
oral administration of streptomycin and neomycin. Using the intestinal flora from
a second group of mice whose intestinal flora consisted exclusively of anaerobic bacteria, the Groningen group contaminated this decontaminated group of mice. The
invading *Enterobactereaceae* were eliminated, and it was concluded that the anaerobic
bacteria played a decisive role in avoiding colonisation. In another study Van der
Waaij et al (1977) showed that human anaerobes increased the capacity to resist colonisation, from nil to almost normal, when given to germ-free mice. The importance
of the anaerobic flora was again suggested in studies with mice giving antibiotics
known to eliminate these flora. Van der Waaij et al (1972) administered ampicillin
or streptomycin to a group of mice and compared the effects of oral (resistant) bacterial
contamination with another group of mice not receiving antibiotics. The antibiotic
treated group showed more heavy and prolonged fecal colonisation, while the spread
of the contaminant organisms into regional lymph nodes and spleen was much more
frequent and extensive in this group.

In an extensive review Van der Waaij (1979) reinforced the suggested role of anaerobic flora in the defence processes of the DT (Colonisation Resistance). The anaerobes,
that are present in much higher number than the aerobes, have four main functions:

1. They surround the aerobes, reducing or impairing their growth.
2. They adhere to and line the mucosa, impairing the adherence of aerobes.
3. They produce bacteriocins and stimulate the secretion of mucin.
4. They stimulate bowel peristalsis.

The presence of anaerobes is thus indispensable to reducing the danger resulting
from aerobic flora.

For Guiot (1982) an important factor in this bacterial antagonism is competition
for substrate under anaerobic conditions such as those observed in the large intestines.
Abrams & Bishop (1966) stated that the mucosa is not directly protected by the
anaerobic flora, but indirectly by their effect upon peristalsis and intestinal emptying.
Other factors contributing to CR are presented in Table 9.3. Concerning the immunological factors it is important to note that IgA covers the majority of GNB in the
intestines but not the anaerobic flora (Bacteroides sp or fusiform bacteria) (Van der
Waaij et al, 1985). The importance of the immunoregulation of the intestinal flora
is extensively discussed by Van der Waaij (1985, 1986).

As Schimpff (1980) states 'the concept of CR may be the new approach needed
for microbial suppression of the non-isolated patient. If the anaerobic flora is undis-
turbed, newly acquired organisms generally cannot colonise the patient'. Accepting
the concept of CR we understand why so often the administration of antibiotics is
associated with the emergence of GNB in the treated host, often leading to severe
infection. This situation is well known in both hospitalised patients (Pollack et al,
1972; Price & Ghonheim, 1981; Rose & Babcok, 1975; Slack, 1983) and in patients

outside hospital (Van Saene et al, 1983a). Yoshioka et al (1982) observed the same phenomenon in children. The emergence of GNB in the oropharynx of children was seen after administration of 50 mg/kg of ampicillin, less extensively after the administration of a similar dose of cephaloxin, and absent after parenteral aminoglycosides. As GNB do not occur in the oropharynx of children under normal conditions, the authors concluded 'Antibiotics should therefore be used with the greatest caution in patients with impaired defence mechanisms'.

Selective decontamination of the digestive tract

In the prevention of infection caused by GNB the following aspects should be considered in clinical management:

1. GNB usually colonise the DT before causing infection in any other organ or system.
2. Anaerobic flora seem to play an important role in maintaining the DT free of GNB.
3. The immunocompromised patient (such as the majority of ICU patients) has impaired, or at least depressed, defence mechanisms.

Selective decontamination of the digestive tract (SDD) is a new technique of infection control aimed at the elimination of all aerobic Gram-negative bacteria and yeasts from the DT, without interference with the indigenous anaerobic flora. This technique is based upon the concept of CR, eliminating the GNB from the DT and helping the depressed defence mechanisms to keep the DT free from these PPMs. To achieve SDD in clinical practice three golden principles should be respected:

1. Antimicrobial agents given systemically should not reach the DT in low concentrations which would stimulate bacterial resistance, and should not interfere with the anaerobic flora in the DT. When choosing an antibiotic to control infection in a given organ, preference should be given to that which attains a higher concentration in the infected organ. However, it is often not realised that the same antibiotic may reach other places in the body in a lower concentration where bacteria also grow. The DT may be reached by antibiotics in several ways, e.g. excreted in the saliva, by the liver or in the intestinal mucus. The administration of such agents will invariably increase the risk of colonisation of the DT by resistant bacteria, and/or yeasts and superinfection, if the local defence mechanisms are not competent or not supported by selective decontamination. In the situation where a patient receiving SDD is given additionally antibiotics which may eliminate the anaerobic flora, such as most (broad-spectrum) penicillins, the therapeutic combination could lead to the state of total decontamination or sterilisation of the DT. This situation, although not always avoidable, places the host in the highest risk of acquisition of resistant microorganisms, requiring strict, expensive and often unsuccessful isolation conditions. In Table 9.4 we present a list of known antimicrobial agents and their proven or suspected effect upon CR in mice with a susceptible intestinal flora. On the one hand, this list aims more to be a reminder of the need for such considerations in the treatment of the critically ill patient than to represent an already proven and comprehensive classification. On the other hand, it is

Table 9.4   Antimicrobial agents and their effect upon CR

Group	Indifferent	Decreasing
Penicillins	Mecillinam (i.v.)	All others
Cephalosporins	Cefaclor	All others
	Cefradine	
	Cefotaxim	
	Ceftazidim	
Aminoglycosides	Tobramycin	All others
Chloranphenicol and tetracyclins	Doxycycline (i.v.)	All others
Erythromycin	—	All
Quinolones	all	—
Anti fungal	all	—
Anti anaerobes	Metronidazole (i.v.)	All others
Polymyxins	all (oral)	—
Miscellaneous	Cotrimoxazole	—
	Vancomycin (i.v.)	—
	Aztreonam	—

exclusively based on normally recommended doses (Van der Waaij, 1984, 1979; Wiegersma et al, 1981).

2. Antimicrobial agents given orally and aimed at producing a systemic effect should be absorbed completely when passing through the small intestine, otherwise low concentrations will reach the large bowel with the same consequences as previously mentioned. The oral administration of antibiotics is generally not indicated in ICU patients. We mention it here because this is the preferred route of administration in other immunocompromised patients (leukemic, etc.) and is indicated in several reports detailing the efficacy of SDD regimens.

3. The DT is rendered free of GNB by means of local application of high concentration of narrow spectrum antimicrobial agents which will not affect the protective (Gram-positive) organisms and will not be absorbed by the DT, thus avoiding toxic side effects and ensuring that no effective concentrations reach other organs or systems which might facilitate the emergence of resistant mutants. In SDD the most frequently utilised antibiotics are polymyxins, (low doses of) tobramycin and lately aztreonam all aimed at the elimination of GNB, with amphothericin B providing antifungal cover. The SDD regimen is normally composed of two antibiotics complementing each other against GNB and one against yeasts. The combination and respective doses vary greatly from centre to centre.

High doses are apparently needed because the drugs bind to food and fecal materials, and the drug-free concentration found in feces is dose dependent (Hazenberg et al, 1983; Van Saene et al, 1985; Veringa & Van der Waaij, 1984). In the light of the spectrum of results presented by the three research groups studying the same compounds the capacity of binding to feces is extremely variable from drug to drug, and apparently from person to person. From these studies it is also not possible to conclude whether binding capacity corresponds to drug inactivation or, on the contrary, to preferential maintenance of antibiotic concentration in feces.

An interesting study, by Mulder et al (1984), measuring beta-aspartylglycine in the stool as an indicator of anaerobic flora activity, showed that volunteers receiving more than 300 mg tobramycin orally per day had an increased excretion of that dipetide.

However, healthy volunteers will achieve lower fecal concentrations following equal doses of a given antibiotic when compared with the majority of ICU patients with adynamic ileus and often distended intestines. SDD has for some years been used in immunocompromised oncology patients, with very good results (Schimpff, 1980; Guiot et al, 1983; Sleijfer et al, 1980). This technique was introduced into our institute in 1980 and adapted to meet the requirements of ICU patients.

Place of SDD in ICU infection control policy

Ventilatory support, hemodynamic support, infection control, metabolic and nutritional support, and neurologic support are the main concerns in any ICU, together with a sound budget and organisational structure. Infection control must be approached within this context in the knowledge that good management of all aspects is indispensable to the achievement of successful infection control. The general infection control in our ICU is as follows:

SELECTIVE DECONTAMINATION OF THE DIGESTIVE TRACT

SDD is preferably a prophylactic measure applied to all patients who are expected to remain longer than 4 days in the unit. Having established the indication for SDD, the regimen is applied daily during ICU stay (Table 9.5). This regimen includes two important features:

1. It covers the most important aerobic gram-negative bacteria (tobramycin in low doses is given to complement polymyxin and to cover Proteus spp) without interfering with the anaerobic flora, and utilising only non-absorbable antimicrobial agents.
2. The oropharynx is considered an important component of the DT (see Table 9.1). It is known that the oropharynx is one of the first sites of GNB colonisation in the critically ill patient (Johanson et al, 1972). Not only is this a major source of pneumonia (Stoutenbeek et al, 1986) but also the existence of GNB in the oropharynx facilitates the emergence of resistant mutants since many antibiotics are secreted in the saliva, often in sub-inhibitory concentrations.

Table 9.5   SDD regimen in the ICU

Oral application:			
Polymyxin E	2% of each in sodium carboxyl methyl cellulose		
Tobramycin	(Orobase[R]), applied locally 4 times a day.		
Amphotericin B			

Gastrointestinal application:		Adult	Children*	
			12–4 years	<4 years
Polymyxin E	4x	100 mg	50 mg	25 mg
Tobramycin	4x	80 mg	40 mg	10 mg
Amphotericin B	4x	500 mg	250 mg	100 mg

* Dose is related to DT volume and not to weight.

To establish an adequate suppressive SDD-antibiotic concentration in the oropharynx a paste with appropriate antibiotics is used. The paste we utilise, (Orobase[R]) containing 2% of each antibiotic, is applied with a gloved finger between the gums and the cheek. It adheres very well to the mucosa and delivers the antibiotics slowly to the saliva. The taste of the compound is unpleasant and this might be the major reason why the technique is less popular among non-ICU patients.

For the intestines the gastrointestinal application is given as a 10 ml antibiotic mixture through the gastric tube (or orally) 4 times daily. When nasogastric suction is being used it is discontinued for half-hour after each administration.

Although we have never observed detectable serum levels of these SDD agents when given as indicated, Rohrbaugh et al (1984) described absorption of oral aminoglycosides following bone marrow transplantation in four cases with severe mucosal inflammation.

In the absence of gastric emptying and of normal bowel peristalsis the SDD delivered to the stomach will—with difficulty—reach the large bowel. Decontamination of the stomach prevents extension of colonisation from the bowel to the upper part of the DT. When considered desirable, (persistent ileus, heavy colonisation of the large bowel, etc.) enemas are given to decontaminate the lower part of the DT. Two to three times daily half the SDD dose is administered in 100 to 200 ml saline retention enema. When surgical procedures have resulted in the creation of blind loops, fistulae etc., (duodenal stump, colostomy, choledostomy, etc.) a variable amount of SDD mixture may, where possible, be administered into those areas, e.g. half the total dose via the gastric tube and the remainder via an ileostomy.

DECONTAMINATION OF COLONISATION SOURCES OTHER THAN DT

SDD will not suffice if other sources of colonisation are present. Continuous surveillance of colonisation in possible body sites other than the DT is necessary and its elimination, when found, is mandatory. The compound utilised for decontamination or sterilisation of these alternative sites depends on the site in question and on the PPMs requiring elimination. We utilise the SDD mixture and sometimes 'oral SDD', for decontaminating the vagina, often a source of heavy colonisation in the ICU patient.

Some disinfectant solutions are also utilised: chlorhexidine 1% in water for wounds and colonisation of body surfaces; Acetic acid 1% when pseudomonas spp. need to be eliminated; Taurolin^R 0.5–1% when contamination occurs in body cavities such as pleura, mediastinum or peritoneum. Taurolin is a new antimicrobial compound formed by the condensation of taurinamide and formaldehyde stabilised with PVP. It is rapidly metabolised and the end-products are carbon dioxide, water and taurine (Pfirrmann, 1985). Its margin of safety is very large and it can also be administered intravenously. It is not toxic, has a marked anti-endotoxic action, does not inactivate leucocyte function (Van Saene, 1984), does not interact with fibrin and its spectrum of action covers all bacteria and fungi.

SYSTEMIC ANTIBIOTIC THERAPY

SDD is designed to cover GNB; gram-positive bacteria (GPB) are outside its scope of action. Prevention of GPB infection is obviously also important. Patients at risk are mostly those in the peroperative period, post trauma, and those subjected to invasive monitoring and therapy. Examination of Table 9.1 indicates that *Staph. aureus* and *epidermidis, Strep. viridans* and *Strep. pneumonia* together with the GNB *H. influenza* and *E. coli* are the organisms most likely to cause infection in a weakened host not colonised by other PPMs. To provide prophylactic cover against microorganisms we utilise cefotaxime i.v. in doses of 50–100 mg/kg/day, not only because of its efficacy but because of its lack of interference with the indigenous flora (Table 9.4). Cefotaxime is given until the risk of colonisation is eliminated and or until the critically ill patient subjected to invasive monitoring/therapy reaches a stable condition. This is usually the situation after 5 days treatment. Rarely has it proved necessary to use additional antibiotics active against Gram-positive organisms. In those situations when GNB infection is to be treated or prevented (severe trauma, soiled wounds, peritonitis etc.) tobramycin is added in the usual doses. Metronidazole is also administered when contamination/infection with anaerobes is suspected (soiled wounds, extensive abdominal surgery, etc.). Although systemic antibiotic therapy will of course be modified according to the bacteriological results and relevant clinical criteria, it is remarkable that in the last five years these three antimicrobial agents have been, with few exceptions, continuously the most utilised agents in our ICU.

In situations of suspected/proven pneumonia we utilise half the intravenous dose of the administered antibiotics by insufflation into the tracheobronchial tree (e.g. 4 times 500 mg cefotaxime, 4 times 40 mg tobramycin), thus increasing the tissue penetration of the agent.

MONITORING

The important difference between the bacteriological monitoring required for the SDD regimen and that traditionally performed, is that, with the new technique, monitoring infection has to occur one step before the risk and evolution of colonisation. The follow-up of every ICU patient has to be done on a regular basis, and the diagnosis of colonisation has to be quantitative in order to give information as to whether it is increasing or responding to SDD. The most relevant aspects of monitoring are described by Van Saene et al 1983. It is an important practical point that this technique represents a much smaller workload in the laboratory than that previously observed in the same unit. The reason is that more than 70% of the samples are now negative for GNB and no further work is therefore necessary (Van Saene et al, 1983). One technician is able to cope with the regular workload of 10 ICU beds.

In the last 5 years we have treated about 2000 patients with the SDD regimen. From this experience the most impressive feature has been the progressive decrease in the clinically significant infection rate. For the first time we have experienced successful infection control; prevention of infection has been brought to similar level of efficacy as prevention of vital function failure.

Stoutenbeek et al (1983) compared 3 groups of polytrauma ICU patients:

1. Without prophylactic antibiotics,
2. With SDD and no systemic antibiotics,
3. With SDD and cefotaxime,

and reported an infection rate of respectively 86%, 55% and 14%.

In another study (Stoutenbeek et al, 1984) a 3 week evaluation of colonisation in the oropharynx and in the rectum was compared between one group (I) of trauma patients without prophylactic antibiotics and another group (II) with SDD regimen. In group I colonisation of the oropharynx by GPB was reduced and by GNB increased to 80% of samples, and in the rectum colonisation with GNB increased to 90%

of the samples, with a high growth density of diverse *Enterobactereaceae* and also *Pseudomonadaeceae*. In group II the incidence of colonisation of both oropharynx and rectum was below 10% of samples, with a very low growth density.

The use of the SDD regimen decreased the emergence of superinfections in our ICU from 24% to 3% as shown in another study (Stoutenbeek et al, 1984). In a group of patients not receiving SDD, 17 different systemic antibiotics were used and the patients required treatment for a mean of 18.3 days. The SDD group of patients used only 6 different antibiotics and the mean duration of treatment was 13.9 days.

A point of concern is whether SDD gives rise, with time, to the emergence of resistant mutants in the ICU. In a study of resistance pattern in 4209 isolates (from 1982 to 1984), Stoutenbeek et al (1985) observed that 4.3% of the isolates were resistant to cefotaxime, 1% to tobramycin and 2.5% to Polymyxin. Not only was the rate of resistance remarkably low but more importantly there was no tendency for resistance to increase in frequency during the study period. This may only be explained by the efficacy of the SDD regimen in eliminating the responsible bacteria from the sites where resistance could develop.

The effect of the SDD regimen upon the environment was also beneficial. Before utilisation of the technique, all accessible places (sinks, lavatories, working tables, etc.) were contaminated in almost 100% of the samples with a high growth density. After SDD was instituted, only 10% of the samples were positive, with a low growth density (Miranda et al, 1983). In other words, the equilibrium between environment and patients has been brought to a much lower 'pressure level' of bacterial contamination.

As in the case of the laboratory technical staff the increase in workload of the SDD regimen for the nursing staff has been largely compensated for by the sharp reduction in the number of heavily infected patients with all their attendant problems.

We have also examined the effect of SDD upon costs in the ICU (Miranda et al, 1983). We calculated a cost saving of about $900 000 per year as a direct consequence of the decrease in extra hospitalisation days, use of disposables, nursing manpower, medication (blood and blood products, antibiotics, cardiovascular drugs, etc.) and laboratory diagnostic examinations.

SDD is probably one of very few hospital innovations which actually reduce cost. Most other technical advances induce an increase of new products and new services.

ACKNOWLEDGEMENTS

The authors thank Professor D. Van der Waaij for his review of this manuscript.

REFERENCES

Abrams G D, Bishop J E 1966 Effects of the normal microbial flora on the resistance of the small intestine to infection. Journal of Bacteriology 92 (6); 1604–1608
Allen J R, Hightower A W, Martin S M, Dixon R E 1981 Secular trends in nosocomial infection: 1970–1979. American Journal of Medicine 70: 389–392
Altemeier W A, Burke J F, Pritt B A, Sandersky W R 1975 Manual on control of infection in surgical patients. By the committee on control of surgical infections and committee on pre- and postoperative care. JB Lippincott, Philadelphia

Bartlett J G, Onderdonk A B, Drude E, Goldstein G, Anderka M, Alpert S, McCormack W M 1977 Quantitative bacteriology of the vaginal flora. Journal of Infectious Diseases 136 (2): 271–277

Bennett J V 1978 Human infections: economic implications and preventions. Annals of Internal Medicine 89 (part 2): 761–763

Bennett R, Erikson M, Nord C E, Zetterstrom R 1982 Suppression of aerobic and anaerobic fecal flora in newborns receiving parenteral gentamycin and ampicillin. Acta Paeditrica Scandinavica 71: 559–562

Boysen P G, Rand K H, Jerkins R T, Murphy E J 1979 Relationship of serial gram strains and cultures of tracheal aspirates to musocomial pneumonia. Critical Care Medicine 7: 142

Brachman P S 1980 Major infectious diseases in the United States. In: II World Congress Antisepsis. H P Publishing, New York

Brachman P S, Dan B B, Haley R W, Hooton T M, Garner J S, Allen J R 1980 Nosocomial surgical infections: incidence and cost. Surgical Clinics of North America 60 (1): 15–25

Bryan C S, Reynolds K L 1984 Bacteremic nosocomial pneumonia. Analysis of 172 episodes from a single metropolian area. American Review of Respiratory Diseases 129: 668–671

Buisson L B, Meakin J L 1983 Host defence mechanisms in the acutely ill patient. In: Ledingham I McA, Hanning C D (eds) Recent advances in critical care medicine—2. Churchill Livingstone, Edinburgh

Buxton A E, Anderson R L, Werdegar D, Atlas E 1978 Nosocomial respiratory tract infections and colonization with Acinetobacter calcoaceticus. Epidemiologic characteristics. American Journal of Medicine 65: 507–513

Casewell M, Phillips I 1977 Hands as route of transmission for Klebsiella species. British Medical Journal 2: 1315–1317

Casewell M, Phillips I 1978a Food as a source of Klebsiella species for colonization and infection of intensive care patients. Journal of Clinical Pathology 31: 845–849

Casewell M W, Phillips I 1978b Epidemiological patterns of Klebsiella colonisation and infection in an intensive care ward. Journal of Hygiene (Camb) 80: 295–300

Clarke G M 1985 Multiple system organ failure. In: Current topics in intensive care. Clinics of Anaesthesiology 3 (4): 1027–1053

Cross A S, Roup B 1981 Role of respiratory assistance devices in endemic nosocomial pneumonia. American Journal of Medicine 70: 681–685

Crossley K, Gardner L C 1981 Antimicrobial prophylaxis in surgical patients. Journal of the American Medical Association 245 (7): 722–726

Damas P 1983 Evaluation of host defense after trauma. Acta Anaesthesiologica Belgica 34 (3): 151

Daschër F D, Frey P, Wolff G, Banmann P C, Suter P 1982 Nosocomial infections in intensive care wards: a multicenter prospective study. Intensive Care Medicine 8: 5–9

Du Moulin G C, Paterson D G, Hedley-Whyte J, Lisbon A 1982 Aspiration of gastric bacteria in antacid treated patients: a frequent cause of postoperative colonization of the airway. Lancet 30: 242–245

Eickhoff T C 1979 Nosocomial respiratory tract infections: the gastro-intestinal tract as a reservoir. In: New criteria for antimicrobial therapy. Proceedings of a symposium in Utrecht. Excerpta Medica, pp. 5–11

Eickhoff T C, Brachman P S, Bennett J V, Brown J F 1969 Surveillance of nosocomial infections in community hospitals. I. Surveillance methods, effectiveness and initial results. Journal of Infectious Diseases 120 (3): 305–317

Feeley T W, Du Moulin G C, Hedley-Whyte J, Bushnell L S, Gilbert J P, Feingold D S 1975 Aerosol polymyxin and pneumonia in seriously ill patients. New England Journal of Medicine 293: 471–475

Finegold S M, Sutter V L, Mathisen G E 1983 Normal indigenous intestinal flora. In: Heutger D J (ed) Human intestinal microflora in health and disease. Academic Press, New York

Fischer R P, Polk H C 1975 Changing etiologic patterns of renal insufficiency in surgical patients. Surgery, Gynaecology and Obstetrics 140: 85–86

Freeman J, McGowan J E Jr 1978 Risk factors for nosocomial infection. Journal of Infectious Diseases 138: 811–819

French G L, Homi J 1979 Insignificance of colonic bacteria in the sputum of patients in a new ICU. Critical Care Medicine 7 (11): 487–491

Freter R 1974 Interaction between mechanisms controlling the intestinal flora. American Journal of Clinical Nutrition 27: 1409–1416

Fry D E, Harbrecht P J, Polk H C Jr06 1981 Systemic prophylactic antibiotics. Need the 'costs' be so high? Archives of Surgery 116: 466–469

Givens C D, Wenzel R P 1980 Catheter-associated urinary tract infections in surgical patients: a controlled study on the excess morbidity and costs. Journal of Urology 124: 646–648

Glinz W, Grob P J, Nydegger V E, Ricklin T, Stamm F, Stoffel D, Lasance A 1985 Polyvalent immunoglobulins for prophylaxis of bacterial infections in patients following multiple trauma. Intensive Care Medicine 11: 288–294

Glover J L, Jolley L 1971 Gram-negative colonization of the respiratory tract in postoperative patients. American Journal of Medical Sciences 261 (1): 24–26

Goldstein E, Green G M 1966 The effect of acute renal failure on the bacterial clearance mechanisms of the lung. Journal of Laboratory and Clinical Medicine 68 (4): 531–542

Goldstein E, Green G M, Seamann C 1970 The effect of acidosis on pulmonary bacterial function. Journal of Laboratory and Clinical Medicine 75: 912–923

Goodman J S, Schaffner W, Collins H A, Battersby E J, Koenig M G 1968 Infection after cardiovascular surgery. Clinical study including examination of antimicrobial prophylaxis. New England Journal of Medicine 278 (3): 117–123

Gould F K, Freeman R, Brown M A 1985 Respiratory complications following cardiac surgery. The role of microbiology in its evaluation. Anaesthesia 40: 1061–1064

Green M S, Rubinstein E, Amit P 1982 Estimating the effects of nosocomial infections on the length of hospitalization. Journal of Infectious Diseases 145 (5): 667–672

Guiot H F L 1982 Role of competition for substrate in bacterial antagonisms in the gut. Infection and Immunity 38 (3): 887–892

Guiot H F L, Van den Broek P J, Van der Meer J W M, Van Furth R 1983 Selective antimicrobial modulation of the intestinal flora of patients with acute nonlymphocytic leukemia: a double blind, placebo-controlled study. Journal of Infectious Diseases 147 (4): 615–623

Haley R W, Culver D H, White J W, Morgan W M, Emori T G, Munn V P, Hooton T M 1985 The efficacy of infection surveillance and control programs in preventing nosocomial infections in US Hospitals. American Journal of Epidemiology 121: 182–205

Haley R W, Hooton T M, Culver D H et al 1981 Nosocomial infections in US Hospitals, 1975–1976. Estimated frequency by selected characteristics of patients. American Journal of Medicine 70: 947–959

Hazenberg M P, Van der Boom M, Bakker M, Van de Merwe J P 1983 Binding to faeces and influence on human anaerobes of antimicrobial agents used for selective decontamination. Antonie van Leeuwenhoek 49: 111–117

Hill G B, Eschenbach D A, Holmes K K 1985 Bacteriology of the vagina. Scandinavian Journal of Urology and Nephrology S86: 24–39

Hillman K M, Riordan T, O'Farrel S M, Tabagchali S 1982 Colonization of the gastric contents in critically ill patients. Critical Care Medicine 10: 444

Holdeman L V, Good I J, Moore W E C 1976 Human fecal flora: variation in bacterial composition within individuals and a possible effect of emotional stress. Applied and Environmental Microbiology 31 (3): 359–375

Holzman B H, Scott G B 1981 Control of infection and techniques of isolation in the pediatric intensive care unit. Pediatric Clinics of North America 28 (3): 703–721

Hooton T M, Haley R W, Culver D H, White J W, Morgan W M, Carrol R J 1981 The joint association of multiple risk factors with the occurrence of nosocomial infections. American Journal of Medicine 70: 960–970

Jemmot III J B, Borysinko J Z, Borysenko M, McClelland D C, Chapman R, Meyer D, Benson H 1983 Academic stress, power, motivation, and disease in secretion rate of salivary secretory immunoglobulin A. Lancet (25 June): 1400–1402

Johanson W G J, Pierce A K, Sanford J P, Thomas G D 1972 Nosocomial respiratory infections with gram negative bacilli, the significance of colonization of the respiratory tract. Annals of Internal Medicine 77: 701–706

Johanson W G, Sanford J P 1968 Problems of infection and antimicrobials relating to anaesthesia and inhalation therapy. In: Jenkins M T (ed) Common and uncommon problems in anesthesiology. F A Davis Co, Philadelphia

Krieger J N, Kaiser D L, Wenzel R P 1983 Nosocomial urinary tract infections: secular trends, treatment and economics in a university hospital. Journal of Urology 130: 102–106

Krivit W, Giebink G S, Leonard A 1979 Overwhelming postsplenectomy infection. Surgical Clinics of North America 59 (2): 223–233

Kunin C M 1982 Urinary tract infection: new information concerning pathogensis and management. Journal of Urology 128: 1233

La Force F M 1981 Hospital-acquired gram-negative rod pneumonias: an overview. American Journal of Medicine 70: 664–669

La Force F M, Eickhoff I C 1977 The role of infection in critical care. Anesthesiology 47: 195–202

Levy S B 1982 Microbial resistance to antibiotics. An evolving and persistent problem. Lancet 83: 88

Mackowiak P A 1982 The normal microbial flora. New England Journal of Medicine 307 (2): 83–93

Maki D G 1981 Nosocomial bacteraemia. An epidemiologic overview. American Journal of Medicine 70: 719–732

Meakins J L, Wicklund B, Forse R A, McLean A P H 1980 The surgical intensive care unit: current concepts in infection. Surgical Clinics of North America 60 (1): 117–132

Meers P D, Ayliffe G A Y, Emmerson A M et al 1981 Report on the national survey of infection in hospitals, 1980. Journal of Hospital Infections 2 (suppl): 1–51

Miller T E 1984 Uraemia—does it affect host resistance to infection disease? European Journal of Clinical Microbiology 3 (5): 383–386

Milligan S L, Luft F C, McMurray S D, Kleit S A 1978 Intraabdominal infections and acute renal failure. Archives of Surgery 113: 467–472

Miranda D R, Van Saene H K F, Stoutenbeek Ch P, Zandstra D F 1983 Environment and cost in surgical intensive care unit. The implication of selective decontamination of the digestive tract (SDD). Acta Anaesthesiologica Belgica 34 (3): 223–232

Molnar J A, Burke J F 1983 Prevention and management of infections in trauma. World Journal of Surgery 7:158–163

Montgomerie J R 1979 Epidemiology of Klebsiella and hospital associated infections. Review of Infectious Diseases 1 (5): 736–753

Morris D H, Bullock F D 1919 The importance of the spleen in resistance to infection. Annals of Surgery 70 (5): 513–521

Mulder J G, Wiersma W E, Welling G W, Van der Waaij D 1984 Low dose oral tobramycin treatment for selective decontamination of the digestive tract: a study in human volunteers. Journal of Antimicrobial Chemotherapy 13: 495–504

Mulholland S G, Bruun J N 1973 A study of hospital urinary tract infections. Journal of Urology 110: 245–248

Noble W C 1983 Microbiology of normal skin. In: Noble W C (ed) Microbial skin disease: its epidemiology. Edward Arnold, London

Northey D, Aders M L, Hartsuk J M, Rhoades E R 1974 Microbial surveillance in a surgical intensive care unit. Surgery, Gynaecology and Obstetrics 139 (3): 321–325

Petersdorf R G, Curtin J A, Hoeprich P D, Peeler R N, Bennett J L Jr 1957 A study of antibiotic prophylaxis in unconscious patients. New England Journal of Medicine 257 (21): 1001–1009

Petrás G, Bognár 1981 Origin and spread of pseudomonas *aeruginosa*, Proteus and Klebsiella during twenty years in an infectious hospital. Acta Microbiologica Academiae Scientiarum Hungariae 28: 367–380

Pfirrman R W 1985 Taurolin: Ein neues Konzept zur antimikrobiellen chemotherapie chirurgischer infektion. Einfuhrung und Ubersicht in Taurolin. Urban & Schwarzenberg, New York, pp 3–23

Pietsch J B, Meakin J L 1979 Predicting infection in surgical patients. Surgical Clinics of North America 59 (2): 185–197

Pollack M, Nieman R E, Reinhardt J A, Charache P, Jett M P, Hardy P H Jr 1972 Factors influencing colonization and antibiotic resistance patterns of gram-negative bacteria in hospital patients. Lancet 2: 668

Price D J, Ghonheuer A T 1981 Dangers of antibiotic therapy in ventilated patients. Critical Care Medicine 9: 260

Rapin M, George C 1983 Management of sepsis. In: Tinker J, Rapin M (eds) Care of the critically ill patient. Springer Verlag, New York

Rohrbaugh T M, Anolik R, August C S, Serota F T, Koch P A 1984 Absorption of oral aminoglycosides following bone marrow transplantation. Cancer 53: 1502–1506

Roitt J 1977 Essential immunology, 3rd edn. Blackwell Scientific Publications, Oxford

Rose H D, Babcok 1975 Colonization of intensive care unit patients with gram-negative bacilli. American Journal of Epidemiology 101 (6): 495–501

Rosendorf L L, Daicoff G, Baer H 1974 Sources of gram negative infection after open heart surgery. Thoracic and Cardiovascular Surgery 67 (2): 195–201

Saba T M 1975 Reticuloendothelial systemic host defense after surgery and traumatic shock. Circulatory Shock 2 (2): 91–108

Sanford J P 1974 Infection control in critical care units. Critical Care Medicine 2: 211–216

Sanford J P, Pierce A K 1979 Lower respiratory tract infections. In: Bennitt J V, Brachnau P S (eds) Hospital infections. Little, Brown, Boston, pp 255–286

Schimpff S C 1979 Infection in acute non-lymphocytic leukemia: the alimentary canal as a major source of pathogenesis. In: New criteria for antimicrobial therapy. Proceedings of a symposium in Utrecht. Excerpta Medica, pp 12–27

Schimpff S C 1980 Infection prevention during profound granulocytopenia. New approaches to alimentary canal microbial suppression. Annals of Internal Medicine 93: 358–361

Scott C F 1982 Length of operation and morbidity: is there a relationship? Surgery 69 (6): 1017–1021

Shapiro M, Townsend T R, Rosner B, Kass E H 1979 Use of antimicrobial drugs in general hospitals. Pattern of prophylaxis. New England Journal of Medicine 301 (7): 351–355

Slack M P E 1983 The use and abuse of antibiotics In: Ledingham I McA, Hanning C D (eds) Recent advances in critical care medicine—2. Churchill Livingstone, Edinburgh

Sleyfer D Th, Mulder N H, de Vries-Hospers H G, Fidler V, Nieweg O, Van der Waaij D, Van Saene
    H K F 1980 Infection prevention in granulocytopenic patients by selective decontamination of the
    digestive tract. European Journal of Cancer 16: 859–869
Smith P J, Brookfield D S K, Shaw D A, Gray J 1984 An outbreak of Serratia Marscescens infection
    in a neonate unit. Lancet (21 Jan): 151–153
Stamm W E, Weinstein R A, Dixon R E 1981 Comparison of endemic and epidemic nosocomial infections.
    American Journal of Medicine 2: 393–397
Stoddart J C 1983 Hospital-acquired infections. In: Tinker J, Rapin M (eds) Care of the critically ill
    patient. Springer Verlag, New York
Stoutenbeek Ch P, Van Saene H K F, Miranda D R, Zandstra D F 1983 A new technique of infection
    prevention in the intensive care unit by selective decontamination of the digestive tract. Acta
    Anaesthesiologica Belgica 34 (3): 209–221
Stoutenbeek Ch P, Van Saene H K F, Miranda D R, Zandstra D F 1984a The effect of selective
    decontamination of the digestive tract on colonisation and infection rate in multiple trauma patients.
    Intensive Care Medicine 10: 185–192
Stoutenbeek Ch P, Van Saene H K F, Miranda D R, Zandstra D F, Binnendijk B 1984b The prevention
    of superinfection in multiple trauma patients. Journal of Antimicrobial Chemotherapy 14 (suppl B):
    203–211
Stoutenbeek Ch P, Van Saene H K F, Miranda D R, Zandstra D F, Langrehr D 1985 The emergence
    of resistance against prophylactically used antibiotics is prevented by selective decontamination of the
    digestive tract. Proceedings of the 14th International Congress of Chemotherapy, Kyoto, Japan, pp 15–
    106
Stoutenbeek Ch P, Van Saene H K F, Miranda D R, Zandstra D F, Langrehr D 1986 The effect of
    oropharyngeal decontamination using topical non-absorbable antibiotics on the incidence of nosocomial
    respiratory tract infections in multiple trauma patients (in press)
Thoburn R, Fekety F R, Cluff L E, Melvin V B 1968 Infections acquired by hospitalized patients. Archives
    of Internal Medicine 121: 1–10
Thorp Y M, Richards W C, Telfer A B M 1979 A survey of infection in an intensive care unit. Anaesthesia
    34: 643–650
Van Saene H K F, Willems F Th G, Zweens J 1983a Influence of amoxycillin and cefaclor on the
    colonization resistance of oropharynx. Scandinavian Journal of Infectious Diseases S49: 97–99
Van Saene H K F, Stoutenbeek Ch P, Miranda D R, Zadstra D F 1983b A novel approach to infection
    control in the intensive care unit. Acta Anaesthesioligica Belgica 34 (3): 193–208
Van Saene J J M 1984 Personal communication.
Van Saene J J M, Van Saene H K F, Stoutenbeek Ch P, Lerk C F 1985 Influence of faeces on the
    activity of antimicrobial agents used for decontamination of the alimentary canal. Scandinavian Journal
    of Infectious Diseases 17: 295–300
Van der Waaij D 1979a The colonisation resistance of the digestive tract in experimental animals and
    its consequence for infection prevention, acquisition of new bacteria and the prevention of spread of
    bacteria between cage water. In: New criteria for antimicrobial therapy; maintenance of digestive tract
    colonisation resistance. Proceedings of a symposium in Utrecht, 1979. Excerpta Medica, pp 43–52
Van der Waaij D 1979b Colonization resistance of the digestive tract as a major lead in the selection
    of antibiotics for therapy. In: New criteria for antimicrobial therapy. Proceedings of a symposium in
    Utrecht. Excerpta Medica, pp 271–280
Van der Waaij D 1984 The digestive tract in immunocompromised patients: importance of maintaining
    its resistance to colonization, especially in hospital in-patients and those taking antibiotics. Antonie
    van Leeuwenhoek 50: 745–761
Van der Waaij 1985 The immunoregulation of the intestinal flora: consequences of decreased thymus
    activity and broad-spectrum antibiotic treatment. Zentralblatt für Bakteriologie Suppl 13: 73–89
Van der Waaij D 1986 The apparent role of the mucous membrane and the gut-associated lymphoid
    tissue in the selection of the normal resident flora of the digestive tract. Clinical Immunology Newsletter
    7 (1): 4–7
Van der Waaij D, Berghuis J M 1974 Determination of the colonization resistance of the digestive tract
    in individual mice. Journal of Hygiene (Camb) 72: 379–387
Van der Waaij D, Berghuis-de Vries J M, Lekkerkerk-van der Wees J E C 1971 Colonization resistance
    of the digestive tract in conventional and antibiotic-treated mice. Journal of Hygiene (Camb) 69: 405–411
Van der Waaij D, Berghuis J M, Lekkerkerk J E C 1972 Colonization resistance of the digestive tract
    of mice during systemic antibiotic treatment. Journal of Hygiene (Camb) 70: 605–610
Van der Waaij D, Cohen B J, Anver M R 1974 Mitigation of experimental inflammatory bowel disease
    in guinea pigs by selective elimination of the anaerobic gram-negative intestinal microflora.
    Gastroenterology 63: 460–472

Van der Waaij D, Tieleman-Speltie T M, De Roeck Houben A M J 1978 Relation between the faecal concentration of various potentially pathogenic microorganisms and infections in individuals (mice) with severely decreased resistance to infection. Antonie van Leeuwenhoek 44: 395–405

Van der Waaij D, Vorsen J M, Korthals Altes C, Hartgrink C 1977 Reconventionalization following antibiotics decontamination in man and animals. American Journal of Clinical Nutrition 30: 1887–1895

Van der Waaij D, de Vries-Hospers H G, Snijder J A M, Halie M R, Nieweg H O 1985 Faecal endotoxin and activity of the gut-associated lymphoid tissue in patients with malignant (B-cell) lymphoma. Zentralblatt für Bakteriologie, Parasitenkunde, Infektionskrankheiten und Hygiene (A) 259: 520–530

Veringa E M, Van der Waaij D 1984 Biological inactivation by faeces of antimicrobial drugs applicable in selective decontamination of the digestive tract. Journal of Antimicrobial Chemotherapy 14: 605–612

Wagner D 1985 Personal communication

Watt I, Ledingham McA 1984 Mortality amongst multiple trauma patients admitted to an intensive therapy unit. Anaesthesia 39: 973–981

Wiegersma N, Jansen G, Van der Waaij D 1982 Effect of twelve antimicrobial drugs on the colonization resistance of the digestive tract of mice and on endogenous potentially pathogenic bacteria. Journal of Hygiene (Camb) 88: 221–230

Yoshioka H, Fujita K, Maruyama S, Oka R 1982 Change in aerobic pharyngeal flora related to antibiotic use and the emergence of gram-negative bacilli. Clinical Pediatrics 21 (8):460–462

Ziegler E J, McCutchan J A, Brande A I 1979 Treatment of gram-negative bacteremia with antiserum to core glycolipid I. The experimental basis of immunity to endotoxin. European Journal of Cancer 15: 71–76

Ziegler E J, McCutchan J A, Fierer J, Glanser M P, Sadoff J C, Douglas H, Brande A I 1982 Treatment of gram-negative bacteremia and shock with human antiserum to a mutant Escherichia coli. New England Journal of Medicine 307 (20): 1225–1230

Zimmermann J E 1971 Respiratory failure complicating post-traumatic acute renal failure; etiology, clinical features and management. Annals of Surgery 174 (1): 12–18

10. Metabolic rate and thermoregulation after injury

Roderick A. Little

INTRODUCTION

It is perhaps appropriate to ask at the outset what a physiologist with an interest in thermoregulation has to offer critical care medicine. The answer may well be nothing but I hope that before reaching such a conclusion the reader who pays me the compliment of reading this short contribution will be rewarded with an increased awareness, if not understanding, of the effect of injury (and sepsis) on thermoregulation.

A discrepancy between tissue oxygen demand and supply is considered to be a major factor in the aetiology of shock (Halmagyi, 1976). Oxygen consumption in the different tissues contributes to whole body metabolic rate the level of which will be determined, in part, by the demands for thermoregulation. There is increasing evidence, both experimental and clinical, that thermoregulation is modified by injury and sepsis and this will form the basis of this chapter.

DEFINITIONS

Sir David Cuthbertson (1942) first suggested that the metabolic response to injury could be divided into the early 'ebb' phase followed by the 'flow' or recovery phase. It needed a pathologist to add a third phase, 'necrobiosis', to describe the pattern of response which precedes death (Stoner, 1961a).

For convenience the terms oxygen consumption, metabolic rate and heat production are used synonymously. This is, of course, not strictly correct because the relationship between oxygen consumption and heat production is determined by the substrate being oxidised, as reflected by the respiratory quotient, RQ (Frayn, 1983). However, the errors involved in assuming a value for the RQ are not large (Wilmore, 1977).

Metabolic rate can be considered to have two components, basal and thermoregulatory (e.g. Mount, 1979). At environmental or ambient temperatures within the thermoneutral range metabolic rate is at its lowest or basal value, although to be sure a value is truly basal a number of other precise conditions relating to nutrition, activity, etc., have to be met (Mitchell, 1962; Little, 1985). The criteria for defining a basal state are so strict and clinically impractical that the term resting energy expenditure is often used instead (Elwyn et al, 1980). As environmental temperature falls below thermoneutrality metabolic rate rises as the organism attempts to maintain the temperature gradient between itself and the outside. This increase in metabolic rate above basal is the thermoregulatory component of heat production (Fig. 1(a)).

THE 'EBB' PHASE

The ebb phase is, as its name implies, said to be characterised by a decline in metabolic rate. The experimental evidence for this is good but the clinical data are, at best, equivocal.

Experimental studies
Most work in this area has been done by Stoner and his colleagues (for reviews see Stoner, 1981, 1986) and can be summarised as follows: after an injury, such as bilateral hind limb ischaemia produced by rubber band tourniquets in the rat, heat production at ambient temperature below the thermoneutral range is reduced. This is due to a central inhibition of thermoregulation and is not secondary to a failure of oxygen transport (Little & Threlfall, 1974). During the period of limb ischaemia shivering thermogenesis is inhibited and the ambient and hypothalamic temperature thresholds for increasing heat production are reduced (Stoner, 1972). There are also changes in the thresholds for the onset of heat loss such that higher temperatures have to be applied to the hypothalamus to increase heat loss. The increasing separation between the hypothalamic temperatures for the onset of heat gain and heat loss means that the effects of injury cannot be explained by an alteration in thermoregulatory set point.

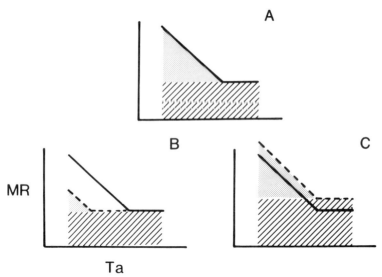

Fig. 10.1 Relationship between metabolic rate (MR) and ambient temperature (T_a) showing the relative contributions of basal (▨) and thermoregulatory heat production (▧) in the uninjured rat (A), injured rat following a period of bilateral hind-limb ischaemia (– – –, B) and endotoxin infused rat (– – –, C).

If the tourniquets are removed and there is fluid loss into the damaged limbs non-shivering thermogenesis is also inhibited and there is further separation between the hypothalamic thresholds. The ambient temperature threshold (the critical temperature) needed to stimulate heat production is further reduced (Fig. 10.1(b)). The impairment of thermoregulation at this time is such that, at ambient temperatures below the normal thermoneutral range, deep body temperature starts to fall. The depression of the critical temperature and the fall in deep body temperature are both directly related to the severity of injury (Stoner, 1961b). During this ebb phase it is only the thermoregulatory component of heat production that is inhibited, whole body oxygen consumption does not fall below basal. This suggests that oxidative metabolism is not being inhibited by toxins released from damaged tissues or by a failure of oxygen transport. In the injured animals the slope of the regression line relating oxygen consumption to ambient temperature is the same as in uninjured animals (Fig. 10.1(b)) suggesting that once thermoregulatory heat production is switched on in the injured rat, the sensitivity of the process is normal.

This central inhibition of thermoregulation depends on the activation of nor-adrenergic neurones in the hind brain from which axons ascend in the ventral nor-adrenergic bundle to liberate noradrenaline in the region of the dorsomedial nucleus of the hypothalamus (Stoner & Marshall, 1977). The hind brain neurones are activated by nociceptive impulses ascending from muscle receptors in C fibres to the deeper laminae of the dorsal horns of the spinal cord. From there long neurones cross to ascend in the opposite ventrolateral columns or spinothalamic tracts (Redfern et al, 1984; Stoner, 1986).

There is no doubt that a central inhibition is the most important factor in the impairment of shivering after injury. However, arterial blood pressure may also have a role (Fig. 10.2). In the anaesthetised cat exposed to a low ambient temperature

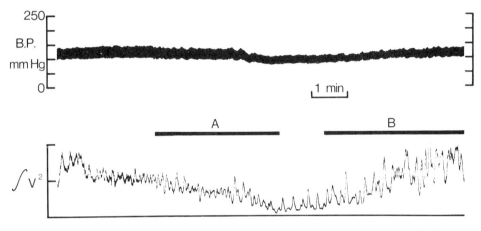

Fig. 10.2   Effect of hemorrhage (A) and reinfusion (B) in the barbitone anaesthetised cat on shivering (shown as the integrated electromyogram volt^2 in arbitrary units: time constant 1.5 s) and arterial blood pressure (mm Hg). $T_a = 8°C$.

shivering can be stopped by haemorrhage and restarted by reinfusion of the withdrawn blood (Little et al, 1980). This effect is mediated by the arterial baroreceptor input to the central nervous system (although the low pressure atrial 'volume' baroreceptors may also be involved) and not by a reduction in, for example, cerebral blood flow. Animals with denervated arterial baroreceptors do not shiver despite having a very high blood pressure and presumably unimpaired cerebral blood flow.

The effects of injury on thermoregulation in the rat can be prevented. Interruption of the relevant central noradrenergic neurones prevents the inhibition of shivering but perhaps of more clinical relevance is the efficacy of the infiltration with local anaesthetic of the muscles of the hind limbs shortly after applying the tourniquets (Stoner & Marshall, 1982). It is of interest that fluid therapy (intraperitoneal saline) which gives 100% survival after an injury normally associated with an 80% mortality does not seem to modify the changes in thermoregulation, although this requires confirmation. Raising the ambient temperature to the thermoneutral range after injury might seem to be a good thing. As expected there is no fall in oxygen consumption or deep body temperature and the good news is reinforced by the fact that arterial blood pressure and blood acid-base status are better maintained. Unfortunately the improvement is more apparent than real as mortality is increased and survival time is markedly reduced (Little & Threlfall, 1974). This observation suggests that the inhibition of thermoregulation in the ebb phase may have a protective role and this is discussed further below.

Clinical studies
It is very difficult to study thermoregulation in the injured patient shortly after an accident when treatment has priority but some studies have been made especially after minor and moderately severe injuries as assessed by the injury severity score (Baker et al, 1974). After severe injuries both mean body and core temperature fall and are negatively related to the severity of injury (Little & Stoner, 1981). The mechanism of the fall in temperature is unclear but in the most severely injured, who will have high plasma lactate concentrations (Stoner et al, 1979), it could be due to an impairment of oxygen transport. A feature of these patients was that they did not shiver despite having mean body temperatures below the normal threshold. The failure to shiver may have been secondary to hypotension (*see above*) but it cannot have been due to hypoglycaemia which also inhibits shivering (Haight & Keatinge, 1973) as the patients would have been hyperglycaemic at this time after injury. A fascinating hypothesis is that there is a central inhibition of thermoregulation shortly after injury in man, just as in the rat.

There is no convincing evidence for a reduction in metabolic rate in man shortly after accidental trauma (e.g. Cuthbertson, 1932) although values as low as 55% of predicted have been measured after severe injuries (Little et al, 1981). Even when such a reduction is found its significance is not clear—it is a reduction from a predicted value and can take no account of the subject's metabolic rate before injury. This may have been low already, for example as part of the adaptation to a reduced food intake (Brown et al, 1984). Also when these measurements are made in, for example, the accident and emergency department, the ambient temperature may be high, close to the thermoneutral range in which metabolic rate is basal and unaffected by all but the most severe trauma which plunges the patient directly into necrobiosis and death (see below). It is very relevant that after accidental haemorrhage in patients oxygen consumption fell but only to basal values (Vladek et al, 1971).

Changes in metabolic rate can be considered as the autonomic component of thermoregulation but there is another pattern of response related to behaviour. Cabanac and his colleagues have shown that the selection of an ambient temperature which maximises thermal comfort or sensory pleasure is a useful test of behavioural thermoregulation (Cabanac, 1969; Cabanac et al, 1972). Such a behavioural test based on the choice of a pleasurable temperature for the hand has been used in patients during the first few hours after sustaining minor or moderately severe injuries (Little et al, 1986).

It was first confirmed, in controls, that a pleasurable temperature for the hand (T_{hand}) was negatively related to core temperature (T_c) (Fig. 10.3(a)). Shortly (0.8–5.0 h)

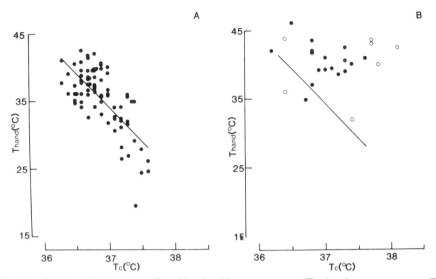

Fig. 10.3   Relationship between preferred hand ambient temperature (T_{hand}) and core temperature (T_c) in control subjects (A) and in injured patients (○ ISS 4; ● ISS 9–10) (B). The regression line shown in (B) is the relationship for control subjects taken from (A). (Reproduced with permission from Little et al, 1986.)

after minor or moderately severe injury (e.g. undisplaced or displaced long bone fracture in one leg) this relationship was lost and in the patients the slope of this regression line was not significantly different from zero and they usually chose a T_{hand} (40–45°C) towards the upper end of the normal range irrespective of T_c (Fig. 10.3(b)). Each patient selected T_{hand} as accurately as the controls and the normal pattern of response returned during recovery 2–4 months after injury. It is of interest that patients recovering from burns will also choose a high ambient temperature which would be uncomfortable for an uninjured person (Wilmore et al, 1975; Wilmore, 1977; Henane et al, 1981). These effects of injury on the selection of T_{hand} can be mimicked by producing tissue ischaemia with a thigh cuff inflated to suprasystolic pressures but not by the blood loss which might be associated with the injuries studied. This is further evidence for the importance of nociceptic afferent impulses in the pathogenesis of the inhibition of homoeostatic reflexes by trauma (Little & Stoner, 1983; Little, 1986).

THE 'NECROBIOTIC' PHASE

If the endogenous homoeostatic mechanisms aided by appropriate therapy are success-ful the ebb phase is followed by the flow phase leading on to recovery. However, if the injury, or subsequent sepsis, is overwhelming and the host, even with help, is unable to compensate for the loss of intravascular volume, etc., then the phase of necrobiosis supervenes. This phase is characterised by a progressive failure of oxygen transport reflected by the progressive rise in plasma lactate concentration (Cowan et al, 1984) and by increases in the lactate/pyruvate and β-hydroxybutyrate/acetoace-tate ratios indicating a fall in the redox state of the cytoplasm and mitochondria respectively. Oxygen consumption falls below basal even in a thermoneutral environment, body temperature also falls and death ensues.

There is no doubt that a sustained fall in oxygen consumption below basal is associated with a grave prognosis and this is recognised by the definition of basal metabolic rate as the minimal rate of energy expenditure compatible with life (Mitchell, 1962). The mortality rate in patients who had undergone major trauma or operation increased from 20% to 80% in those who had an oxygen consumption below normal (Wilson et al, 1972).

This phase is mentioned because it is the one beloved of many research teams whose models of haemorrhage or sepsis produce fulminant irreversible shock which bears little or no resemblance to clinical reality. Such studies have yielded useful information on the relative resistance of different organs to hypoxia or anoxia but the point of diminishing returns has long been passed and the need is for better more 'realistic' models (Stoner, 1979).

THE 'FLOW' PHASE

Thus it seems that in the 'ebb' phase of the response to an injury in which the integrity of the central nervous system is preserved there is good evidence for a change in the central control of thermoregulation. The situation after direct injury to the brain is unknown and warrants further investigation. The question arises—what is happening to these control mechanisms in the 'flow' phase? There is little controversy that the flow phase is characterised by an increase in metabolic rate which is usually accompanied by an increase in core temperature. This hypermetabolism is not necessarily secondary to infection or sepsis and can be compared to the traumatic fever following abdominal surgery, described by Malcolm at the end of the last century (Malcolm, 1893). There have not been many experimental studies perhaps reflecting the difficulty of finding a suitable 'model' although some progress has been made recently in the development of a model for chronic sepsis. There have been a number of clinical studies especially after burning injury (see Davies, 1982).

Experimental studies
The magnitude of the increase in metabolic rate depends on the type and severity of injury, the time after injury and the ambient temperature. A 40% full thickness scald in the rat leads to a 23% increase in metabolic rate (Arturson & Hjelm, 1984) whereas a smaller scald of 30% body surface area increases metabolic rate by only 15% (Threlfall et al, 1980) (Fig. 10.4). The increase in metabolic rate, which is not dependent on thyroid activity, can be abolished by raising the ambient temperature to 32°C which is higher than the critical temperature for uninjured rats (28–30°C) (Caldwell et al, 1959). The increase in critical temperature can be explained by the demands imposed by the increased evaporative heat loss from the burned area. Raising ambient temperature does not change the evaporative heat loss but reduces dry heat loss and so thermoneutrality can be re-established for the burned animal when the increased evaporative heat loss is balanced by the reduced dry heat loss (Caldwell et al, 1965; Caldwell, 1970). The importance of evaporative water loss is confirmed by the finding that the excessive oxygen consumption in the burned rat can be abolished by covering the wound with an impermeable material (Moyer, 1962). The change

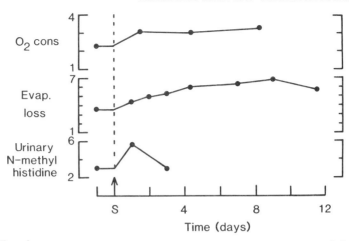

Fig. 10.4 Effect of a 30% scald (at the arrow) in the rat on oxygen consumption (L(STP)/h/kg body weight), evaporative weight loss (g/h/kg body weight) and urinary N-methylhistidine excretion (μmol/d). Mean values only are shown for clarity. (Redrawn from data in Threlfall et al, 1980.)

in critical temperature in the flow phase of the response to burn injury in the rat is not, therefore, necessarily secondary to a change in central control.

An increase in evaporative heat loss is not, however, essential for stimulating hypermetabolism in the flow phase in the rat. Unilateral femur fracture which does not affect evaporative water loss increases oxygen consumption by some 10% over a 14-day period (Cairnie et al, 1957) an effect which is more than doubled by bilateral femur fracture (Miksche & Caldwell, 1967). Perhaps surprisingly the increase in metabolic rate is reduced by raising the environmental temperature (Campbell & Cuthbertson, 1967). Feeding the animals a protein-free diet before injury also reduced the hypermetabolism and the protein catabolic response (Carnie et al, 1957) a coincidence which led to the general hypothesis that the increase in heat production in the flow phase could be fully explained by the thermic effect of protein catabolism (Cuthbertson, 1980). However, others calculated that protein catabolism can only account for a part of the response (Miksche & Caldwell, 1967), a point that will be discussed again (see below). Further evidence against a major role for protein breakdown in hypermetabolism in the rat is shown in the response to scalding where the phase of skeletal muscle protein breakdown is transient and occurs early in the prolonged phase of increased whole body oxygen consumption (Threlfall et al, 1980 (Fig. 10.4).

The hypermetabolic state associated with clinical sepsis can be produced experimentally by the infusion of live *E. coli* in dogs (Shaw & Wolfe, 1984) or the infusion for 2 h of endotoxin in Rhesus monkeys (Houtchens & Westenskow, 1984). An essential step in both procedures is resuscitation with intravenous fluids such as Ringer's lactate. A prolonged hypermetabolic response can also be produced in the unanaesthetised rat by the intravenous infusion of *E. coli* endotoxin from a subcutaneously implanted osmotic mini-pump (Fish & Spitzer, 1984; Goran et al, 1985; Little et al, 1986). This technique produces an increase in oxygen consumption when compared with pair-fed saline infused controls for at least the 7-day period of infusion. The need for pair-feeding in this study emphasises that care must be taken to ensure that results obtained in injured animals or patients are compared with valid controls (e.g. Gump et al, 1973). The chronic endotoxin infusion produced a significant increase in oxygen consumption at ambient temperatures within the thermoneutral range indicating an increase or upward resetting of basal metabolic rate (see Fig. 10.1(c)). The mechanism of this is, as yet, unresolved but it is tempting to speculate that stimulated macrophages produce the lymphokine interleukin-1 (IL-1 or endogenous pyrogen) which, via the release of prostaglandins, raises the hypothalamic thermoregulatory set-point. Evidence in support of this is that the cyclo-oxygenase inhibitor, indomethacin, significantly reduces oxygen consumption within the thermoneutral range in these endotoxin infused rats.

Clinical studies

The resting energy expenditure increases in the flow phase in man and the magnitude and duration of the rise are directly related to the severity of injury (e.g. Wilmore, 1977). Surgical operations lead to a surprisingly small response (at least to a non-surgeon) for example, total-hip replacement increases metabolic rate by only some 5% (Michelsen et al, 1979). Multiple long-bone fractures increase metabolic rate some 10–20% above predicted values for some 1–2 weeks after injury (Roe & Kinney, 1965; Frayn et al, 1984) (Fig. 10.5). Sepsis as a complication of gastrointestinal surgery

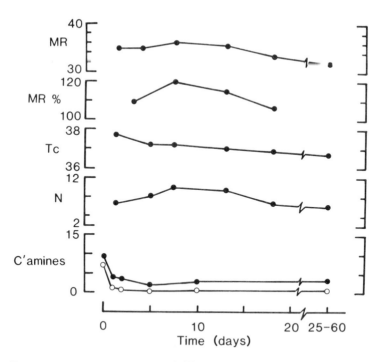

Fig. 10.5   Changes in metabolic rate (MR—kcal/m²/h corrected to a normal core temperature of 36.7°C), metabolic rate (MR%—expressed as a percentage of predicted from arm muscle circumference—Brown et al, 1984), core temperature (T_c—°C), urinary nitrogen loss (N—g/m²day) and plasma catecholamine concentration (C'amines—● noradrenaline, ○ adrenaline—nmol/l) in patients after musculoskeletal injuries with Injury Severity Scores ranging from 9–43. (Redrawn from data in Frayn et al, 1984; Frayn, 1986.)

or penetrating wounds can increase metabolic rate even after correction for any elevation in core temperature (Brown et al, 1984) but the increases are often small (Askanazi
et al, 1980a). The greatest increases, up to 100%, are found after major full-thickness
burns involving more than 50% of the body surface (Davies et al, 1977; Davies,
1982). It seems that doubling of the metabolic rate is a maximal response subject
to the limitations imposed by the cardiovascular and respiratory systems (e.g. Little,
1985).

It is important to realise that not only are the increases in metabolic rate less than
were once believed but so too are the actual levels of energy expenditure. Measured
energy expenditures above 3000 kcal/day are unusual (Askanazi et al, 1980a; Stoner
et al, 1983) an important consideration when help with feeding is indicated. It is,
perhaps, worth briefly considering why the measured metabolic rates are often so
low in the injured and septic patient. Such people may have suffered a loss of weight
and adjustment to a reduced calorie intake before the operation and subsequent sepsis
and they are often acutely fasted or starved and immobilised in bed, all of which
reduce metabolic rate (e.g. Cuthbertson, 1929; Keys et al, 1950; Brown et al, 1984).
Thus the flow phase response to injury is superimposed on a falling background
level of 'normal' metabolic activity. This is well illustrated by the following example:

'Patients undergoing major elective orthopedic surgery (total hip replacement)
showed a similar lack of change in energy expenditure. However the data presented
here suggest that this lack of change in metabolic rate was actually a twofold phenomenon. Since in normal, bedridden subjects, there was a drop in resting energy
expenditure with 5% dextrose, the lack of change in the hip patients indicated
a compensatory effect of surgery to increase resting energy expenditure'. (Azkanazi
et al, 1981)

What is the mechanism of this increase in heat production in the flow phase? First
consider the situation after burning injury where there is a large increase in water
loss from the damaged area and the energy cost of the latent heat of evaporation
has to be met by an increase in metabolic rate (Little, 1985). The problems imposed
by a large obligatory evaporative fluid loss are not confined to burning injury but
can also occur when a laparostomy is performed, in cases of severe intraabdominal
sepsis, exposing a large area of granulation tissue (Mughal et al, 1986). Evaporative
water loss can be reduced by covering the burned surface with an impermeable dressing
(e.g. Lamke et al, 1977; Zawacki et al, 1971) but there is no agreement on the effect
this has on metabolic rate (see Davies, 1982). There is also little agreement on the
effects of offsetting the increase in evaporative heat loss by the reduction in dry heat
loss produced by a rise in ambient temperature. While all agree that exposure to
a warm, dry environment is beneficial for the patients, some claim that the hypermetabolism is abolished (e.g. Arturson, 1978), some that it is markedly reduced (e.g.
Barr et al, 1968) while others have been able to demonstrate only a small reduction
(e.g. Aulick et al, 1979).

Wilmore has argued that the dissociation between evaporative water loss and hypermetabolism and the persistence of an elevated metabolic rate at a raised environmental
temperature (Fig. 10.6) are evidence for a change in hypothalamic thermoregulatory
control. He suggests that rather than being the cause of the hypermetabolism the
obligatory evaporative water loss provides a convenient route for the dissipation of

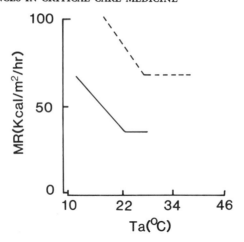

Fig. 10.6   Relationship between metabolic rate (MR) and ambient temperature (T_a) in control subjects
(————) and in thermally injured patients (>60% body surface area, – – –). (Redrawn from Wilmore,
1977.)

the excess calories produced by the resetting of metabolic activity (Wilmore, 1977).
The hypermetabolism after burns is not driven by a peripheral cold stimulus as mean
skin temperature is elevated in such patients (Wilmore et al, 1975). Elimination of
all routes of heat loss by immersing the burned patient in warm water does not reduce
the hypermetabolism. Indeed they do all they can to maintain their elevated heat
production by reducing blood flow through intact skin (Wilmore, 1977). The resetting
of hypothalamic thermoregulatory function after thermal injury leads to an increase
in sympathetic nervous activity and the increase in catecholamine release mediates
the increase in heat production. There is a positive relationship between the rate
of urinary catecholamine excretion and metabolic rate which can be reduced by combined adrenergic blockade (Wilmore et al, 1974). The importance of catecholamines
has, however, been questioned by results obtained in burned children, anaesthetised
for skin grafting, where plasma catecholamine concentrations decreased at a time
when the rate of heat production was increasing (Crabtree et al, 1980). There is
also some doubt about a primary role for catecholamines in mediating the increase
in metabolic rate after non-thermal injury. In such patients the peak in metabolic
rate and catabolic response occurs some 7–10 days after injury at a time when plasma
catecholamine concentrations have returned to normal (Frayn et al, 1984; Frayn,
1986) (see Fig. 10.5).

   It is perhaps useful at this stage to consider the link between injured tissues and
the host. Neural afferent activity after injury is important in initiating the stimulation
of the pituitary–adrenal axis (Hume & Egdahl, 1959) and the 'ebb' phase changes
in thermoregulatory and cardiovascular reflex activity (Redfern et al, 1984; Little
et al, 1986). However, denervation of the wound or interruption of the sensory input
to the brain does not diminish the hypermetabolic response to thermal injury (Wilmore,
1977). The production of interleukin-1 by activated macrophages in the wound is
a candidate for the role of a humoral mediator. It is involved in the pathogenesis
of fever and also mediates a number of the metabolic changes associated with injury
and sepsis (Wilmore, 1986; Frayn, 1986).

The increase in protein catabolism characteristic of the flow phase may contribute to the hypermetabolism but, just as in experimental studies, it can only be responsible for some 20% of total heat production even after severe soft tissue injury (Duke et al, 1970; James, 1981). Protein synthesis is also increased at this time after severe injury (e.g. James, 1981) and may also contribute to the hypermetabolism; the amount of protein synthesis is an important factor in determining metabolic rate in children (Brooke & Ashworth, 1972).

There may be an iatrogenic component of the increase in heat production in injured or septic patients who are being fed parenterally. An infusion of glucose increases metabolic rate in normal subjects (Jequier & Tiebaud, 1982) and this is increased in the depleted patients with sepsis (Askanazi et al, 1980). Also in some patients glucose-based total parenteral nutrition increases minute ventilation more than expected from the increased metabolic load. The respiratory distress can be ameliorated by reducing the amount of glucose or replacing some of it with a fat emulsion suggesting that the increased CO_2 load produced by the glucose infusion is a major factor (Askanazi et al, 1980b; Stoner et al, 1981). The increased CO_2 load is, however, not the only factor mediating the increase in ventilation, amino acid infusions also increase ventilatory drive. This may be due to the low pH of many such mixtures but it has also been suggested that it is secondary to a decrease in the serotoninergic suppression of central respiratory drive following an inhibition of tryptophan uptake into the brain by increased levels of branched chain amino acids in the plasma (Elwyn et al, 1983).

Much of our thinking about the pathogenesis of the hypermetabolic response to injury has been conditioned by the idea that the increase in heat production is being driven or 'pushed' by, for example, a central upward resetting of metabolic control. Wilmore (1986) and Stoner (1986) have developed the idea of the wound, whether it is a fracture site, abscess or burned surface, as an organ and they suggest that the changes are being 'pulled' by the demands of the new organ. There is a positive correlation between whole-body oxygen consumption and cardiac output in burned patients and most of the increase in blood flow is directed to the burn the circulation of which is not under reflex control (Gump et al, 1970; Aulick et al, 1977). There is an increase in oxygen consumption by the wound which consumes glucose and releases lactate into the circulation. This lactate is reconverted to glucose in the liver by an energy consuming process.

Thus, in summary, it seems that much of the increased energy expenditure in the 'flow' phase can be accounted for by a combination of (1) the oxygen consumption of the wound, (2) the increased energy expenditure by the heart, (3) the energy required for the conversion of lactate to glucose in the liver, (4) the Q^{10} effect of the raised body temperature during this period, (5) the energy cost of protein catabolism and (6) the need to provide the latent heat of evaporation of water when there is an evaporative loss from the burn or wound surface (Stoner, 1986).

VALUE OF THE 'EBB' AND 'FLOW' PHASES

In conclusion it is, perhaps, worth considering whether any beneficial effects can be ascribed to the changes in metabolic rate described above. The optimum ambient temperature for survival in the 'ebb' phase after injury in laboratory animals is below thermoneutral, that is low enough to permit a fall in core temperature. Preventing or reversing this hypothermia by raising ambient temperature or pharmacological stimulation of heat production, reduces survival time and increases mortality. The response is therefore of survival value and a teleological argument can be advanced that a fall in heat production coupled with a switch from carbohydrate to fat as the substrate for energy production (Frayn, 1985) allows the animal to conserve its energy reserves at a time when it cannot forage or hunt. However if, as happens clinically, treatment is superimposed the situation may be somewhat different, for example the optimum environmental temperature for survival of mice after limb ischaemia is increased by treatment with saline (Tabor & Rosenthal, 1947).

The hypermetabolism in the 'flow' phase may also be of benefit. The elevated body temperature will increase enzyme activity in, for example, the liver and the wound which may aid reparative processes. A fever is associated with increased survival in infected lizards and rabbits (Kluger et al, 1975). Lymphokine production and IL-1 induced T cell proliferation and antibody production are all enhanced at an elevated temperature (reviewed by Atkins, 1983). It is intriguing that interleukin-1 which stimulates a number of host defence processes and perhaps also muscle proteolysis (Clowes, 1983) creates the optimal body temperature for such reactions.

CONCLUSION

In conclusion it seems that the changes in heat production or metabolic rate in both the 'ebb' and 'flow' phases have some protective value. It is tempting to speculate that the 'ebb' phase evolved to enable an animal to survive relatively minor injuries. The changes in central control at this time probably reflecting a continuation of the alerting or defence reaction which occurs as part of the preparation for fight or flight at the appreciation of danger. More severe injuries were, perhaps, always fatal but now treatment has been superimposed by man and as survival has improved the 'flow' phase changes are seen more clearly. These changes possibly dependent, at least in part, on the stimulation of macrophages evolved primarily as a host defence mechanism against infection and for the healing of minor injuries. Previously they were self limiting as homoeostasis was quickly restored or overwhelmed. Now they proceed unbated, sustained by many of the advances in critical care medicine. The challenge is to identify the stimuli which trigger the flow phase and the mechanism of the interaction between those stimuli and homoeostasis.

REFERENCES

Arturson M G S 1978 Metabolic changes following thermal injury. World Journal of Surgery 2: 203
Arturson M G S 1984 Concentration of adenine nucleotides and glycolytic intermediates in erythrocytes, liver and muscle tissue in rats after thermal injury. Scandinavian Journal of Plastic and Reconstructive Surgery 19: 21
Askanazi J, Carpentier Y A, Elwyn D H, et al 1980a Influence of total parenteral nutrition on fuel utilization in injury and sepsis. Annals of Surgery 191: 40
Askanazi J, Rosenbaum S H, Hyman A I, et al 1980b Respiratory changes induced by the large glucose loads of total parenteral nutrition. Journal of the American Medical Association 243: 1444
Askanazi J, Carpentier Y A, Jeevanandam M, Michelson C B, Elwyn D H, Kinney J M 1981 Energy expenditure, nitrogen balance, and norepinephrine excretion after injury. Surgery 89: 478
Atkins E 1983 Fever—new perspectives on an old phenomenon. The New England Journal of Medicine 308: 958

Aulick L H, Hander E H, Wilmore D W, Mason A D, Pruitt B A 1979 The relative significance of thermal and metabolic demands on burn hypermetabolism. Journal of Trauma 19: 559

Aulick L H, Wilmore D W, Mason A D, Pruitt B A 1977 Influence of burn wound on peripheral circulation in thermally injured patients. American Journal of Physiology 233: H520

Baker S P, O'Neill B, Haddon W, Long W B 1974 The Injury Severity Score: a method for describing patients with multiple injuries and evaluating emergency care. Journal of Trauma 14: 187

Barr P-O, Birke G, Liljedahl S-O, Plantin L-O 1968 Oxygen consumption and water loss during treatment of burns with warm dry air. Lancet i: 164

Brooke E O, Ashworth A 1972 The influence of malnutrition on the postprandial metabolic rate and respiratory quotient. British Journal of Nutrition 27: 407

Brown R, Gross E, Little R A, Stoner H B, Tresadern J 1984 Whole body oxygen consumption and anthropometry. Clinical Nutrition 3: 11

Cabanac M 1969 Plaisir ou déplaisir de la sensation thermique et homeothermial. Physiology and Behaviour 4: 359

Cabanac M, Massonnet B, Belaiche R 1972 Preferred skin temperature as a function of internal and mean skin temperature. Journal of Applied Physiology 33: 699

Cairnie A B, Campbell R M, Pullar J D, Cuthbertson D P 1957 The heat production consequent on injury. British Journal of Experimental Pathology 38: 504

Caldwell F T 1970 Changes in energy metabolism during recovery from injury. In: Porter R, Knight J (eds) Energy metabolism in trauma. Churchill, London, p 23

Caldwell F T, Hammel H T, Dolan F 1965 Determination of energy balance following thermal burns by using gradient calorimetry. Surgical Forum 16: 486

Caldwell F T, Osterholm J L, Sower N D, Moyer C A 1959 Metabolic response to thermal trauma of normal and thyroprivic rats at three environmental temperatures. Annals of Surgery 150: 976

Campbell R M, Cuthbertson D P 1967 Effect of environmental temperature on the metabolic response to injury. Quarterly Journal of Experimental Physiology 52: 114

Clowes G H A, George B C, Villee C A, Saravis C A 1983 Muscle proteolysis induced by a circulating peptide in patients with sepsis or trauma. The New England Journal of Medicine 308: 545

Cowan B N, Burns H J G, Boyle P, Ledingham I McA 1984 The relative prognostic value of lactate and haemodynamic measurements in early shock. Anaesthesia 39: 750

Crabtree J H, Bowser B H, Campbell J W, Guinee W S, Caldwell F T 1980 Energy metabolism in anesthetized children with burns. American Journal of Surgery 140: 832

Cuthbertson D P 1929 The influence of prolonged muscular rest on metabolism. Biochemical Journal 23: 1328

Cuthbertson D P 1932 Observations on the disturbance of metabolism produced by injury to the limbs. Quarterly Journal of Medicine 1: 233

Cuthbertson D P 1942 Post-shock metabolic response. Lancet i: 433

Cuthbertson D P 1980 Alterations in metabolism following injury: part 1. Injury 11: 175

Davies J W L 1982 Physiological responses to burning injury. Academic Press, New York

Davies J W L, Lamke L-O, Liljedahl S-O 1977 Treatment of severe burns. II. Metabolic studies during successful treatment of three adult patients with burns covering 80–85% of the body surface. Acta Chirurgica Scandinavica (Supplementum) 468: 25

Duke J H, Jørgensen S B, Broell J R, Long C L, Kinney J M 1970 Contribution of protein to caloric expenditure following injury. Surgery 68: 168

Elwyn D H, Kinney J M, Gump F E, Askanazi J, Rosenbaum S H, Carpentier Y A 1980 Some metabolic effects of fat infusions in depleted patients. Metabolism 29: 125

Elwyn D H, Askanazi J, Weissman C, Kinney J M 1983 Respiratory effects of amino acids: implications for therapy. In: Kleinberger G, Deutsch E (eds) New Aspects of Clinical Nutrition. Karger, Basel, p 428

Fish R E, Spitzer J A 1984 Continuous infusion of endotoxin from an osmotic pump in the conscious, unrestrained rat: a unique model of chronic endotoxemia. Circulatory Shock 12: 135

Frayn K N 1983 Calculation of substrate oxidation rates in vivo from gaseous exchange. Journal of Applied Physiology 55: 628

Frayn K N 1983 Substrate turnover after injury. British Medical Bulletin 41: 232

Frayn K N 1986 Hormonal control of metabolism in trauma and sepsis. Clinical Endocrinology 24: 577

Frayn K N, Little R A, Stoner H B, Galasko C S B 1984 Metabolic control in non-septic patients with musculo-skeletal injuries. Injury 16: 73

Goran M I, Frayn K N, Little R A 1985 Intravenous endotoxin infusion by osmotic mini-pump in the rat. Biochemical Society Transactions 13: 528

Gump F E, Martin P, Kinney J M 1973 Oxygen consumption and caloric expenditure in surgical patients. Surgery, Gynecology and Obstetrics 137: 499

Gump F E, Price J B, Kinney J M 1970 Blood flow and oxygen consumption in patients with severe burns. Surgery, Gynecology and Obstetrics 130: 23

Haight J S J, Keatinge W R 1973 Failure of thermoregulation in the cold during hypoglycaemia induced by exercise and ethanol. Journal of Physiology 229: 87

Halmagyi D F J 1976 Blood flow, oxygen transport and metabolic rate in experimental shock. In: Ledingham I McA (ed) Shock, Clinical and Experimental Aspects. Monographs in Anaesthesiology 4. Excerpta Medica. Elsevier, New York, p 43

Henane R, Bittel J, Banssillon V 1981 Partitional calorimetry measurements of energy exchanges in severely burned patients. Burns 7: 180

Houtchens B A, Westenskow D R 1984 Oxygen consumption in septic shock: collective review. Circulatory Shock 13: 361

Hume D M, Egdahl R H 1959 The importance of the brain in the endocrine response to injury. Annals of Surgery 150: 697

James W P T 1981 Protein and energy metabolism after trauma: old concepts and new developments. Acta Chirurgica Scandinavica (Supplementum) 507: 1

Jequier E, Tiebaud D 1983 Effects of glucose and lipid infusions on energy expenditure in man. In: Kleinberger G, Deutsch E (eds) New Aspects of Clinical Nutrition. Karger, Basle, p 23

Keys A, Brozek J, Henschel A, et al 1950 The Biology of Human Starvation. University of Minnesota Press, Minneapolis

Kluger M J, Ringler D H, Anver M R 1975 Fever and survival. Science 188: 166

Lamke L-O, Nilsson G E, Reithner H L 1977 The evaporative water loss from burns and the water vapour permeability of grafts and artificial membranes used in the treatment of burns. Burns 3: 159

Little R A 1985 Heat production after injury. British Medical Bulletin 41: 226

Little R A 1986 Homeostatic reflexes after injury. In: Vincent J L (ed) Update in Intensive Care and Emergency Medicine. Springer-Verlag, Berlin, p 377

Little R A, Threlfall C J 1974 Effect of nonhemorrhagic injury on blood acid base status, erythrocyte 2, 3-diphosphoglycerate concentrations and hemoglobin–oxygen affinity. Circulatory Shock 1: 209

Little R A, Goran M I, Frayn K N, Jones R O, Foggard G J W 1986 The effect of chronic endotoxin infusion on oxygen consumption in the rat. Circulatory Shock 19: 111

Little R A, Marshall H W, Reynolds M I, Stoner H B 1980 Effect of changes in baroreceptor input on the intensity of shivering in the anaesthetised cat. Pflügers Archiv 384: 261

Little R A, Stoner H B 1981 Body temperature after accidental injury. British Journal of Surgery 68: 221

Little R A, Stoner H B 1983 The modification of homoeostatic reflexes by trauma. In: Lewis D H, Haglund U (eds) Shock Research. Elsevier, Amsterdam, p 101

Little R A, Stoner H B, Frayn K N 1981 Substrate oxidation shortly after accidental injury in man. Clinical Science 61: 789

Little R A, Stoner H B, Randall P, Carlson G 1986 An effect of injury on thermoregulation in man. Quarterly Journal of Experimental Physiology 71: 295

Malcolm J D 1893 The Physiology of Death from Traumatic Fever—A Study in Abdominal Surgery. Churchill, London

Michelsen C B, Askanazi J, Gump F E, Elwyn D H, Kinney J M, Stinchfield F E 1979 Changes in metabolism and muscle composition associated with total hip replacement. Journal of Trauma 19: 29

Miksche L W, Caldwell F T 1967 The influence of fever, protein metabolism, and thyroid function on energy balance following bilateral fracture of the femur in the rat. Surgery 62: 66

Mitchell H H 1962 Comparative Nutrition of Man and Domestic Animals. Vol 1. Academic Press, New York

Mount L E 1979 Adaptation to Thermal Environment: Man and his Productive Animals. Edward Arnold, London

Moyer C A 1962 The metabolism of burned mammals and its relationship to vaporizational heat loss and other parameters. In: Artz C P (ed) Research In Burns. Davis, Philadelphia, p 113

Mughal M, Bancewicz J, Irving M H 1986 'Laparostomy': a technique for the management of intractable intra-abdominal sepsis. British Journal of Surgery 73: 253

Redfern W S, Little R A, Stoner H B, Marshall H W 1984 Effect of limb ischaemia on blood pressure and the blood pressure–heart rate reflex in the rat. Quarterly Journal of Experimental Physiology 69: 763

Roe C F, Kinney J M 1965 The caloric equivalent of fever. II. Influence of major trauma. Annals of Surgery 161: 140

Shaw J H F, Wolfe R R 1984 A conscious septic dog model with hemodynamic and metabolic responses similar to responses of humans. Surgery 95: 553

Stoner H B 1961a Critical analysis of trauma and shock models. Federation Proceedings 20: 38

Stoner H B 1961b The biochemical response to injury. Scientific basis of medicine. Annual Reviews. Athlone Press, London, p 172

Stoner H B 1972 Effect of injury on the responses to thermal stimulation of the hypothalamus. Journal of Applied Physiology 33: 665

Stoner H B 1979 Responses to injury—past research and future plans. In: Schumer W, Spitzer J J, Marshall B E (eds) Advances in Shock Research. Vol 2. Liss, New York, p 1

Stoner H B 1981 Thermoregulation after trauma. Advances in Physiological Science 26: 25

Stoner H B 1986 A role for the central nervous system in the responses to trauma. In: Little R A, Frayn K N (eds) The Scientific Basis of the Care of the Critically Ill. Manchester University Press, Manchester, p 215

Stoner H B, Marshall H W 1977 Localization of the brain regions concerned in the inhibition of shivering by trauma. British Journal of Experimental Pathology 58: 50

Stoner H B, Marshall H W 1982 Neural pathways mediating the inhibition of shivering by nonthermal afferent impulses from ischemic limbs. Experimental Neurology 78: 275

Stoner H B, Frayn K N, Barton R N, Threlfall C J, Little R A 1979 The relationships between plasma substrates and hormones and the severity of injury in 277 recently injured patients. Clinical Science 56: 563

Stoner H B, Little R A, Elebute E A, Gross E, Tresadern J, Frayn K N 1981 Some metabolic problems in patients with injury and sepsis. In: Wesdorp R I C, Soeters P B (eds) Clinical Nutrition. Churchill Livingstone, Edinburgh, p 297

Stoner H B, Little R A, Frayn K N, Elebute E A, Tresadern J, Gross E 1983 The effect of sepsis on the oxidation of carbohydrate and fat. British Journal of Surgery 70: 32

Tabor H, Rosenthal S M 1947 Body temperature and oxygen consumption in traumatic shock and hemorrhage in mice. American Journal of Physiology 149: 449

Threlfall C J, Little R A, Frayn K N 1980 The post-scald metabolic response in the growing rat: evidence for a transient phase of muscle protein breakdown. Burns 7: 25

Vladek B C, Bassin R, Kark R E, Shoemaker W C 1971 Rapid and slow hemorrhage in man—II. Annals of Surgery 173: 331

Wilmore D W 1977 The metabolic management of the critically ill. Plenum Medical, New York

Wilmore D W 1986 The wound as an organ. In: Little R A, Frayn K N (eds) The Scientific Basis for the Care of the Critically Ill. Manchester University Press, Manchester, p 45

Wilmore D W, Long K M, Mason A D, Skreen R W, Pruitt B A 1974 Catecholamines: mediator of the hypermetabolic response to thermal injury. Annals of Surgery 180: 653

Wilmore D W, Orcutt T W, Mason A D, Pruitt B A 1975 Alterations in hypothalamic function following thermal trauma. Journal of Trauma 15: 697

Wilson R F, Christenson C, LeBlanc L P 1972 Oxygen consumption in critically ill surgical patients. Annals of Surgery 176: 801

Zawacki B C, Spitzer K W, Mason A D, Johns L A 1970 Does increased evaporative water loss cause hypermetabolism in burned patients? Annals of Surgery 171: 801

11. Endogenous Opioids in Shock

Charles J. Hinds   Michael D. J. Donaldson

Opium has been used for medicinal purposes at least since the third millennium BC. In the 16th century AD the use of laudanum, an opiate derivative, was popularised by Paracelsus, and currently opiates remain amongst the most effective and widely prescribed analgesic agents. Although the ability of poppy seed extracts to produce analgesia, relaxation and euphoria, as well as prevent diarrhoea and suppress the cough reflex, has long been recognised, the mechanisms underlying these actions were not understood until recently.

A number of observations, however, implied that exogenously administered opiates might be interacting with specific receptors. These included the structural similarities of synthetic and naturally occurring opiates, the stereospecificity of opiate agonists and antagonists, and the phenomenon of 'natural analgesia'. The latter is characteristically seen in those subjected to extreme stress, for example in battle or on the playing field, and has been vividly described by the explorer Livingstone in an account of his travels in Africa:

> 'I heard a shout and looking half round I saw the lion in the act of springing upon me. He caught me by the shoulder and we both came to the ground together. Growling horribly, he shook me as a terrier dog does a rat. The shock produced a stupor similar to that which seems to be felt by a mouse after the first gripe of the cat; it caused a sort of dreaminess in which there was no sense of pain nor feeling of terror, though I was quite conscious of all that was happening. It was like what patients partially under the influence of chloroform describe. They see the operation but do not feel the knife.'

ENDOGENOUS OPIOID PEPTIDES

Opiate receptors were finally demonstrated in nervous tissue in the early 1970s (Pert & Synder, 1973) and in 1975 it was reported that two naturally occurring ligands for these receptors, with potent opiate activity, had been isolated from pig brain. These were the pentapeptides leucine (leu-) and methionine (met-) enkephalin (enkephalin from the Greek 'in the head') (Hughes et al, 1975). Later it was recognised that the terminal five amino-acids of the larger pituitary derived peptide β-lipotrophin (β-LPH) were identical to those of met-enkephalin. Opiate bioactivity was then demonstrated in a variety of β-LPH fragments, the most potent of which was β-endorphin (endorphin from endogenous morphine). Subsequently, many other peptides with opiate activity have been isolated from biological tissue, the majority of which incorporate an enkephalin amino-acid sequence, although they may vary considerably in length. Examples include met-enkephalin-Arg-Phe, Peptide E which contains the met-enkephalin sequence, and dynorphin which incorporates the leu-enkephalin sequence

(Table 11.1). It has also become apparent that these 'endogenous opioid peptides' (EOPs) originate from a variety of precursors, that they are differently distributed, that different mechanisms regulate their release and that they probably subserve distinct functions.

Table 11.1 Endogenous opioid peptides

Name	Amino acid sequence
Met-enkephalin	*Tyr-Gly-Gly-Phe-Met*
Leu-enkephalin	*Tyr-Gly-Gly-Phe-Leu*
β-Endorphin (human)	*Tyr-Gly-Gly-Phe-Met*-Thr-Ser-Glu-Lys-Ser-Gln- Thr-Pro-Leu-Val-Thr-Leu-Phe-Lys-Asn-Ile- Ile-Lys-Asn-Ala-Tyr-Lys-Lys-Gly-Glu-Ala-
Met-enkephalin-Arg[6]-Phe[7]	*Tyr-Gly-Gly-Phe-Met*-Arg-Phe
Peptide E	*Tyr-Gly-Gly-Phe-Met*-Arg-Arg-Val-Gly-Arg-Pro- Glu-Trp-Trp-Met-Asp-Tyr-Gln-Lys-Arg-Tyr- Gly-Gly-Phe-Leu
Dynorphin	*Tyr-Gly-Gly-Phe-Leu*-Arg-Arg-Ile-Arg-Pro-Lys- Leu-Lys-Trp-Asn-Asp-Gln

β-endorphin

In contrast to the extensive distribution of the enkephalins (see below) most of the β-endorphin-containing nerve terminals appear to arise from cell groups in and around the hypothalamic arcuate nucleus, with long axonal projections extending to the brainstem as well as reticular, midbrain and limbic regions (Watson et al, 1978). This distribution suggests that within the brain β-endorphin may have a role in the regulation of hypothalamopituitary function and that it may play a part in the integration of hypothalamic, brainstem and limbic activity. Moreover this distribution is consistent with the possibility that activation of this system could affect cardiovascular function, and it has been suggested that β-endorphin may have an inhibitory role in central cardiovascular regulation (Petty et al, 1982). More recently, immunoreactive β-endorphin has been identified in peripheral sites, including the gastrointestinal tract (Orwoll & Kendall, 1980).

Circulating β-endorphin is derived, together with a number of other peptides including adrenocorticotrophic hormone (ACTH) and β-LPH, from the large precursor molecule pro-opiomelanocortin (POMC) (Fig. 11.1) which is found in the anterior and intermediate lobes of the pituitary gland. Secretion of these POMC-derived peptides is regulated by corticotrophin-releasing factor (CRF) and β-endorphin is released from the pituitary concomitantly with ACTH in response to stress (Guillemin et al, 1977) as well as exhibiting a similar circadian rhythm in normal subjects (McIntosh et al, 1985).

The role of circulating β-endorphin is uncertain although it probably plays a role in the biological response to stress. It has a relatively long half-life and therefore probably mediates more prolonged neuronal and, possibly, endocrine changes. Direct effects on the heart or peripheral vasculature cannot be ruled out and it is possible that β-endorphin may interact with the opiate receptors on the chromaffin cells of the adrenal medulla, for which this peptide has a high affinity, to inhibit their secretory activity. It has also been suggested that circulating β-endorphin (and possibly enkephalins) may gain access to autonomic centres in the brain via circumventricular sites

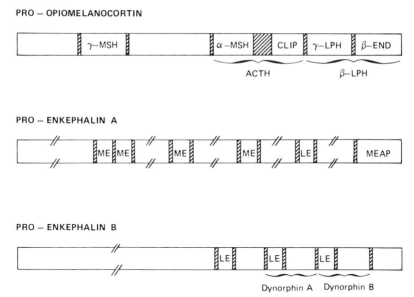

Fig. 11.1 MSH = melanocyte stimulating hormone. CLIP = corticotrophin-like intermediate lobe peptide. LPH = lipotrophin. ACTH = adrenocorticotrophic hormone. END = endorphin. ME = met-enkephalin. MEAP = met-enkephalin-Arg-Phe. LE = leu-enkephalin.

where there is no effective blood-brain barrier, such as the area postrema which contains a high concentration of opiate receptors (Holaday, 1983).

The enkephalins

These are located in the central nervous system, sympathetic ganglia and the adrenal glands, as well as in the gut. Within the central nervous system enkephalins are widely distributed and have been identified in the brainstem, the striatum, the limbic system and the hypothalamus, as well as in areas involved in the regulation of autonomic function. Moreover, significant amounts of this peptide have been identified in the substantia gelatinosa of the spinal cord. The enkephalins may act as neurotransmitters at opiate receptors, and it appears that their subsequent neuronal actions are usually inhibitory (North, 1979). The presence of enkephalins in the dorsal horn of the spinal cord and thalamus suggests that they may modulate pain perception, while their distribution in the hypothalamus and brainstem suggests a role in the control of autonomic functions.

Peptides containing the enkephalin sequence are also concentrated in sympathetic ganglia and the adrenal medulla where they appear to be stored together with catecholamines in the chromaffin cells (Schultzberg et al, 1978; Viveros et al, 1979). These enkephalins are derived from a large precursor molecule (proenkephalin A) (Fig. 11.1) which incorporates both the pentapeptides, as well as larger enkephalin-containing peptides, within its amino-acid sequence (Noda et al, 1982; Comb et al, 1982). Enkephalins have been shown to be released, together with catecholamines, from isolated adrenal glands (Viveros et al, 1979; Corder et al, 1982) as well as cultured adrenal chromaffin cells (Kumakura et al, 1980), and stimulation of the splanchnic nerve results in increased plasma levels of immunoreactive met-enkephalin (Govoni et al, 1981). Thus it seems that activation of the sympathetic nervous system releases not only catecholamines but also enkephalins, and other peptides (Corder, 1982), from the adrenal medulla. Since the adrenal chromaffin cells have been shown to contain specific opioid binding sites it is possible that the enkephalins inhibit their secretory activity by modulating the effects of splanchnic nerve activity at nicotinic receptors (Kumakura et al, 1980). This may represent a negative feedback mechanism which limits further secretion of catecholamines and other peptides from the adrenal medulla in response to sustained sympathetic stimulation. It may be that similar mechanisms are also operative at peripheral sympathetic nerve terminals since met-enkephalin inhibits, presynaptically, the exocytotic release of noradrenaline at the postganglionic sympathetic nerve terminal (Gaddis & Dixon, 1982).

The role of circulating enkephalins, which have an extremely short half-life, is at present unclear. Nevertheless, because adrenal enkephalins enter the inferior vena cava directly they could reach opiate receptors in the heart and lungs in sufficient concentrations to elicit a physiological response. It has been suggested that enkephalins might be rapidly degraded by peptidases in the lung following actions at sites such as the pulmonary 'J' receptors (Holaday, 1983). However, using a canine model of endotoxin shock, we were unable to demonstrate any transpulmonary gradient or biochemical modification of enkephalins across the lungs (Watson et al, 1986).

Dynorphins

A third class of EOPs has been described more recently — the dynorphins ('dynos' is Greek for 'power'). These are variable sized peptides containing the leu-enkephalin sequence at the N-terminus, and are among the most potent opioid peptides so far described. They are derived from a separate large precursor peptide — proenkephalin B (Fig. 11.1), and dynorphin immunoreactivity is present in a number of central nervous system sites (including the hypothalamus, posterior pituitary, brainstem, spinal cord and prevertebral sympathetic ganglia), as well as the myenteric and submucosal enteric ganglia.

The precise role of the dynorphins is not yet known. However, the coexistence of dynorphin and vasopressin in the neurosecretory vesicles of magnocellular neurons projecting from the hypothalamus to the posterior pituitary (Watson et al, 1982; Whitnall et al, 1983) raises the possibility of a neuromodulatory role in the release of vasopressin (Maysinger et al, 1984). The secretion of dynorphin from the posterior pituitary into the circulation is regulated in a manner similar to that of vasopressin (Holaday et al, 1985; Hollt et al, 1981).

MULTIPLE OPIATE RECEPTORS (Table 11.2)

Soon after the identification of stereospecific opiate receptors (Pert & Snyder, 1973), Martin and his colleagues (1976) postulated that the wide variety of effects produced by different opiate agonists could be explained by their preferential binding to at least three distinct opioid receptor subtypes. These were designated μ, κ and σ. Within this framework μ receptors are involved in the production of supraspinal analgesia, respiratory depression, euphoria and physical dependence. The action of κ receptors is to induce spinal analgesia, miosis and sedation. Activation of σ receptors causes dysphoria and hallucinations, as well as respiratory and vasomotor excitation.

Table 11.2 Multiple opioid receptor subtypes

Opioid receptor subtype	Possible physiological function	Agonists	Antagonists
μ (Mu)	Analgesia Bradycardia Euphoria Respiratory depression Miosis Catalepsy Baroflex inhibition Seizure threshold elevation Hypothermia Gastrointestinal motility	Morphine β-Endorphin	Naloxone β-Funaltrexamine Naloxazone
δ (Delta)	Analgesia Respiratory depression Cardiovascular depression Seizure threshold elevation	Leu-Enkephalin D-Ala^2-D-Leu^5 Enkephalin β-Endorphin	ICI 154,129 ICI 174,864 Naloxone, high doses
κ (Kappa)	Spinal Analgesia Miosis	Nalorphine Ethylketocyclazocine Dynorphin	?
σ (Sigma)	Dysphoria (may be the phencyclidine receptor)	Cyclazocine Phencyclidine (nonopioid)	?
ε (Epsilon)	Functions common to μ and δ	β-Endorphin	?

Since all the actions of known opioids cannot be explained within this model, other subspecies of receptor are presumed to exist, including the δ receptor which has been defined in the mouse vas deferens using leu-enkephalin as the ligand (Lord et al, 1977). Moreover, it has been suggested that β-endorphin has its own ε receptor, as well as serving as a good ligand for both μ and δ receptors. The enkephalins have a high affinity for the δ receptors (Lord et al, 1977; Wood et al, 1981), while it has been proposed that dynorphin acts as the native ligand for the κ receptor as well as having an affinity for the δ receptor.

The discovery and further characterisation of endogenous opiate receptors, as well as their naturally occurring ligands, has produced a wealth of new information with important implications for many branches of medicine. Apart from the obvious relevance of these findings to endocrinologists, therapeutic possibilities have arisen in the management of psychiatric illnesses, cerebrovascular accidents, opiate addiction and the control of pain. Moreover, activation of endogenous opioid systems may at least partly explain the mechanism of acupuncture analgesia. In this review, however, we will concentrate on the importance of EOPs in the pathogenesis of shock and consider the therapeutic implications of this involvement.

ROLE OF ENDOGENOUS OPIOID PEPTIDES IN SHOCK

The observation that there are a number of similarities between the signs of narcotic overdose and those of circulatory shock, combined with the knowledge that endogenous opioid mechanisms are activated by stress, prompted Holaday and Faden to investigate the possible involvement of EOPs in the pathogenesis of this condition. They found that the administration of a large bolus dose of naloxone (10 mg/kg) could both prevent and reverse endotoxin-induced hypotension in rats (Holaday & Faden, 1978), and later showed that the dextrorotatory stereosisomer of the drug was ineffective (Faden & Holaday, 1980). (Since only the levorotatory form binds to opiate receptors the latter observation implied that naloxone was acting by competitively displacing EOPs from receptor sites.) Moreover, subsequent studies demonstrated that other opiate antagonists, such as naltrexone, could also produce haemodynamic improvement in experimental shock (Gurll et al, 1982a). Since similar doses of naloxone do not produce a pressor response in the absence of stress (i.e. when opioid systems are known to be quiescent), these findings imply that endogenous opioids are at least partly responsible for cardiovascular depression in shock.

This hypothesis is consistent with studies showing that EOPs can cause hypotension when administered centrally (Florez & Mediavilla, 1977; Laubie et al, 1977; Moss & Scarpelli, 1981; Petty & DeJong, 1982; Sitsen et al, 1982) or systemically (Lemaire et al, 1978). It is also compatible with the presumed role of these peptides in the regulation of autonomic function as outlined above.

β-endorphin

Because β-endorphin is released from the pituitary together with ACTH in response to stress (Rossier et al, 1977; Guillemin et al, 1977), and since systemic administration of this peptide can cause hypotension (Lemaire et al, 1978), it was initially suggested that increased plasma levels of β-endorphin might be contributing to cardiovascular depression in shock. Certainly circulating levels of β-endorphin-like immunoreactivity are elevated in experimental shock (Carr et al, 1982; Faden et al, 1981a; Thijs et al, 1983; Hinshaw et al, 1984) and human sepsis (Hinds et al, 1985; Weissglas, 1983), although similar increases have been described in post-cardiac surgery patients who were not shocked (Hinds et al, 1985), as well as during labour (Thomas et al, 1982), in response to surgery (McIntosh et al, 1985; Smith et al, 1985) and in hypoxaemic intensive care patients (Yanagida & Corssen, 1981). Moreover, animal studies have shown that adrenalectomised rats, in which plasma β-endorphin is elevated, are sensitised to shock hypotension and yet fail to respond to naloxone (Holaday et al, 1983a), while studies on isolated papillary muscles suggest that circulating β-endorphin is unlikely to be responsible for myocardial depression in shock (Weissglas, 1983). It seems unlikely, therefore, that increases in circulating levels of β-endorphin are an important cause of cardiovascular depression in shock.

Nevertheless, in view of the distribution of β-endorphin-containing neurones outlined previously as well as the cardiovascular depression which follows injection of β-endorphin into the central nervous system (Laubie et al, 1977; Moss & Scarpelli, 1981; Petty & DeJong, 1982; Sitsen et al, 1982) it remains possible that increases in β-endorphin activity within the central nervous system may contribute to the haemodynamic disturbance in shock.

Enkephalins

Circulating immunoreactive met-enkephalin levels have also been shown to be elevated in endotoxin shock (Evans et al, 1984a; Watson et al, 1986) and in response to haemorrhage (Farrell et al, 1983; Bruckner et al, 1984). The close relationship between the enkephalins and the sympathetic nervous system described previously, as well as the localisation of enkephalins in central areas involved in the control of autonomic function, together with the hypotension which can follow central administration (Florez & Mediavilla, 1977), suggest that these EOPs may be of particular importance in the cardiovascular manifestations of shock. Moreover, there is some evidence that circulating enkephalins can produce haemodynamic effects. Hanbauer and colleagues (1982), for example, have shown that in the anaesthetised dog depleted of adrenal catecholamines by reserpine pretreatment, splanchnic nerve stimulation releases adrenal enkephalins and that this is associated with a reduction in arterial pressure which can be reversed by naloxone. Furthermore, it has been suggested that circulating enkephalins can modulate the effects of other pressor substances since as little as 10^{-7} M enkephalin can antagonise the chronotropic effect of noradrenaline on isolated rat atria (Eiden & Ruth, 1982).

Dynorphins

Although the dynorphins are probably involved in central cardiovascular regulation, the exact nature of their actions in shock is unclear. For example, microinjection of dynorphin into the preoptic nucleus of the rat hypothalamus produces significant cardiovascular depression (Feuerstein & Faden, 1984), and following haemorrhage, dynorphin immunoreactivity is reduced in brain nuclei involved in cardiovascular regulation (Feuerstein et al, 1984b). It has been suggested therefore that inhibition of vasopressin release by dynorphin is reduced in response to haemorrhage, and that this represents one of the mechanisms for the maintenance of blood pressure in shock (Feuerstein et al, 1984c).

Dynorphins may also act at peripheral sites since the administration of dynorphin into the coronary arteries of dogs produces a depression of left ventricular contractile force (Caffrey et al, 1985), and in pithed rats intravenous dynorphin induces a fall in heart rate (Gautret & Schmitt, 1985). Other studies suggest that dynorphin may act presynaptically on neuronal κ receptors in blood vessels, thereby inhibiting noradrenaline release and producing vasodilatation (Sun & Zang, 1985).

OPIATE ANTAGONISTS IN EXPERIMENTAL SHOCK

A large number of studies have now been published which confirm haemodynamic improvement following administration of opiate antagonists in a variety of models of septic (Reynolds et al, 1980; Evans et al, 1984b; Raymond et al, 1981; Gahhos et al, 1982; Gurll et al, 1981; Hinshaw et al, 1984; Fettman et al, 1984; Schrauwen & Houvenaghel, 1985), haemorrhagic (Vargish et al, 1980; Faden & Holaday, 1979; Gurll et al, 1982a, c; Curtis & Lefer, 1980), spinal (Holaday & Faden, 1980) and other forms of circulatory shock (for example anaphylaxis, splanchnic mesenteric arterial occlusion, burns) (Holaday, 1983).

The efficacy of naloxone in endotoxin shock in dogs was first demonstrated by Reynolds and his colleagues in 1980. They showed that naloxone attenuated the decrease in left ventricular contractility and mean arterial pressure, as well as reversing the decline in cardiac output and stroke volume. Since heart rate, pulmonary artery pressures and total peripheral resistance were unchanged, these findings suggested that the haemodynamic improvement following naloxone was mediated primarily by an improvement in myocardial contractility. Using a canine model of severe, persistent endotoxin shock it has been shown that naloxone produces only limited and transient haemodynamic improvement in the absence of volume replacement. When the circulating volume was expanded in both control and treated animals, however, significant and sustained increases in mean arterial pressure, cardiac output and maximum rate of rise of left ventricular pressure were observed in those animals given naloxone; calculated total peripheral resistance was essentially unchanged. These findings therefore also suggested a primary myocardial effect of naloxone (Evans et al, 1984b). Similarly, in dogs subjected to acute haemorrhage, naloxone increased cardiac output and mean arterial pressure by improving myocardial performance (Vargish et al, 1980). More recent studies have also confirmed that naloxone increases myocardial contractility in experimental shock (Lechner, Gurll & Reynolds, 1985b, c).

As well as haemodynamic improvement a number of other potentially beneficial effects of naloxone administration in shock have been described. Thus in mice, naloxone prevented the decrease in body temperature, circulating white cells and platelets which normally follows endotoxin administration in this species (Wright & Weller, 1980), while in endotoxaemic dogs naloxone significantly attenuated hypotension, haemoconcentration, acidosis and hypoglycaemia (Raymond et al, 1981). In cats subjected to haemorrhage naloxone not only produced haemodynamic improvement but also reduced the release of lysosomal enzymes and decreased circulating levels of myocardial depressant factor (Curtis & Lefer, 1980). Rees and colleagues (1982) showed that naloxone reversed gastric epithelial hypoxia and prevented the development of systemic acidosis in dogs infused with live E. coli. Following acute spinal cord injury naloxone significantly reduced subsequent neurological impairment (Faden et al, 1981b), possibly by antagonising the effects of local increases in opioid activity on blood flow within the cord, as well as by improving systemic blood pressure.

In some studies, however, the response to naloxone has been unimpressive (Thijs et al, 1983; Carr et al, 1982; Gahhos et al, 1982), in others no improvement occurred (Gurll et al, 1982b) and in some the effects were detrimental (Hinshaw et al, 1984; Schrauwen & Houvenaghel, 1985; Traverso et al, 1985). Moreover, naloxone is most efficacious when given in the early stages of experimental shock (Holaday, 1983) and most studies have only evaluated its cardiovascular effects during this period.

It must also be appreciated that the beneficial effects of naloxone in shock are very dose-dependent and that, although some cardiovascular improvement may occur following as little as 0.1 mg/kg, optimal effects are seen when doses of more than 1 mg/kg are administered (Faden & Holaday, 1980; Gurll et al, 1982c). Thus, for example, Gurll et al (1982c) showed that low doses of naloxone (0.5 mg/kg) produced little cardiovascular improvement and did not influence survival time, whereas at higher doses (1 or 2 mg/kg) there was a dose-related haemodynamic response and prolonged survival time. Moreover, there are also important species differences in the optimal dose of naloxone in shock. Both acidosis and a reduction in body temperature (Gurll et al, 1982b) can inhibit the cardiovascular effects of naloxone, and this may partly explain the poor response to opiate antagonists administered in the later stages of shock (Gahhos et al, 1982).

Experimental data concerning the effects of naloxone administration on survival in shock are conflicting (Hinshaw et al, 1984). Although a number of studies have demonstrated increased survival times in naloxone-treated animals (Reynolds et al, 1980; Raymond et al, 1981; Gurll et al, 1981; Gurll et al, 1982a, c; Faden & Holaday, 1979; Vargish et al, 1980) others have failed to show improvements in survival (Koyama et al, 1983), and in some studies naloxone even decreased short-term survival (Fettman et al, 1984; Schrauwen & Houvenaghel, 1985; Traverso et al, 1985). Moreover, there are considerable species differences in both the haemodynamic responses to naloxone administration and its effects on survival. Thus, Hinshaw and his colleagues (1984) found that in dogs infused with live *E. coli* naloxone prevented severe haemorrhagic necrosis of the gastrointestinal tract and increased permanent survival rates, whereas in baboons (also infused with live *E. coli*) naloxone precipitated marked vasoconstriction and all the treated animals died within 42 hours.

SITES AND MECHANISMS OF ACTION OF OPIATE ANTAGONISTS IN SHOCK

Most of the evidence suggests that activation of endogenous opioid systems within the central nervous system is the most important cause of cardiovascular depression in shock and that the haemodynamic effects of opiate antagonists are predominantly centrally mediated (Holaday, 1984). Thus Janssen & Lutherer (1980) have shown that ventriculocisternal administration of naloxone protects against severe hypotension during endotoxin shock in dogs, while Holaday and his colleagues have demonstrated that the low doses of naloxone which are beneficial when administered centrally are ineffective when given intravenously to rats subjected to endotoxic, haemorrhagic or spinal shock (Holaday, 1984; Holaday & Faden, 1980). Since micro-injections of D-Ala-D-leu-enkephalin (a relatively selective δ agonist) into the third ventricle of anaesthetised rats produced profound hypotension without significant effects on heart rate, whereas morphine (a μ agonist) produced only profound bradycardia when injected into the fourth ventricle, it has been suggested that opioid effects on the hypothalamus during shock may involve enkephalin actions at δ receptors (Holaday, 1982). Others, however, consider that these agonists are only relatively selective for the δ receptor and that their cardiovascular effects may be mediated by activity at μ receptors (Faden & Feuerstein, 1983). In addition, microinjections of δ-selective agonists into the anterior hypothalamic region of unanaesthetised animals can produce a hypertensive response (Pfeiffer et al, 1983). The suggestion that δ receptors are involved in the cardiovascular manifestations of shock is supported, however, by studies investigating the haemodynamic response to a variety of selective opiate antagonists (see below). It is postulated, therefore, that naloxone releases autonomic centres within the brain from inhibitory tone by antagonising endogenous opioid activity at the δ receptor. (Since naloxone has a twenty- to thirty-fold greater affinity for the μ than the δ receptor (Chang & Cuatrecasas, 1979), this may partly explain why such large doses of naloxone are required to produce beneficial effects in shock.)

A number of studies provide further evidence that the cardiovascular effects of opiate antagonists are at least partly due to a centrally mediated increase in autonomic outflow and sympathomedullary activity. For example, both intravenous and intracisternal administration of naloxone can increase preganglionic splanchnic nerve activity (Manugian et al, 1981), while the pressor response to naloxone in stressed cats can be attenuated by cutting the splanchnic nerves (Dashwood & Feldberg, 1979). Moreover, the haemodynamic improvement which follows naloxone administration in feline endotoxin shock is associated with an increase in preganglionic splanchnic nerve activity (Koyama et al, 1983).

Both direct and indirect evidence suggests that the pressor response to opiate antagonists is mediated via an increase in sympathomedullary activity. For example, α-adrenergic blockade attenuates the pressor response to naloxone administration in haemorrhagic shock (Schadt & York, 1982) and adrenalectomy, as well as selective adrenal demedullectomy, can abolish the beneficial effects of naloxone in endotoxin (Holaday et al, 1983a) and haemorrhagic (Patten et al, 1983) shock. Moreover, increases in plasma levels of noradrenaline, but not adrenaline, have been demonstrated in response to naloxone in rabbits subjected to haemorrhage (Schadt & Gaddis, 1985) (suggesting an increase in peripheral sympathetic nerve activity), while in human septic shock, naloxone administration significantly increased circulating adrenaline levels (Hughes, 1984).

Conversely, however, Feuerstein and colleagues (1981) failed to demonstrate any relationship between plasma levels of dopamine, noradrenaline or adrenaline and naloxone's haemodynamic effects in a rat model of haemorrhagic shock. In feline spinal injury only changes in plasma dopamine levels correlated with the rise in mean arterial pressure which followed naloxone administration (Faden et al, 1981c). Moreover, others have shown that naloxone (in doses which caused a pressor response) did not further augment the already elevated catecholamine levels in endotoxaemic rats (Bernton, Long & Holaday, 1985), or in canine haemorrhagic shock (Lechner, Gurll & Reynolds, 1985a). In an uncontrolled study in human septic shock naloxone did not further increase the elevated plasma catecholamine levels (Bonnet et al, 1985).

It has been suggested, therefore, that naloxone acts peripherally in shock to enhance the effects of existing adrenergic discharge, rather than by increasing sympathoadrenal activity (Lechner et al, 1985a, b)—a theory which is attractive in as much as it provides an explanation for the persistent hypotension which may occur in shock despite markedly elevated catecholamine levels. The same group have also produced evidence that this effect is exerted primarily by interaction at cardiac opiate receptors (Lechner et al, 1985c).

Finally, in spinal shock naloxone may improve cardiovascular function via a different mechanism since, in the rat model of spinal shock employed by Holaday & Faden (1980), the cervical spinal cord is severed, interrupting supraspinal regulation of the sympathetic nervous system. In these circumstances it is suggested that endogenous opioids act centrally to increase parasympathetic outflow and that this, combined with the loss of sympathetic tone, causes cardiovascular depression which can be reversed by naloxone (Faden et al, 1980).

In conclusion, it remains unclear which of the EOPs is primarily responsible for cardiovascular depression in shock and the site, or sites, at which naloxone exerts its beneficial effects have not been precisely established. Nevertheless, the various suggested mechanisms are by no means mutually exclusive and the discrepancies between experimental studies may be explained by species differences, the influence of anaesthesia, and the aetiology of the shock. In summary, therefore, it seems likely that naloxone can act both centrally and peripherally to antagonise opioid-induced inhibition of sympathomedullary outflow, and to enhance the actions of catecholamines at receptor sites.

OPIATE-STEROID INTERACTIONS IN SHOCK

The role of large doses of corticosteroids in the treatment of shock remains controversial (Kass, 1984). One possible beneficial action of glucocorticoids in shock could be to suppress β-endorphin synthesis and/or release via a negative feedback mechanism (Simantov, 1979). The resulting reduction in β-endorphin activity might then reduce the endogenous opioid component in shock, thus leaving naloxone with little opioid effect to antagonise. Evidence for this antagonism of naloxone's efficacy by high doses of steroids has come from Lutz et al (1981) and Vargish et al (1983) in canine haemorrhagic shock as well as Peters et al (1981) in septic patients. More recently, however, others have demonstrated that steroids enhance the beneficial effects of naloxone in porcine septic shock (Weissglas et al, 1982), in canine hypovolaemic shock (Beamer & Vargish, 1986) and in patients with septic shock (Hughes, 1984). Furthermore, relatively low doses of hydrocortisone restore the therapeutic effects of naloxone in adrenalectomised dogs with haemorrhagic shock (Patton et al, 1983).

It is important to note, however, that the dosage and timing of administration of steroids used in the above studies varied considerably, and discrepancies in results may be related to a higher-dose suppressant effect and a lower-dose potentiation of naloxone's therapeutic action. Moreover, the initial assumption that β-endorphin plays a primary role in shock pathophysiology (Holaday & Faden, 1978) must be re-evaluated in the light of more recent work (see above).

CLINICAL EXPERIENCE

Despite these generally encouraging experimental findings, and the increased understanding of the mechanisms of action of opiate antagonists in shock, the role of these agents in the clinical management of this condition remains unclear.

A number of uncontrolled studies (Peters et al, 1981; Groeger et al, 1983) as well as some early anecdotal reports (Tiengo, 1980; Dirksen et al, 1980; Wright et al, 1980) have suggested that naloxone can produce haemodynamic improvement in some patients with septic shock provided that it is administered relatively early (Groeger et al, 1983) and that there is no chronic adrenocortical suppression (Peters et al, 1981). In these studies naloxone was given in relatively low doses (0.02–0.3 mg/kg) compared to those which have been found to produce optimal cardiovascular improvement and increase survival in animal studies. In another uncontrolled study, therefore, Rock and his colleagues (1985) administered much larger doses of naloxone (increments of 0.1, 0.2, 0.4, 0.8 and 1.6 mg/kg to a maximum total dose of 3.1 mg/kg) to patients in established septic shock who had failed to respond to volume replacement, appropriate antibiotics and inotropic support. They concluded that naloxone did not reliably improve blood pressure and that it could cause significant adverse effects. Although it should be noted that in this study naloxone was administered on average 20 hours after the onset of hypotension, it does suggest that naloxone is ineffective in just that group of patients who are in greatest need of improvements in therapy. A more recent uncontrolled study (Bonnet et al, 1985) also found that lower doses of naloxone (0.01–0.1 mg/kg) failed to modify cardiac index, blood pressure, heart rate or systemic vascular resistance in patients with septic shock.

In a complicated, randomised, double-blind study with matched groups, Hughes (1984) compared conventional treatment with low-dose naloxone, methylprednisolone or combined naloxone and methylprednisolone. In this study blood pressure increased significantly only when naloxone treatment was combined with steroids. More recently naloxone was compared with placebo in a prospective, double-blind, randomised study in patients with septic shock. Mean systolic blood pressure increased to a similar extent in both groups and survival rates were not significantly different at 48 hours and seven days after treatment (DeMaria et al, 1985). Once again, however, the doses of naloxone used (0.4–1.2 mg intravenously) were considerably less than those shown to be beneficial in animal studies.

Not only are the results of these studies unimpressive, but the introduction of naloxone into routine clinical practice is further inhibited by its potential for producing a number of adverse effects. Most importantly, naloxone administration reverses opiate (and natural) analgesia and consequently some studies have specifically excluded patients receiving narcotics (DeMaria et al, 1985; Rock et al, 1985; Groeger et al, 1983). Naloxone treatment may also be associated with an analeptic effect and, in one patient with septic shock, apparently precipitated a grand mal seizure (Rock et al, 1985). Other reported complications of naloxone therapy, presumably related to activation of the sympathetic nervous system, have included pulmonary oedema (Taff, 1983; Rock et al, 1985; Flacke et al, 1977) and ventricular fibrillation (Cuss et al, 1984), as well as hypertension and dysrhythmias (Azar & Turndorf, 1979). Unexpected hypotension has also been attributed to the use of this agent (Rock et al, 1985). Nevertheless, a large, prospective, placebo-controlled, randomised, double-blind investigation of the effects of larger doses of naloxone (for example 1 mg/kg, possibly followed by a continuous intravenous infusion) in shock is required before a final conclusion can be reached. More detailed studies of the effects of this agent on cardiovascular and respiratory function in shocked patients, as well as its influence on survival, are also required.

ALTERNATIVES TO NALOXONE

In view of the complications of naloxone treatment, in particular reversal of analgesia, alternative means of manipulating the endogenous opioid system in shock are being investigated. Interesting possibilities include the use of selective or partial opiate antagonists and thyrotrophin releasing hormone (TRH).

Selective opiate receptor antagonists

The recent development of more selective opioid receptor agonists and antagonists (Corbett et al, 1984) has led to further clarification of the receptor types responsible for the cardiovascular changes seen in shock (Curtis & Lefer, 1983a). For example, the short-acting δ antagonist ICI 154,129 (a synthetic enkephalin analogue) reverses endotoxic shock in rats following intravenous administration in doses that do not antagonise morphine analgesia (Holaday et al, 1982b). Moreover, the selective μ antagonist, naloxazone (Holaday et al, 1983b), failed to reverse hypotension at doses that significantly antagonised morphine analgesia.

These findings, together with other evidence discussed previously, suggest that endogenous opioids evoke their cardiovascular responses via an action at central δ opiate receptors. However, it is worth noting that other receptors (i.e. κ) have been implicated in the opioid component of spinal shock (Faden et al, 1985) and that

κ receptor agonists have a beneficial effect in haemorrhagic shock (Curtis & Lefer, 1983b). Also, prior occupancy of the μ receptor by irreversible μ antagonists such as naloxazone or β-funaltrexamine, while without effect by themselves in shock, prevented the usual therapeutic actions of subsequent naloxone or ICI M154,129 (D'Amato & Holaday, 1984; Holaday et al, 1983b). Similarly, pretreatment with the κ receptor agonist Dynorphin 1–13 is without effect upon endotoxic shock in the rat and yet prevents the pressor effects of both naloxone and ICI 174,864 (a putative δ receptor antagonist) (Long et al, 1984). These results indicate that certain κ agonists and μ antagonists may selectively alter the actions of δ receptor antagonists, suggesting that μ, κ and δ binding sites may be part of the same opiate receptor macromolecule that functionally interacts through allosteric mechanisms.

Opiate agonist–antagonists (partial opiate agonists)
A further alternative to naloxone in the treatment of shock is the use of opiate agonist-antagonist drugs — a title that has evolved to describe the complex spectrum of effects caused by the different affinity and activity of these drugs at the various opiate receptors. Thus some drugs are competitive antagonists at one receptor, but are agonists at others, and an ideal drug for use in shock might combine μ, or possibly κ, receptor mediated analgesia and sedation with the cardiovascular benefits of δ receptor antagonism.

Meptazinol (a partial agonist with relative selectivity for μ receptor sites) has been shown to elevate blood pressure in rats and cats with haemorrhagic shock (Chance et al, 1985) in a comparable manner to naloxone; this effect appears to be due to an increase in peripheral resistance as cardiac output is not significantly changed. Likewise, in anaphylactic (Paciorek et al, 1985) and endotoxic (Paciorek & Todd, 1982) shock in rats, meptazinol increased blood pressure to a similar or greater degree than did naloxone. It seems likely that the pressor effect of meptazinol in anaphylactic shock is mediated via the sympathetic nervous system, since it can be blocked by either reserpine or phentolamine pretreatment (Paciorek et al, 1985). In human relapsing fever treated with tetracycline, meptazinol reduced the clinical severity of the Jarisch-Herxheimer reaction (which is presumably due to the release of endotoxin-like substances), particularly its febrile component, and also diminished the leucocytosis and prevented rises in respiratory rate and pulse rate. Naloxone and high-dose methylprednisolone had no effect (Teklu et al, 1983).

In the case of nalbuphine (a competitive antagonist of μ receptors and a partial agonist at κ and σ receptors) a dose-dependent improvement in mean arterial pressure, cardiac output, left ventricular contractility, heart rate and survival of dogs subjected to haemorrhagic shock was achieved with the intravenous administration of 0.5–4.0 mg/kg; at the latter dose the response was maximal. Larger doses, however, were found to be detrimental (Hunt et al, 1984). In hypovolaemic rats, nalbuphine (1–5 mg/kg) improved both cardiac function and mean arterial pressure (McKenzie et al, 1985).

Thyrotrophin releasing hormone (TRH)
Since its isolation in 1969, the tripeptide TRH has been shown to be widely distributed within the central nervous system and in peripheral organs. It has numerous pharmaco-

logical actions including potent actions on autonomic, somatic and behavioural systems which are independent of its effects on the pituitary–thyroid axis.

The ability of TRH to antagonize certain of the physiological actions of the EOPs, combined with its total lack of effect on opiate analgesia and its failure to bind to opioid receptors, has led to its use in experimental shock as a 'physiological antagonist' of opioid effects. Like naloxone, pharmacological doses of TRH improve blood pressure and, in some cases, survival in septic and haemorrhagic shock in a variety of different species (Holaday, 1983; Reynolds et al, 1982; Gurll et al, 1982d; Sugiura et al, 1986). The beneficial effects of naloxone and TRH in shock are also additive, even when each is given at an optimal or supraoptimal dose (Holaday & Faden, 1981). Unlike naloxone, however, TRH is also effective in a variety of shock models that do not appear to respond to opiate antagonists, including shock produced by leukotrienes (Lux et al, 1983a), lipoxygenase (Faden et al, 1983b), platelet activating factor (Feuerstein et al, 1984a) and systemic anaphylaxis (Lux et al, 1983b).

TRH is also beneficial in treating traumatic spinal cord injury in the cat, and is superior both to naloxone and to high-dose corticosteroids (Faden et al, 1983a). In this model, TRH improved blood pressure, reduced the severity and incidence of pulmonary oedema and decreased mortality and chronic neurological deficit (Faden et al, 1981d).

The beneficial effects of TRH appear to be largely centrally mediated, possibly via regulation of sympathomedullary outflow (Holaday et al, 1982a), since doses of TRH that have little or no effect when given systemically reverse shock following central intraventricular administration (Lux et al, 1983a; Feuerstein et al, 1984a) and destruction of central autonomic pathways blocks its therapeutic action (Feuerstein et al, 1983a). The effect of TRH on the cardiovascular system seems to result mainly from an increase in total peripheral resistance, rather than from improved cardiac function (Zaloga et al, 1984).

Knowledge of the peripheral mechanisms by which the central actions of TRH produce a pressor response remains incomplete, although data thus far suggest several possible mechanisms. For example, TRH administration produces significant increases in circulating catecholamines (Lux et al, 1983a), as well as a pressor response antagonised by adrenergic blocking agents (Feuerstein et al, 1983b). However, intravenous TRH can also increase blood pressure and heart rate independently of sympathomedullary activity (Holaday & Faden, 1983; Holaday et al, 1982a; Zaloga et al, 1982), and others have shown the cardiovascular effects of intracerebroventricular TRH to be relatively unaffected by treatment with phenoxybenzamine or ganglion blockers or pretreatment with reserpine (Horita et al, 1979). Moreover, in endotoxaemia in rats TRH failed to further increase plasma levels of catecholamines at doses that caused a pressor response (Bernton et al, 1985; Long et al, 1983). Also, TRH-stimulated vasopressin release (Horita et al, 1979; Weitzman et al, 1979) may well be compatible with the observed increase in systemic vascular resistance, without ionotropic or chronotropic effects (Zaloga et al, 1984). Finally, it has been suggested that many of the pharmacological effects of TRH can be explained by widespread interactions of TRH with cholinergic systems, and that TRH may regulate the excitability of central cholinergic neurones (Yarbrough, 1983).

Controlled clinical studies evaluating the efficacy of TRH in human acute spinal cord injury are now under way, as are clinical studies of new, more potent, longer lasting TRH analogues, which may, in due course, replace TRH in the treatment of shock (Faden & Jacobs, 1985).

CONCLUSION

Since Holaday's initial work, subsequent studies have considerably enhanced our understanding of the mechanisms involved in the pathogenesis of shock. Nevertheless, at present, it appears that naloxone is simply another rather more dangerous and less predictable means of supporting cardiovascular function in shock. Moreover, there is only limited information concerning its cardiorespiratory effects in man, no comparative studies with currently available inotropes have been performed, and neither the indications for its use in shock nor the optimum dose have been established. Finally, the influence of naloxone therapy on survival has not yet been investigated in man. The routine use of naloxone in the treatment of shock cannot therefore be recommended until further controlled studies have resolved some of these questions. On the basis of anecdotal reports (Furman et al, 1984) it might be argued that it is worthwhile giving naloxone when other measures have failed, even though it seems that naloxone is least effective when administered late in the evolution of shock. In the future, the use of selective opiate antagonists, partial agonists, or TRH may prove to be a more satisfactory means of antagonising the endogenous opioid system in shock.

REFERENCES

Azar I, Turndorf H 1979 Severe hypertension and multiple atrial premature contractions following naloxone administration. Anesthesia and Analgesia 58: 524–525
Beamer K C, Vargish T 1986 Effect of methylprednisolone on naloxone's haemodynamic response in canine hypovolaemic shock. Critical Care Medicine 14: 115–119
Bernton E W, Long J B, Holaday J W 1985 Opioids and neuropeptides: mechanisms in circulatory shock. Federation Proceedings 44: 290–299
Bonnet F, Bilaine J, Lhoste F, Mankikian B, Kerdelhue B, Rapin M 1985 Naloxone therapy of human septic shock. Critical Care Medicine 13: 972–975
Bruckner U B, Lang R E, Ganten D 1984 Release of opioid peptides in canine hemorrhagic hypotension: effects of naloxone. Research in Experimental Medicine 184: 171–178
Caffrey J L, Gaugl J F, Jones C E 1985 Local endogenous opiate activity in dog myocardium: receptor blockade with naloxone. American Journal of Physiology 248: H382–388
Carr D B, Bergland R, Hamilton A, et al 1982 Endotoxin-stimulated opioid peptide secretion: two secretory pools and feedback control in vivo. Science 217: 845–848
Chance E, Paciorek P M, Todd M H, Waterfall J F 1985 Comparison of the cardiovascular effects of meptazinol and naloxone following hemorrhagic shock in rats and cats. British Journal of Pharmacology 86: 45–53
Chang K J, Cuatrecasas P 1979 Multiple opiate receptors: enkephalins and morphine bind to receptors of different specificity. Journal of Biological Chemistry 254: 2610–2618
Comb M, Seeburg P H, Adelman J, Eiden L, Herbert E 1982 Primary structure of the human met- and leu-enkephalin precursor and its mRNA. Nature 295: 663–666
Corbett A D, Gillan M G C, Kosterlitz H W, McKnight A I, Paterson S J, Robson L E 1984 Selectivities of opioid peptide analogues as agonists and antagonists at the δ-receptor. British Journal of Pharmacology 83: 271–279
Corder R, Mason D F J, Perrett D, et al 1982 Simultaneous release of neurotensin, somatostatin, enkephalins and catecholamines from perfused cat adrenal glands. Neuropeptides 3: 9–17
Curtis M T, Lefer A M 1980 Protective actions of naloxone in hemorrhagic shock. American Journal of Physiology 239: H416–H421
Curtis M T, Lefer A M 1983a Actions of opiate antagonists with selective receptor interactions in hemorrhagic shock. Circulatory Shock 10: 131–145
Curtis M T, Lefer A M 1983b Effectiveness of ethylketocyclazocine in hemorrhagic shock. Advances in Shock Research 10: 101–109

Cuss F M, Colaco C B, Baron J H 1984 Cardiac arrest after reversal of effects of opiates with naloxone. British Medical Journal 288: 363–364

D'Amato R J, Holaday J W 1984 Multiple opiate receptors in endotoxic shock: evidence for delta involvement and mu-delta interactions in vivo. Proceedings of the National Academy of Science 81: 2898–2901

Dashwood M R, Feldberg W 1979 Central inhibitory effect of released opiate peptides on adrenal medulla, revealed by naloxone in the cat. Journal of Physiology 290: 22P–23P

DeMaria A, Craven D E, Heffernan J J, McIntosh T K, Grindlinger G A, McCabe W R 1985 Naloxone versus placebo in treatment of septic shock. Lancet i: 1363–1365

Dirksen R, Otten M H, Wood G J, et al 1980 Naloxone in shock. Lancet ii: 1360–1361

Eiden L E, Ruth J A 1982 Enkephalins modulate the responsiveness of rat atria in vitro to norepinephrine. Peptides 3: 475–478

Evans S F, Medbak S, Hinds C J, Tomlin S J, Varley J, Rees L H 1984a Plasma levels and biochemical characterization of circulating metenkephalin in canine endotoxin shock. Life Sciences 34: 1481–1486

Evans S F, Hinds C J, Varley J G 1984b Effects of intravascular volume expansion on the cardiovascular response to naloxone in a canine model of severe endotoxin shock. British Journal of Pharmacology 83: 443–448

Faden A I, Feuerstein G 1983 Hypothalamic regulation of the cardiovascular and respiratory systems: Role of specific opiate receptors. British Journal of Pharmacology 79: 997–1002

Faden A I, Holaday J W 1979 Opiate antagonists: a role in the treatment of hypovolaemic shock. Science 205: 317–318

Faden A I, Holaday J W 1980 Naloxone treatment of endotoxin shock: stereospecificity of physiologic and pharmacologic effects in the rat. Journal of Pharmacology and Experimental Therapeutics 212: 441–447

Faden A I, Jacobs T P 1985 Effect of TRH analogs on neurologic recovery after experimental spinal trauma. Neurology 35: 1331–1334

Faden A I, Jacobs T P, Holaday J W 1980 Endorphin-parasympathetic interaction in spinal shock. Journal of Autonomic Nervous System 2: 295–304

Faden A I, Jacobs T P, Mougey E, Holaday J W 1981a Endorphins in experimental spinal injury: therapeutic effect of naloxone. Annals of Neurology 10: 326–332

Faden A I, Jacobs T P, Holaday J W 1981b Opiate antagonist improves neurologic recovery after spinal injury. Science 211: 493–494

Faden A I, Jacobs T P, Feuerstein G, Holaday J W 1981c Dopamine partially mediates the cardiovascular effects of naloxone after spinal injury. Brain Research 213: 415–421

Faden A I, Jacobs T P, Holaday J W 1981d Thyrotropin releasing hormone improves neurological recovery after spinal trauma in cats. New England Journal of Medicine 305: 1063–1067

Faden A I, Jacobs T P, Smith M T, Holaday J W 1983a Comparison of thyrotropin releasing hormone (TRH), naloxone and dexamethasone treatments in experimental spinal injury. Neurology 33: 673–678

Faden A I, Feuerstein G, Hayes E, Lux W E 1983b Leukotrienes and anaphylactic shock: a therapeutic role for thyrotropin releasing hormone. Circulatory Shock 10: 246

Faden A I, Molineaux C J, Rosenberger J G, Jacobs T P, Cox B M 1985 Increased dynorphin immunoreactivity in spinal cord after traumatic injury. Regulatory Peptides 11: 35–41

Farrell L D, Harrison T S, Demers L M 1983 Immunoreactive metenkephalin in the canine adrenal: response to acute hypovolaemic stress. Proceedings of the Society for Experimental Biology and Medicine 173: 515–518

Fettman M, Hand M, Chandrasena L, et al 1984 Naloxone therapy in awake endotoxemic yucatan minipigs. Journal of Surgical Research 37: 208–225

Feuerstein G, Faden A I 1984 Cardiovascular effects of Dynorphin A (1–8), Dynorphin A (1–13) and Dynorphin A (1–17) microinjected into the preoptic medialis nucleus of the rat. Neuropeptides 5: 295–298

Feuerstein G, Chiueh C C, Kopin I J 1981 Effect of naloxone on the cardiovascular and sympathetic response to hypovolaemic hypotension in the rat. European Journal of Pharmacology 75: 65–69

Feuerstein G, Zukowska-Grojec Z, Bayorh M, Kopin I J, Faden A I 1983a Leukotriene D4-induced hypotension is reversed by thyrotropin releasing hormone. Prostaglandins 26: 711–724

Feuerstein G, Hassen A H, Faden A I 1983b TRH: Cardiovascular and sympathetic modulation in brain nuclei of the rat. Peptides 4: 617–620

Feuerstein G, Lux W E, Snyder F, Ezra D, Faden A I 1984a Hypotension produced by platelet-activating factor is reversed by thyrotropin releasing hormone. Circulatory Shock 13: 255–260

Feuerstein G, Molineaux C J, Rosenberger J G, Zerbe R L, Cox B M, Faden A I 1984b Vasopressin and opioid peptide relationships in discrete cardiovascular nuclei of rats exposed to hypovolaemic hypotension. Society for Neuroscience Abstracts 10: 301

Feuerstein G, Molineaux C J, Rosenberger J G, Zerbe R L, Cox B M, Faden A I 1984c Effect of haemorrhage on vasopressin, dynorphin A, and leu-enkephalin in the hypothalamo-pituitary system of the rat. Clinical and Experimental Hypertension Part A, Theory and Practice 6 (10 & 11): 1973–1976

Flacke J W, Flacke W E, Williams G D 1977 Acute pulmonary oedema following naloxone reversal of high-dose morphine anesthesia. Anesthesiology 47: 376–378

Florez J, Mediavilla A 1977 Respiratory and cardiovascular effects of met-enkephalin applied to the ventral surface of the brain stem. Brain Research 138: 585–590

Furman W L, Menke J A, Barson W J, Miller R R 1984 Continuous naloxone infusion in two neonates with septic shock. Journal of Paediatrics 105: 649–651

Gaddis R R, Dixon W R 1982 Modulation of peripheral adrenergic neurotransmission by methionine-enkephalin. Journal of Pharmacology and Experimental Therapeutics 221: 282–288

Gahhos F M, Chiu R C J, Hinchey E J, Richards G K 1982 Endorphins in septic shock. Archives of Surgery 117: 1053–1057

Gautret B, Schmitt H 1985 Central and peripheral sites for cardiovascular actions of dynorphin (1–13) in rats. European Journal of Pharmacology 111: 263–266

Govoni S, Hanbauer I, Hexum T D, Yang H-Y T, Kelly G D, Costa E 1981 In vivo characterization of the mechanisms that secrete enkephalin-like peptides stored in dog adrenal medulla. Neuropharmacology 20: 639–645

Groeger J S, Carlon G C, Howland W S 1983 Naloxone in septic shock. Critical Care Medicine 11: 650–654

Guillemin R, Vargo T, Rossier J, et al 1977 Beta-endorphin and adrenocorticotrophin are secreted concomitantly by the pituitary gland. Science 197: 1367–1369

Gurll N J, Reynolds D G, Vargish T, Lutz S A, Ganes E 1981 Primate endotoxemic shock reversed by opiate receptor blockade with naloxone. Physiologist 24: 543

Gurll N J, Reynolds D G, Vargish T, Lechner R 1982a Naltrexone improves survival rate and cardiovascular function in canine hemorrhagic shock. Journal of Pharmacology and Experimental Therapeutics 220: 625–628

Gurll N J, Reynolds D G, Vargish T, Ganes E 1982b Body temperature and acid base balance determine cardiovascular responses to naloxone in primate hemorrhagic shock. Federation Proceedings 41: 1135

Gurll N J, Reynolds D G, Vargish T, Lechner R 1982c Naloxone without transfusion prolongs survival and enhances cardiovascular function in hypovolaemic shock. Journal of Pharmacology and Experimental Therapeutics 220: 621–624

Gurll N J, Reynolds D G, Holaday J W, Ganes E 1982d Improved cardiovascular function and survival using thyrotropin releasing hormone (TRH) in primate haemorrhagic shock. Physiologist 25: 342

Hanbauer I, Govoni S, Majane E A, Yang H-Y T, Costa E 1982 In vivo regulation of the release of met-enkephalin-like peptides from dog adrenal medulla. In: Advances in Biochemical Psychopharmacology. Raven Press, New York 33: 209–215

Hinds C J, Evans S F, Varley J G, Tomlin S, Rees L H 1985 Neuroendocrine and cardiovascular changes in septic shock and after cardiac surgery: Effect of high dose corticosteroid therapy. Circulatory Shock 15: 61–72

Hinshaw L B, Beller B K, Chang A C K, et al 1984 Evaluation of naloxone for therapy of Escherichia coli shock. Archives of Surgery 119: 1410–1418

Holaday J W 1982 Cardiorespiratory effects of μ and δ opiate agonists following third or fourth ventricular injections. Peptides 3: 1023–1029

Holaday J W 1983 Cardiovascular effects of endogenous opiate systems. Annual Review of Pharmacology and Toxicology 23: 541–594

Holaday J W 1984 Neuropeptides in shock and traumatic injury: sites and mechanisms of action. Neuroendocrine Perspectives 3: 161–199

Holaday J W, Faden A I 1978 Naloxone reversal of endotoxic hypotension suggests role of endorphins in shock. Nature 275: 450–451

Holaday J W, Faden A I 1980 Naloxone acts at central opiate receptors to reverse hypotension, hypothermia and hypoventilation in spinal shock. Brain Research 189: 295–299

Holaday J W, Faden A I 1981 Naloxone and thyrotropin releasing hormone have addictive effects in reversing endotoxic shock. In: Advances in Endogenous and Exogenous Opioids (Proceedings of the International Narcotic Research Conference, Kyoto, Japan, 26–30 July). Elsevier Biomedical Press, Amsterdam, pp 367–369

Holaday J W, Faden A I 1983 Thyrotropin releasing hormone: Autonomic effects upon cardiorespiratory function in endotoxic shock. Regulatory Peptides 7: 111–125

Holaday J W, D'Amato R J, Ruvio B A, Faden A I 1982a Action of naloxone and TRH on the autonomic regulation of circulation. In: Advances in Biochemical Psychopharmacology. Raven Press, New York, 33: 353–361

Holaday J W, Ruvio B A, Robles L E, Johnson C E, D'Amato R J 1982b M154, 129, A putative delta antagonist, reverses endotoxic shock without altering morphine analgesia. Life Sciences 31: 2209–2212

Holaday J W, D'Amato R J, Ruvio B A, Feuerstein G, Faden A I 1983a Adrenalectomy blocks pressor
    responses to naloxone in endotoxin shock: evidence for sympathomedullary involvement. Circulatory
    Shock 11: 201–210
Holaday J W, Pasternak G W, D'Amato R J, Ruvio B A, Faden A I 1983b Naloxazone lacks therapeutic
    effects in endotoxic shock yet blocks the effects of naloxone. European Journal of Pharmacology 89:
    293–296
Holaday J W, Black L E, Long J D 1985 Neuropeptides in shock and trauma. In: Endocrine Aspects
    of Acute Illness. Churchill Livingstone, New York, pp 257—284
Hollt V, Haarman I, Seizinger B R, Herz A 1981 Levels of dynorphin- (1–13) immunoreactivity in rat
    neurointermediate pituitaries are concomitantly altered with those of leu-enkephalin and vasopressin
    in response to various endocrine manipulations. Neuroendocrinology 33: 333–339
Horita A, Carino M A, Weitzman R E 1979 Role of catecholamine and vasopressin release in the TRH-
    induced vasopressor response. In: Catecholamines: Basic and Clinical Frontiers. Vol 2. Pergamon Press,
    New York, pp 1140–1142
Hughes G S 1984 Naloxone and methylprednisolone sodium succinate enhance sympathomedullary
    discharge in patients with septic shock. Life Sciences 35: 2319–2326
Hughes J, Smith T W, Kosterlitz H W, Fothergill L, Morgan B A, Morris H R 1975 Identification
    of two related pentapeptides from the brain with potent opiate agonist activity. Nature 258: 577–579
Hunt L B, Gurll N J, Reynolds D G 1984 Dose dependent effects of nalbuphine in canine hemorrhagic
    shock. Circulatory Shock 13: 307–318
Janssen H F, Lutherer L O 1980 Ventriculo-cisternal administration of naloxone protects against severe
    hypotension during endotoxin shock. Brain Research 194: 608–612
Kass E H 1984 High dose corticosteroids for septic shock. New England Journal of Medicine 311: 1178–
    1179
Koyama S, Santiesteban H L, Ammons W S, Manning J W 1983 The effects of naloxone on the peripheral
    sympathetics in cat endotoxin shock. Circulatory Shock 10: 7–13
Kumakura K, Karoum F, Guidotti A, Costa E 1980 Modulation of nicotine receptors by opiate receptor
    agonists in cultured adrenal chromaffin cells. Nature 283: 489–492
Laubie M, Schmitt H, Vincent M, Remond G 1977 Central cardiovascular effects of morphinomimetic
    peptides in dogs. European Journal of Pharmacology 46: 67–71
Lechner R B, Gurll N J, Reynolds D G 1985a Role of the autonomic nervous system in mediating the
    response to naloxone in canine hemorrhagic shock. Circulatory Shock 16: 279–295
Lechner R B, Gurll N J, Reynolds D G 1985b Naloxone potentiates the cardiovascular effects of
    catecholamines in canine hemorrhagic shock. Circulatory Shock 16: 347–361
Lechner R B, Gurll N J, Reynolds D G 1985c Intracoronary naloxone in hemorrhagic shock: dose-
    dependent stereospecific effects. American Journal of Physiology 249: H272–H277
Lemaire I, Tseng R, Lemaire S 1978 Systemic administration of β-endorphin: Potent hypotensive effect
    involving a serotonergic pathway. Proceedings of the National Academy of Sciences 75: 6240–6242
Long J B, Lake C R, Reid A, Ruvio B A, Holaday J W 1983 Effects of naloxone and TRH on plasma
    catecholamines and arterial pressure in normal and endotoxaemic rats. Society for Neuroscience
    Abstracts 9: 107
Long J B, Ruvio B A, Glatt C E, Holaday J W 1984 ICI 174864, a putative δ opioid antagonist, reverses
    endotoxemic hypotension: pretreatment with dynorphin 1–13, a κ agonist, blocks this action.
    Neuropeptides 5: 291–294
Lord J A H, Waterfield A A, Hughes J, Kosterlitz H W 1977 Endogenous opioid peptides: multiple
    agonists and receptors. Nature 267: 495–499
Lutz S A, Vargish T, Reynolds D G, Ganes E M, Gurll N J 1981 Steroid and naloxone interaction
    in canine hemorrhagic shock. Circulatory Shock 8: 212
Lux W E Jr, Feuerstein G, Faden A I 1983a Alteration of leukotriene D4 hypotension by thyrotropin
    releasing hormone. Nature 302: 822–824
Lux W E Jr, Feuerstein G, Faden A I 1983b Thyrotropin releasing hormone reverses experimental
    anaphylactic shock through non-endorphin-related mechanisms. European Journal of Pharmacology 90:
    301–302
McKensie J E, Anselmo D M, Muldoon S M 1985 Nalbuphine's reversal of hypovolemic shock in the
    anesthetized rat. Circulatory Shock 17: 21–23
McIntosh T K, Bush H L, Palter M, et al 1985 Prolonged disruption of plasma β-endorphin dynamics
    following surgery. Journal of Surgical Research 38: 210–215
Manugian V, Koyama S, Santiesteban H L, Ammons W S, Manning J W 1981 Possible role of naloxone
    on sympathetic activity and blood pressure in cat. Federation Proceedings 40: 522
Martin W R, Eades C G, Thompson J A, Hyppler R E, Gilbert P E 1976 The effects of morphine-
    and nalorphine-like drugs in the non-dependent and morphine-dependent chronic spinal dog. Journal
    of Pharmacology and Experimental Therapeutics 197: 517–532

Maysinger D, Vermes I, Tilders F, Seizinger B R, Gramsch C, Hollt V, Herz A 1984 Differential effects of various opioid peptides on vasopressin and oxytocin release from the rat pituitary in vitro. Naunyn-Schmiedeberg's Archives of Pharmacology 328: 191–195

Moss I R, Scarpelli E M 1981 β-endorphin central depression of respiration and circulation. Journal of Applied Physiology 50: 1011–1016

Noda M, Furutani Y, Takahashi H, et al 1982 Cloning and sequence analysis of cDNA for bovine adrenal preproenkephalin. Nature 295: 202–208

North R A 1979 Opiates, opioid peptides and single neurones. Life Sciences 24: 1527–1546

Orwoll E S, Kendall J W 1980 β-endorphin and adrenocorticotropin in extrapituitary sites: gastrointestinal tract. Endocrinology 107: 438–442

Paciorek P M, Todd M H 1982 A comparison of the cardiovascular effects of meptazinol and naloxone following endotoxic shock in anaesthetized rats. British Journal of Pharmacology 75: 128P

Paciorek P M, Todd M H, Waterfall J F 1985 The effects of meptazinol in comparison with pentazocine, morphine and naloxone in a rat model of anaphylactic shock. British Journal of Pharmacology 84: 469–475

Patton M L, Gurll N J, Reynolds D G, Vargish T 1983 Adrenalectomy abolishes and cortisol restores naloxone's beneficial effects on cardiovascular function and survival in canine hemorrhagic shock. Circulatory Shock 10: 317–327

Pert C B, Snyder S H 1973 Opiate receptor: Demonstration in nervous tissue. Science 179: 1011–1014

Peters W P, Johnson M W, Friedman P A, Mitch W E 1981 Pressor effect of naloxone in septic shock. Lancet i: 529–532

Petty M A, de Jong W 1982 Cardiovascular effects of β-endorphin after microinjection into the nucleus tractus solitarii of the anaesthetised rat. European Journal of Pharmacology 81: 449–457

Petty M A, de Jong W, de Wied D 1982 An inhibitory role of β-endorphin in central cardiovascular regulation. Life Sciences 30: 1835–1840

Pfeiffer A, Feuerstein G, Kopin I J, Faden A I 1983 Cardiovascular and respiratory effects of mu-, delta-, and kappa-opiate agonists microinjected into the anterior hypothalamus brain area of awake rats. Journal of Pharmacology and Experimental Therapeutics 225: 735–741

Raymond R M, Harkema J M, Stoffs W V, Emerson T E 1981 Effects of naloxone therapy on hemodynamics and metabolism following a super lethal dosage of escherichia coli endotoxin in dogs. Surgery, Gynecology and Obstetrics 152: 159–162

Rees M, Payne J G, Bowen J C 1982 Naloxone reverses tissue effects of live Escherichia coli sepsis. Surgery 91: 81–86

Reynolds D G, Gurll N J, Vargish T, Lechner R, Faden A I, Holaday J W 1980 Blockade of opiate receptors with naloxone improves survival and cardiac performance in canine endotoxic shock. Circulatory Shock 7: 39–48

Reynolds D G, Gurll N J, Holaday J W, Ganes E 1982 Thyrotropin releasing hormone (TRH) in primate endotoxic shock. Physiologist 25: 309

Rock P, Silverman H, Plump D, Keeala Z, Smith P, Michael J R, Summer W 1985 Efficacy and safety of naloxone in septic shock. Critical Care Medicine 13: 28–33

Rossier J, French E D, Rivier C, Ling N, Guillemin R, Bloom F E 1977 Foot-shock induced stress increases β-endorphin levels in blood but not brain. Nature 270: 618–620

Schadt J C, Gaddis R R 1985 Endogenous opiate peptides may limit norepinephrine release during hemorrhage. Journal of Pharmacology and Experimental Therapeutics 232: 656–670

Schadt J C, York D H 1982 Involvement of both adrenergic and cholinergic receptors in the cardiovascular effects of naloxone during hemorrhagic hypotension in the conscious rabbit. Journal of Autonomic Nervous System 6: 237–251

Schrauwen E, Houvenaghel A 1985 Haemodynamic evaluation of endotoxic shock in anaesthetized piglets: antagonism of endogenous vasoactive substances. Circulatory Shock 16: 19–28

Schultzberg M, Hokfelt T, Lundberg J M, Terenius L, Elfvin L-G, Elde R 1978 Enkephalin-like immunoreactivity in nerve terminals in sympathetic ganglia and adrenal medulla and in adrenal medullary gland cells. Acta Physiologica Scandinavica 103: 475–477

Simantov R 1979 Glucocorticoids inhibit endorphin synthesis by pituitary cells. Nature 280: 684–685

Sitsen J M A, Van Ree J M, De Jong W 1982 Cardiovascular and respiratory effects of β-endorphin in anesthetized and conscious rats. Journal of Cardiovascular Pharmacology 4: 883–888

Smith R, Besser G M, Rees L H 1985 The effect of surgery on plasma β-endorphin and methionine-enkephalin. Neuroscience Letters 55: 17–21

Sugiura A, Smith R A, Shatney C H 1986 Thyrotropin-releasing hormone increases survival in canine haemorrhagic shock. Journal of Surgical Research 40: 63–68

Sun F Y, Zhang Z A 1985 Dynorphin receptor in the blood vessel. Neuropeptides 5, 595–598

Taff R H 1983 Pulmonary edema following naloxone administration in a patient without heart disease. Anesthesiology 59: 576–577

Teklu B, Habte-Michael A, Warrell D A, White N J, Wright D J M 1983 Meptazinol diminishes the Jarisch-Herxheimer reaction of relapsing fever. Lancet i: 835–839

Thijs L G, Balk E, Tuynman H A R E, Koopman P A R, Bezemer P D, Mulder G H 1983 Effects of naloxone on haemodynamics, oxygen transport, and metabolic variables in canine endotoxin shock. Circulatory Shock 10: 147–160

Thomas T A, Fletcher J E, Hill R G 1982 Influence of medication, pain and progress in labour on plasma β-endorphin-like immunoreactivity. British Journal of Anaesthesia 54: 401–408

Tiengo M 1980 Naloxone in irreversible shock. Lancet ii: 690

Traverso W L, Bellamy R F, Hollenbach S J, O'Benar J D 1985 Naloxone does not prevent death after rapid haemorrhage in swine. Surgery, Gynecology and Obstetrics 161: 229–239

Vargish T, Reynolds D G, Gurll N J, Lechner R J, Holaday J W, Faden A I 1980 Naloxone reversal of hypovolemic shock in dogs. Circulatory Shock 7: 31–38

Vargish T, Gurll N J, Reynolds D G, Lutz S A, Ganes E M 1983 Hemodynamic changes following corticosteroid and naloxone infusion in dogs subjected to hypovolemic shock without resuscitation. Life Sciences 33: 489–493

Viveros O H, Diliberto E J, Hazum E, Chang K J 1979 Opiate-like materials in the adrenal medulla: evidence for storage and secretion with catecholamines. Molecular Pharmacology 16: 1101–1108

Watson J D, Varley J G, Tomlin S J, Medbak S, Rees L H, Hinds C J 1986 Biochemical characterization of circulating met-enkephalins in canine endotoxin shock. Journal of Endocrinology 111: 329–334

Watson S J, Akil H, Richard C W, Barchas J D 1978 Evidence for two separate opiate peptide neuronal systems. Nature 275: 226–228

Watson S J, Akil H, Fischli W, Goldstein A, Zimmerman E, Nilaver G, Van Wimersma Greidanus T B 1982 Dynorphin and vasopressin: common localization in magnocellular neurons. Science 216: 85–87

Weissglas I S 1983 The role of endogenous opiates in shock: Experimental and clinical studies in vitro and in vivo. Advances in Shock Research 10: 87–94

Weissglas I S, Hinchey E J, Chiu R C J 1982 Naloxone and methylprednisolone in the treatment of experimental septic shock. Journal of Surgical Research 33: 131–135

Weitzman R E, Firemark H M, Glatz T H, Fisher D A 1979 Thyrotropin releasing hormone stimulates release of Arginine vasopressin and oxytocin in vivo. Endocrinology 104: 904–907

Whitnall M H, Gainer H, Cox B M, Molineaux C J 1983 Dynorphin A (1–8) is contained with vasopressin neurosecretory vesicles in rat pituitary. Science 222: 1137–1138

Wood P L, Charleson S E, Lane D, Hudgin R L 1981 Multiple opiate receptors: differential binding of mu, kappa and delta agonists. Neuropharmacology 20: 1215–1220

Wright D J M, Weller M D I 1980 Inhibition by naloxone of endotoxin-induced reactions in mice. British Journal of Pharmacology 70: 99P–100P

Wright D J M, Phillips M, Weller M D I 1980 Naloxone in shock. Lancet ii: 1361

Yanagida H, Corssen G 1981 Respiratory distress and beta-endorphin-like immunoreactivity in humans. Anesthesiology 55: 515–519

Yarbrough G G 1983 Mini-review; Thyrotropin releasing hormone and cholinergic neurones. Life Sciences 33: 111–118

Zaloga G P, Chernow B, Zajtchuk R, Chin R, Rainey T G, Lake R 1984 Diagnostic doses of protirelin (TRH) elevate BP by non catecholamine mechanisms. Archives of Internal Medicine 144: 1149–1152

12. Recent advances in the management of acute renal failure

Victor Parsons

DIAGNOSTIC PROCEDURES

Most acute renal failure (ARF) seen in the intensive care situation follows surgery in high-risk patients, with multiple organ failure (secondary to hypotension and sepsis), affecting the heart, lungs and kidneys. The warning signs of a falling urine output, falling urine plasma osmolarity ratios and a rising urine sodium with a cellular urinary deposit herald established ARF. We have adopted a diagnostic sequence to make sure that the routine measures are taken to correct on the one hand fluid deficit and to achieve effective cardiac output on the other (Fig. 12.1). Some of the logic of the measures of crystalloid versus colloid administration have been over-simplified (Sturm & Wisner, 1985; Macintyre et al, 1985), but colloids are best avoided unless ultrafiltration and dialysis are quickly available to deal with fluid recruited from extra-vascular spaces. If no improvement is noticed within a couple of hours the question of further investigation may be warranted in a proportion of patients. There is a variety of techniques available (Table 12.1).

The choice may depend on what is available quickly with the minimum of disturbance for the patient. Ultrasound has risen in popularity because it can be done at the bedside and does not require contrast administration which can in certain groups of patients (diabetics, myeloma or nephrotics), precipitate further renal tubular damage (Porter & Bennett, 1980). An immediate estimation of renal size, often increased in ARF, and the absence of obstructive uropathy is obtained (Talner et al, 1981; Rosenfield & Siegal, 1981). Occasionally comments can be made about the patency of the renal veins and the presence of extra renal masses or cysts. Ultrasound can also detect the presence of multiple echogenic areas in the kidney consistent with interstitial nephritis or micro-abscesses.

Intravenous urography is reserved for those patients who, following trauma or surgery to the pelvis, are suspected of having vascular or ureteric damage. We are increasingly aware of vascular occlusion to the renal arteries in the patient who has had vascular surgery to the heart or aorta, and then selective angiograms have revealed unilateral and bilateral stenotic and/or thrombotic lesions (Thul Hupp et al, 1986).

Isotope renography using ^{123}I hippuran has been used regularly in transplant renal failure and has spread to be used in ARF, particularly if the vascular supply is in doubt following extensive aneurysm surgery. [99m]Tc Medronate scanning has been used to delineate the degree of muscle damage in rhabdomyolysis (Frymoyer et al, 1985).

Renal biopsy in ARF

For the majority of postoperative patients, the cause of ARF is all too obvious, but where the patient has presented as acutely ill with no obvious period of hypotension or previous renal disease, renal failure may be part of a systemic illness and biopsy

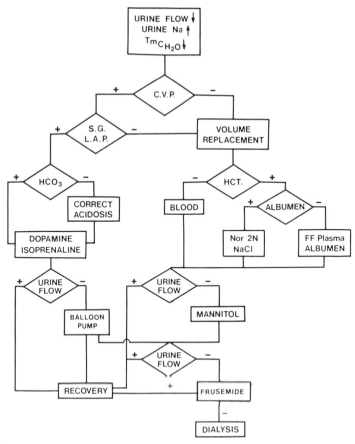

Fig. 12.1   Diagram showing the diagnostic and treatment steps to be taken when oliguria sets in before dialysis is considered. Volume replacement is matched by cardiac support to achieve recovery of urinary output. Obstructive uropathy has previously been excluded.

Table 12.1   Diagnostic techniques in ARF

Ultrasound
CAT scan
IV urography
Vascular imaging
Isotope scanning

may be extremely helpful in sorting out the pathology, and may be resorted to in 10–15% of patients. Various renal units have developed a policy on biopsy in ARF, which although not without risks in the patient with a bleeding tendency, is now regarded as 'good practice' (Gault & Muehrcke, 1983; Richet, 1985). The indications are shown in Table 12.2. The list can be extended but a few examples are given to illustrate the value of a quick biopsy which may influence management immediately. Of the inflammatory causes, acute bacterial interstitial nephritis has been recognised due to mycobacteria and *E. coli*, and biopsy seems the only way of diagnosis, and

Table 12.2   Renal biopsy in ARF complicated by systemic symptoms and signs

Diagnosis	Disease
ARDS and pulmonary purpura	Goodpasture's syndrome; arteritis
Skin and pulmonary lesions	Polyarteritis; vasculitis, granulomata; e.g. sarcoidosis
Fever, pneumonia, myopathy, CNS signs	Legionnaires' disease
Fever, white cells in the urine	Acute interstitial nephritis (bacterial, granulomatous and chemical)
Muscle stiffness, fever	Myoglobinuria of various aetiologies
Malignant disease	Associated glomerulo nephritis; hypercalcaemia
Hepatitis and acute renal failure	Occasionally toxic nephritis and IgA glomerulonephritis
Tuberculosis treated by Rifampicin	Drug-induced renal failure
Haemolytic anaemia ± thrombocytopaenia + evidence of DIC	Renal failure accompanying haemolytic uraemia syndrome

appropriate treatment reverses the situation (Cattell et al, 1985). Legionella infections seem to be on the increase, and although serology may be diagnostic the presence of pulmonary shadows and ARF, if Goodpasture's syndrome has been excluded, makes Legionella infection highly likely and therapy needs to start as soon as possible (Woodhead & MacFarlane, 1985; Fennes, 1985). Rhabdomyolysis is increasingly recognised as a complication of trauma, marathon running, hyperpyrexia, alcoholism, drug abuse and the biopsy appearances are helpful.

Drug-induced ARF provides a difficult problem in the ITU setting where multiple management occasionally leads to mixtures of therapy which the nephrologist would rather not see used. The medicolegal aspects of this problem has as yet to reach the United Kingdom but is already in process in the USA, and here biopsy may be both precautionary and force changes in therapy (Table 12.3), where it is possible.

Table 12.3   Drugs and poisons associated with ARF

Drugs:
    Aminoglycosides ± diuretics, rifampicin
    CIS platinum, mercury
    Cyclosporin A, methotrexate
    Non-steroidal anti-inflammatory drugs
    Allopurinol

Poisons:
    Arsine and arsenic compounds
    Cadmium
    Ethylene glycol
    Phenol
    Paracetamol
    Amphetamine (polyarteritis nodosa picture)

Even more important are the rare but clear-cut toxic ARFs due to poisoning with a variety of agents, some of which can be detected by biopsy (Table 12.3). With advances in the detection of nanograms of such toxic material, the kidney biopsy may be a valuable confirmatory source of the toxin where plasma levels have declined.

A small proportion of patients may warrant a further series of investigations because of symptom clusters (Table 12.4).

Table 12.4   Plasma or serum investigations in ARF which may add more information

Pulmonary shadows ± haematuria cluster:
  (a) Anti GBM antibodies (Goodpasture and other types of acute glomerulonephritis)
  (b) Legionella titres (infection in hospital patients)
  (c) ESR- and C-reactive proteins, WBC antibodies (raised in vasculitis)

Hypotensive hypocalcaemic hypophosphataemic clusters:
  (a) Amylase—?pancreatitis
  (b) Endotoxin—?*E. coli* septicaemia
  (c) Autoantibodies—liver and kidney involvement in SLE and Sjogrens

Hypercalcaemic hyperphosphataemic ± muscle tenderness cluster:
  (a) CPK > 10 000 u in rhabdomyolysis
  (b) Bone marrow:
        Myeloma
        Hairy T-cell leukaemia
  (c) Parathyroid scan—parathyrotoxicosis

NEWER CONCEPTS OF THE CONTROL OF RENAL BLOOD FLOW AND ITS BEARING ON ARF

Besides the renal vasodilator action of small quantities of dopamine and prostaglandins PGE_2 and PGI (Paines Ho & James, 1985), encephalins, kinins (Scicli & Carretero, 1986), atrial naturetic factor (Richards et al, 1985) and possibly hepatic glomerulo-trophin (Alverstand & Bergstrom, 1984) all play a role in the control of blood flow. Intrinsic autoregulation nevertheless seems to take priority over these extrinsic mechanisms for the maintenance of glomerular filtration (Fig. 12.2).

Within the kidney are three contractile groups of cells which control blood flow: the afferent and efferent arteriolar myoneural paracrine cells and the mesangial cells. On contraction, blood flow (QA) and blood pressure within the glomerulus and capillary filtration (K_f) can be manipulated. Interactions based on neural and endocrine signals can also regulate flow from the cortical nephrons to the juxtamedullary glomeruli, whose environment seems to be relatively hypoxic at all times (Epstein, 1985). Kidney perfusion, albeit intermittent and patchy as shown by CAT scanning, in ARF (Ishikawa et al, 1981), is maintained despite severe oliguria.

If one is to attempt to allocate priorities of action, angiotensin, adrenergic, dopaminergic and prostaglandin mechanisms seem to be the main agonists in maintaining both blood flow and its distribution within the kidney to retain viability of cells irrespective of urine production. By using a variety of blockers, phenoxybenzamine, beta-blockers, peripheral AII blockers (Saralasin), angiotensin converting enzyme blockers (Captopril and Enalapril) and prostaglandin synthesis inhibitors (e.g., Indomethacin), the part played by each has been dissected out to give a fragmentary view of the control of blood flow (Blantz & Pelayo, 1984; Navar & Rosivall, 1984; Garella & Matarese, 1984; Paines et al, 1985).

The intensivist faced with such evidence can only be on safe ground by eliminating such therapies which the patient may already be receiving, and introduce some after the basic physiological mechanisms have been allowed to exert their protective role.

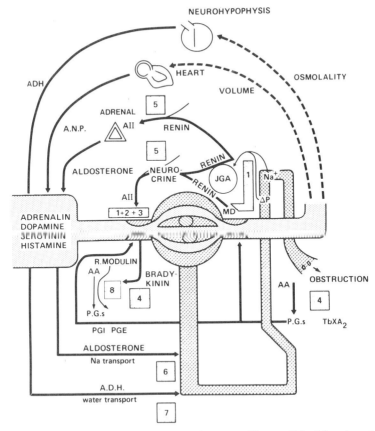

NEUROHYPOPHYSIS

Fig. 12.2 A schematised diagram to show the mechanisms controlling renal blood flow through the glomerulus (dotted pathway). Contractile elements are shown (hatched areas) involving afferent and efferent arteriolar muscle and mesangial cells within the glomerulus. The urinary pathway is cross-hatched. Stimuli arise from within the blood stream, the macula densa (MD) and the juxta glomerular apparatus (JGA) to influence the release of renin, antidiuretic hormone (ADH) and atrial naturetic peptides (ANP), which in turn influence the release of angiotensin II (AII) and aldosterone. Some of these factors and local stimuli lead to the release of bradykinin in turn influencing the release of prostaglandins, PGI, PGE and TBXA$_2$ (thromboxane A$_2$). Blocking agents such as beta-blockers (1), AII (2) and dopaminergic blockers (3) influence the release of renin and the effects of these amines on the circulation. Kinin blockers and prostaglandin blockers (4) interfere with the release of prostaglandins. Renin and angiotensin converting enzyme blockers (5) interfere with the action of AII. Aldosterone blockers (6) and ADH blockers (7) interfere with the elaboration of urine while steroids affect the production of renomodulin (8) in turn interfering with the production of PGs.

The kidney contains the highest quantities of dopamine of any organ in the body and trial of repletion of these stores seems physiologically justified (Henderson et al, 1980; Graziani et al, 1984).

Figure 12.2 attempts to produce a broad view of the various factors involved and the possible blocking agents used or available for altering the responses. Prostaglandin E$_2$ seems to be at the end of several pathways being stimulated by ADH, ANP, bradykinin and angiotensin II, and inhibited by non-steroidal antiinflammatory drugs by their action on the cyclo- and lipooxygenase pathways and steroids by their inhibition of phospholipase activation by the synthesis of macrocortin or renomodulin (Codde & Beilin, 1985).

USE OF DIURETICS, DOPAMINE AND BALLOON PUMPING

From this newer understanding several practical points emerge.

To keep renal blood flow and filtration going as long as possible in the face of systemic influences shutting it down, the following measures need to be taken:

1. Sodium and fluid loading not only encourages a high CVP and adequate cardiac output, but may well ensure the continuing production of atrial naturetic peptides (ANP), which override the effects of locally produced angiotensin (Laragh, 1985; Myers & Moran, 1986).
2. Sodium bicarbonate loading may allow a sustained normal urine pH in the face of metabolic/toxic acidosis that allows the prostaglandin and dopaminergic actions to continue, and divert oxygen for ATP production and cellular maintenance rather than acid production (Chan et al, 1980; Kopp & Mullerthul, 1982).
3. Dopamine, aminophylline and prostacyclin all act synergistically and can be used in physiological dosage (Graziani et al, 1984; Lelcuk et al, 1985), although there is evidence in septic shock that PGI and its breakdown products are already elevated (Halushka et al, 1985).
4. Drugs that affect prostaglandin metabolism (e.g. aspirin, steroids and non-steroidal antiinflammatory drugs), and adrenergic receptors (e.g. beta-blockers), used together or separately may well produce severe reductions in renal blood flow and tip the resorption of filtrate into uraemic ARF (Stoff, 1984; Weinberg et al, 1985). Such mixtures of antihypertensive and non-steroidal anti-inflammatory drugs are commonly used in the elderly whose functioning glomeruli are already on the wane. There is animal experimental evidence that alpha-blockade with phenoxybenzamine can reverse some of the vasoconstriction induced by cyclosporin A (Murray et al, 1985) which may be of use in oliguric transplant patient treated with this agent.
5. The use of aminoglycosides in the septic shocked patient must be weighed against their effects on nephron filtration rate, K_f and plasma flow (Moore et al, 1984).
6. It is against this background that the controversy of using diuretics in the management of incipient ARF is sustained. Diuretics affect renal blood flow by changing the delivery of sodium to the distal tubule by paralysing sodium transport in the proximal tubule and thereby indirectly reducing oxygen demands of the medullary thick limb. This may well also flush out tubular debris in the tubular lumen. Clearly, their use is not going to be effective where vasoconstrictive and other mechanisms have reduced filtration to a low rate. This is the reason for delaying their use until other factors have been corrected or other agents been given a chance to act to produce a filtrate on which the diuretic can have an effect (see Fig. 12.1). It does seem from animal models of ARF that diuretics, and other toxins, such as aminoglycosides, can be additive in their effect. The common use of an aminoglycoside for presumed sepsis and frusemide for a flagging urine output is not the most logical procedure and may make tubular damage worse. On the other hand, once urine is flowing again diuretics do

decrease the period of oliguria and render dialysis less necessary (Brown et al, 1981; Graziani et al, 1984).

7. Obstruction profoundly affects renal blood flow, probably via a thromboxane A_2 pathway, and every effort must be made to relieve it at the earliest opportunity (Morrison, 1982).

8. If inotropes and diuretics have failed to produce a diuresis and where the cardiac output is poor following cardiac surgery or in profound endotoxic shock, aortic balloon pumping has been known to improve renal blood flow and produce a diuresis, but the decision to balloon pump is more likely to be based on the cardiac status of the patient and the need to generate an effective coronary artery filling pressure in the face of profound cardiac muscle depression (Dhainaut et al, 1982).

HEPATORENAL FAILURE

One very recalcitrant variety of ARF which merges with the earlier functional renal failure is that accompanying fulminant hepatic failure (FHF) through a variety of aetiologies (hepatitis, advanced cirrhosis, paracetamol poisoning, extensive metastases).

Given that there is often a bleeding hypovolaemic septic component to these patients' presentation, a proportion of cortical vascular shut-down seen on angiography and renography is presumed to be due to substances which are either not produced by the failing liver or substances which are not detoxified by the liver by the usual routes. This has given rise to the suggestion of a lack of hepatic glomerulotrophin on the one hand (Alverstrand & Bergstrom, 1984) and false vasoconstrictor substances on the other (Fraser & Arieff, 1985). Characterisation of the latter substances has still to be established, but clinically this is the basis for the use of plasma exchange/pheresis/charcoal absorption on the one hand to remove false transmitters, and the strict avoidance of hepatotoxic drugs and attempts to improve the hepatic circulation on the other (Gimson et al, 1982). One particularly serious complication in the haemolytic uraemia syndrome is intravascular and by inference intrahepatic, as well as intrarenal vascular occlusion by platelet thrombi and plasmapheresis, plasma exchange and the use of prostacyclin has led to improvement in individual uncontrolled observations (Weston, 1983).

After an initial enthusiasm for the use of absorption techniques for the treatment of encephalopathy and acute renal failure, the evidence that they achieve a reduction in mortality in FHF is not available yet. Dialysis is indicated for whatever the cause of the oliguria. If there are false transmitters, myocardial depressant factors and substances which alter pulmonary and cerebral capillary permeability, the more permeable dialysis membranes used in ultrafiltration dialysers, such as polyacrylonitrile AN69 (Hospal) seem indicated. The use of mannitol to reduce cerebral oedema in such patients is of proven use (Canalese et al, 1982). Trials of CAVH have still to demonstrate a clear-cut benefit (Coratelli et al, 1985).

A recent review of the types of renal failure accompanying hepatic disease showed that of 69 patients presenting in 1984–85 to the Liver Failure Unit at King's College Hospital, 83% had FHF: 60% due to paracetamol overdosage, the remaining 23% had a variety of causes which included hepatic failure following transplantation using cyclosporin A (9%), alcoholic liver disease (3%), viral hepatitis (3%), chronic liver disease and/or obstructive jaundice (3%) (O'Grady et al, 1986). Of 640 patients admitted with hepatoencephalopathy survival was adversely affected by the presence of renal failure (Table 12.5).

Table 12.5   Prevalence of types of hepatic encephalopathy in 640 patients admitted to King's College Hospital liver failure unit, 1973–1985

	Survival	
Type of hepatic disease	Without ARF	With ARF
Paracetamol overdosage	63%	25%
Viral hepatitis Type A	66%	40%
Viral hepatitis Type B	30%	20%
Viral hepatitis Non A Non B	12%	4%

Renal failure accompanying the more prolonged hepatic insult (non A non B > type B > type A) had the more serious prognosis due to cerebral oedema, pulmonary complications, sepsis, haemorrhage and irreversible hypotension which dialysis did little to reverse. The more sudden and reversible the hepatic insult the better the chance of recovery.

RECENT ADVANCES IN HAEMODIALYSIS AND HAEMOFILTRATION TECHNIQUES:

1. Access.
2. Anticoagulants.
3. Acetate versus bicarbonate.
4. Less complement and WBC activating membranes.
5. Slow daily ultrafiltration (CAVF) coupled with haemodialysis (HD) 'AVID'.
6. Total replacement of haemodialysis by haemofiltration.
7. Haemodialysis ± haemofiltration + plasmapheresis (PP).
8. Continuous ultrafiltration plus intermittent dialysis (CUPID).

Access
With the advent of better double lumen catheters that can be inserted into subclavian veins (Vascath, Haemocath and Permcath Quinton), or with the use of single-lumen catheters with double-headed pumps, the need for routine insertion of shunts has lessened. However, this has led to a series of complications using such catheters from haemopneumothorax, haemomediastinum and problems of persistent sepsis from the catheter site (Vanherweghem et al, 1986). When ultrafiltration is also used shunt insertion, usually in a brachial site, is still carried out.

Anticoagulants
In the complicated patient with multiple operative sites, vascular access or a tracheostomy coupled with the risk of GI haemorrhage, the choice of anticoagulants other than heparin even with regional heparisation becomes important. The alternatives are several (Table 12.6).

The very patients who are bleeding from various sites are those in whom it is most difficult to decide whether anticoagulants are required for dialysis at all. Where there are few platelets, increased prothrombin time and low fibrinogen, anticoagulation is clearly not required given reasonable flow rates across the dialyser after a simple

Table 12.6 Alternatives to heparin as anticoagulant in haemodialysis

No anticoagulant at all
Low molecular weight heparin
Prostacyclin
Citrate

saline heparin flush (500 U/500 ml saline) through the lines and coil. However, in some situations bleeding has led to a highly activated coagulation system which will soon thrombose the whole circuit. We routinely use the Kaolin Activated Clotting Time using the Haemocron in all acute dialysis, and this gives a reliable measure of the thrombotic tendencies of the patients' blood at the commencement of dialysis. Where there is evidence of DIC, ARDS, mental confusion or peripheral vascular stasis (e.g. toxic shock syndrome, severe bacterial septicaemia, malaria or ARF complicating accidental placental haemorrhage), then prostacyclin has been our anticoagulant of choice (Weston, 1983; Keogh et al, 1984).

Flushing, gastrointestinal cramps and hypotension due to vasodilatation are common at an infusion rate of 5 ng/kg/minute, but these soon settle down with a slower rate of 2 ng/kg/min and fluid replacement (Casati & Ponticelli, 1981). Initial priming of the circuit with heparin prevents clotting in this early phase (Rylance et al, 1984).

Low molecular weight heparin has a less profound effect on clotting mechanisms and has been the preferred type of heparin used when long infusions involving CAVF is used in addition (Ljungberg, 1985).

Citrate has been used when plasmaphoresis is coupled with dialysis as the plasma replacement is anticoagulated with citrate. Downstream calcium infusions are used to prevent total body anticoagulation and tetany.

Acetate versus bicarbonate dialysis

Acetate is rapidly metabolised to produce bicarbonate in the liver, and usually this is rapid enough to prevent acute rises in circulating acetate. However, in children, patients with a low cardiac output and in those with advanced hepatic failure significant quantities of acetate gain access to the periphery producing vasodilatation, cardiac depression from a negative inotropic effect, and occasionally brisk hypotension (Mastrangelo et al, 1985). Bicarbonate has also been shown to improve cardiac contractility when compared with acetate using echocardiographic measurements (Chen et al, 1983; Ruder et al, 1985).

Bicarbonate dialysis is now routinely used in the hypotensive shocked patient whose circulation is being maintained on inotropes (Leunissen et al, 1986).

Biocompatible membranes

Activation of complement and WBC and platelet aggregation are frequent side effects of dialysis due to the membranes used which neither prostacyclin nor steroids will reduce (Dodd et al, 1983). Cellulose acetate fibres and the polyacrylonitrile membranes are less activating. Where the patient's pulmonary function is already at risk from increased permeability, platelet and white cell embolism can only add to the vascular perfusion problems and to the respiratory difficulty even on a ventilator. In these circumstances switching dialysers can overcome the additional burden.

ARTERIOVENOUS HAEMOFILTRATION

This technique using high-flux dialysers with much more permeable membranes (up to 10 000 kilodaltons) has been used in three different ways:

1. Total replacement of haemodialysis with large volume ultrafiltration (20–30 l/24 hours) and large volume replacement (continuous arteriovenous haemofiltration, CAVH) (Kramer, 1985).
2. Continuous arteriovenous ultrafiltration with relatively smaller volumes of ultra-filtrate (6–8 l/24 hours). Smaller volumes of replacement fluid (mainly crystalloid and IV feeding regimens) with intermittent haemodialysis. Arteriovenous haemo-filtration with intermittent (every other day), haemodialysis 'AVID' (Dodd et al, 1983).
3. Continuous A-V haemofiltration with intermittent use of the same cartridge for intermittent dialysis using the same membrane, continuous ultrafiltration plus intermittent dialysis CUPID (Simpson & Allison, 1986).

The first technique requires accurate measurement of ultrafiltration volumes with simultaneous calculation of replacement volumes to prevent hypovolaemia. The ultra-filters have large areas, require pumped blood with appropriate monitoring and on-line replacement fluid which is metered in and is best done in intensive care areas. Anti-coagulation needs constant monitoring as applies to haemodialysis.

The second technique can be carried out simply by using a shunt with adequate arterial pressure, a side arm for anticoagulation and a simple venous return to the patient with no pumps, alarms or monitors. The replacement fluid is best given by a central line and usually includes up to 3 litres of intravenous concentrated crystalloid and more rarely colloid. The process can be carried out in the intensive care unit or a ward setting, the patient returning to have haemodialysis as appropriate. Daily weighing is the only extra monitoring required.

The third technique has used the ultrafiltrate compartment of the cartridge to act for several hours a day as a dialyser and ultrafilter. Depending on the source of dialysis fluid, warming and balance monitoring are the only extras required. Some units have used warmed sterile CAPD fluid for such manoeuvres.

Each technique has advantages over haemodialysis, the chief being the ability to remove large quantities of isosmotic fluid without provoking the hypotension, cardiac or pulmonary side effects of haemodialysis. Figure 12.3 shows the removal of a massive quantity of fluid over a short period of time in a very oedematous fluid overloaded patient without recourse to dialysis. A secondary advantage is that removal of fluid by daily dialysis to 'make space' for intravenous fluid in patients following abdominal surgery or aortic aneurysm repair is not necessary. Figure 12.4 shows a patient with multiple gut fistulae continuously fed for 4 months with regular dialysis two or three times a week and CAVH.

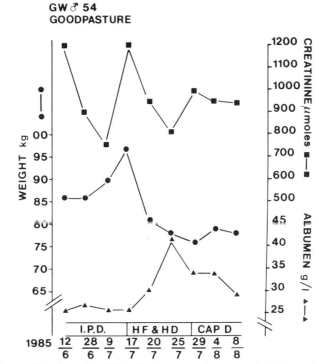

Fig. 12.3 A 54-year-old patient with ARF and pulmonary oedema treated with intermittent peritoneal dialysis (IPD) leading to increasing weight gain and hypoalbuminaemia. Haemofiltration and haemodialysis (HF & HD) led to a 19 kg loss in weight and total correction of the hypoalbuminaemia. Continuous ambulatory peritoneal dialysis (CAPD) maintained the patient after this 10-day period.

Clearances of uraemic waste products entirely by CAVH gives a simulated GFR of approximately 20 ml/min. AVID and CUPID (6 l/day plus three 5-h dialyses per week with clearances of 150 ml/min) give slightly more as each dialysis will be the equivalent of 40 l of ultrafiltrate.

Replacement fluid must contain enough NA^+Cl^- and HCO_3^- to replace the ultra-filtered ions bearing in mind that intravenous feeding regimens will contribute limited amounts of electrolytes and add to the acid carbon dioxide load of the patient, particu-larly if oxygen utilisation by the periphery is low.

Evidence is accumulating to indicate that CAVH may remove substances such as endotoxin, endorphins or prostaglandins, and postulated myocardial depressant factors that haemodialysis does not remove well and then only intermittently. The technique is now being used for ARDS and septic shock before there is any clear indication for haemodialysis and early trials are encouraging (Schetz et al, 1984; Gotloib et al, 1984, 1985).

HAEMOABSORPTION AND PLASMAPHERESIS

The possible removal of large molecular weight toxic antibodies, autoantibodies such as anti-GBM antibodies and anticholinergic receptor site antibodies adds to the range

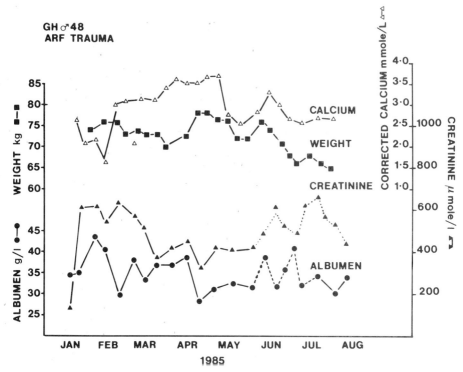

Fig. 12.4   A 48-year-old patient with extensive abdominal trauma maintained on a ventilator for 4 months and AVID with total parenteral nutrition for 5 months showing control of creatinine and albumen concentrations. He had seven explorations and finally replacement of an aortic valve for endocarditis. He is now maintained on intermittent haemodialysis alone and lives at home.

of techniques for treating patients who also have renal failure. Sequential plasma-pheresis and dialysis has been used to remove antibodies to HLA antigens prior to transplantation in patients with renal failure (Shapiro & Shapiro, 1985).

The long sessions required are well tolerated by patients if the fluid shifts are kept to a minimum by careful monitoring of plasma replacement and ultrafiltration. Machines that contain pumps that monitor flows accurately are essential to prevent fluxes and disequilibrium. Prolonged heparinisation has been found to be unnecessary and can be replaced by citrate which is used in the plasmaphoresis cycle.

Haemoabsorption of antigens by the passage of blood across sepharose linked specific antibodies opens up much more accurately designed techniques which will probably replace plasmaphoresis where the toxin or antibody is known (Baumgartner et al, 1985). Advances in these techniques will hold out a better chance of helping the older septic shocked patient with ARF who at the moment suffers such high mortality.

REDUCING THE MORTALITY OF ARF

Various reviews of ARF have used discriminant analysis of the clinical risk factors which predict outcome. Despite increasing agreement about scoring such factors there are still unquantifiable factors which make prediction of a fatal outcome uncertain, and hence a large amount of time and expensive therapy is expended in trying to improve on an overall mortality which still exceeds 50% (Lien & Chan, 1985; Rasmussen et al, 1985; Cameron & Taube, 1986).

Agreement on some factors which worsen prognosis is however emerging and these need the greatest attention in the future:

1. *Persistent sepsis*—thorough and repeated search needs to be made for the removal of necrotic tissue, drainage of septic collections and meticulous attention to all invasive tubing which might be sources of fresh sepsis. Milligan et al (1978) have emphasised the importance of re-exploration of the abdomen.

2. *Multiple organ failure*—prolonged hypotension, cardiac failure of various aetiologies, CNS depression and pulmonary complications, singly or compounded, greatly increase mortality (Routh et al, 1980; Sweet et al, 1981; Pine et al, 1983). Two advances, CAVH and prolonged extracorporeal membrane oxygenation, may reduce the need for high FIO_2 used in ventilated patients with ARF, and hence reduce permanent pulmonary damage when hyperoxygenation is continued for longer than a week.

3. Avoidance of nephrotoxic drugs which may delay recovery (Hollenberg et al, 1976).

4. Correct supply of nutrition matched to oxygen consumption on the one hand and generated CO_2 loads on the other.

Surprisingly, age has not been a predictor of outcome and although pre-existing renal disease may worsen the prognosis in some series, the ability to take on the patients (some 10% in large series) for renal replacement therapy long term has removed this poor prognostic factor (Bullock et al, 1985; Cioffi et al, 1984).

Acute renal failure and its metabolic consequences can now be controlled well with a variety of techniques. The future lies in correcting other organ failure with multiple support systems until irreversible pathological processes remain the sole source of mortality.

REFERENCES

Alverstrand A, Bergstrom J 1984 Glomerular hyperfiltration after protein ingestion during glucagon infusion and insulin dependent diabetes is induced by a liver hormone. Lancet i: 195–196

Baumgartner J D, Glauser M P, McCutchan J A, et al 1985 Prevention of gram negative shock and death in surgical patients by antibody to endotoxin core glycolipid. Lancet ii: 59–62

Blanz R C, Pelayo J C 1984 A functional role for the tubuloglomerular feedback mechanism. Kidney International 24: 739–746

Brown C B, Ogg C S, Cameron J S 1981 High dose frusemide acute renal failure: a controlled trial. Clinical Nephrology 15: 90–96

Bullock M L, Umen A J, Finkelstein M, Keane W F 1985 The assessment of risk factors in 462 patients with acute renal failure. American Journal of Kidney Diseases 5: 97–103

Cameron J S, Taube D 1986 Acute Renal Failure. In: Martin A M, Hanning C (eds) Proceedings of the Acute Respiratory and Renal Failure Workshop, Lincoln College, Oxford. Gambro UMEA, Sweden

Canalese J, Gimson A E S, Davis, Mellon P J, Davis M, Williams R 1982 Controlled trial of dexamethazone for the cerebral oedema of fulminant hepatic failure. Gut 23: 625–629

Casati S, Ponticelli C 1981 Haemodialysis in patients with a risk of bleeding. New England Journal of Medicine 305: 521–522

Cattel W R, Greenwood R N, Baker L R I 1985 Severe reversible renal failure due to chronic interstitial infection in the kidney. In: Proceedings of the 14th International Congress of Chemotherapy, Kyoto SY-10-4, p 20

Chan L, Thulborn K R, Waterton J C, Ledingham J G G, Ross B D, Radda G K 1980 Prevention of ischaemic acidosis, a new approach to acute renal failure. In: Proceedings of the European Dialysis and Transplant Association 17: 681–685. Pitman Medical

Chen T S, Friedman H S, Smith A J, Delmonte M L 1983 Haemodynamic changes during haemodialysis. Role of the dialysate. Clinical Nephrology 20: 190–196

Cioffi W G, Ashikaga T, Gamelli R L 1984 Probability of surviving post-operative acute renal failure. Development of a prognostic index. Annals of Surgery 200: 205–211

Codde J P, Beilin L J 1985 Dietary fish oil prevents dexamethazone induced hypertension in the rat. Clinical Science 69: 691–669

Coratelli P, Passavanti G, Munno I, Fumarol A D, Amerio A 1985 New trends in hepatorenal syndrome. Kidney International 28 (suppl 7):5143–5147

Dhainaut J F, Huet Y, Kahan A, Bricard C, Neveux E, Dallot J-Y, Bachet J, Carli A, Monsaliier F J 1982 Acute myocardial failure during Yersunia enterocolitica infection. Intensive Care Medicine 8: 51–53

Dodd N J, O'Donovan R M, Bennett-Jones D N, Rylance P B, Bewick M, Parsons V, Weston M J 1983 Arteriovenous haemofiltration, a recent advance in the management of renal failure. British Medical Journal 287: 1008–1010

Epstein F H 1985 Hypoxia of the renal medulla. Quarterly Journal of Medicine 57: 807–810

Fennes Z 1985 Legionnaires Disease associated with acute renal failure. A report of two cases and review of the literature. Clinical Nephrology 23: 96–100

Fraser C L, Arieff A I 1985 Hepatic encephalopathy. New England Journal of Medicine 313: 865–873

Frymoyer P A, Giammaria R, Farrar F M, Schroeder E T 1985 Technetium ^{99m}Tc medronate bone scanning in rhabdomyolysis. Archives of Internal Medicine 145: 1991–1995

Garella S, Materese R A 1984 Renal effects of prostaglandins and chemical adverse effects of non-steroidal anti-inflammatory agents. Medicine 63: 165–181

Gault M H, Muehrcke R C I 1983 Renal Biopsy. Current views and controversies. Nephron 34: 1–34

Gimson A E S, Braude S, Mellon P I, Canalese J, Williams R 1982 Earlier charcoal haemoperfusion in fulminant hepatic failure. Lancet 2: 681–683

Gotloib L, Barzilay E, Shustak A, Lev A 1984 Sequential haemofiltration in non-oliguric high capillary permeability pulmonary oedema of severe sepsis. Critical Care Medicine 12: 997–1000

Gotloib L, Barzilay E, Shustak A, Waiss Z, Lev A 1984 Haemofiltration in severe septic adult respiratory distress syndrome associated with varicella. Intensive Care Medicine 11: 319–322

Graziani G, Cantaluppi A, Casati S, et al 1984 Dopamine and Frusemide in oliguric acute renal failure. Nephron 37: 39–42

Halushka P V, Reines H D, Barron S E, et al 1985 Elevated plasma 6-keto prostaglandin $F_{1\alpha}$ in patients in septic shock. Critical Care Medicine 13: 451–453

Henderson I S, Beattioe T J, Kennedy A C 1980 Dopamine hydrochloride in oliguric states. Lancet ii: 827–829

Hollenberg N K, Adams D F, Oken D E, Abrams K L, Merrill J P 1976 Acute renal failure due to nephrotoxins. New England Journal of Medicine 282: 1329–1334

Iaina I, Serban I, Gavendo S, Kapuler S, Eliahou H E 1980 Alleviation of ischaemic acute renal failure by beta blockers. Specific tubular receptor blockade or membrane stabilising effect. In: Proceedings of the European Dialysis and Transplant Association 17: 686–689

Ishikawa I, Saito Y, Shonida A, Onouchi Z 1981 Evidence for patchy renal vasoconstriction in man. Nephron 27: 31–34

Keogh A M, Rylance P B, Weston M J, Parsons V 1984 Prostacyclin (Epoprostenol) haemodialysis in patients at risk of haemorrhage. In: Stevens E, Monkhouse P (eds) Proceedings of the European Dialysis and Transplant Nurses Association 13: 51–54. Pitman, London

Kopp K F, Mullerthul G 1982 Prophylaxis and emergency treatment of acute renal failure by acute iv bicarbonate loading. In: Eliahou H E (ed) Acute Renal Failure. John Libbey, London

Kramer P (ed) 1985 Arteriovenous haemofiltration. Springer-Verlag, Berlin

Laragh J H 1985 Atrial natriuretic hormone, the renin aldosterone axis and blood pressure electrolyte homeostasis. New England Journal of Medicine 313: 1330–1340

Lelcuk S, Alexander F, Kobzik L, Valen C R, Hechtman H B 1985 Prostacyclin and thromboxane A_2 moderate post ischaemic renal failure. Surgery 98: 207–212

Leunissen K M L, Hoorntije S J, Fierrs H A, Dekkers W T, Mulder A W 1986 Acetate versus bicarbonate haemodialysis in critically ill patients. Nephron 42: 146

Lien J, Chan V 1985 Risk factors influencing survival in acute renal failure treated by haemodialysis. Archives of Internal Medicine 145: 2067–2072

Ljungberg B 1985 A low molecular heparin fraction as an anticoagulant during haemodialysis. Clinical Nephrology 24: 15–20

Macintyre E, Bullen C, Machin S J 1985 Fluid replacement in hypovolaemia. Intensive Care Medicine 11: 231–233

Mastrangelo F, Rizelli S, Corliano C, Montinaro A M, Blasi V de, Alfonso L, Aprile M, Napoli M, Laforgiar F 1985 Benefits of bicarbonate dialysis. Kidney International 28 (S17): S188–S193

Milligan S L, Luft F C, McMurray S D, Kleit S A 1978 Intraabdominal infection in acute renal failure. Archives of Surgery 113: 467–471

Moore R D, Smith C R, Lipsky J J, Mellitus D, Lietman P S 1984 Risk factors for nephrotoxicity in patients treated with aminoglycosides. Annals of Internal Medicine 100: 352–357

Morrison A R 1982 Alterations in intrarenal hormones in urinary tract obstruction. Seminars in Nephrology 2: 40–45

Murray B M, Paller M S, Ferris T F 1985 Effect of cyclosporin administration on renal haemodynamics. Kidney International 28: 767–774

Myers B D, Moran S M 1986 Haemodynamically mediated acute renal failure. New England Journal of Medicine 314: 97–104

Navar L G, Rosivall L 1984 Contribution of the renin angiotensin system to the control of intrarenal haemodynamics. Kidney International 25: 857–868

O'Grady, O'Brien, Williams R S 1986 The prevalence of hepatic and renal failure and the effects of dialysis and haemoperfusion on prognosis (In press)

Paines A D, Ho P, James H 1985 Metabolic control of renal vascular resistance and glomerulotubular balance. Kidney International 27: 848–854

Pine R W, Wertz M J, Lennard E S, Dellinger E D, Carnico C J, Minshaw B H 1983 Determinants of organ malfunction or death in patients with intra-abdominal sepsis. A discriminant analysis. Archives of Surgery 118: 242–249

P... .. O A , D...... 1990 Neph.......in indu.ed ..... renal failure. In: D......... B , S.... J H (.....) Acute Renal Failure, Chapter 6. Livingstone, New York

Rasmussen H H, Pitt E A, Ibeis L S, McNeill D R 1985 Prediction of outcome in acute renal failure by discrimination analysis of clinical variables. Archives of Internal Medicine 145: 2015

Richards A M, Nicholls M G, Ikram H, Webster M W I, Espiner E A 1985 Renal haemodynamic and hormonal effects of human alpha naturetic peptide in healthy volunteers. Lancet i: 545–549

Richet G 1985 When should renal biopsy be done in acute uraemia, tomorrow could be too late. Kidney International 28 (suppl 17): S152–S153

Rosenfield A T, Siegal N J 1981 Renal parenchymal disease, histopathologic senographic correlation. American Journal of Radiology 137: 793–798

Routh G S, Briggs J D, Mone J G, Ledingham I McA 1980 Survival from acute renal failure with and without multiple organ dysfunction. Postgraduate Medical Journal 56: 244–247

Ruder M A, Albert M A, Vanstone J 1985 Comparative effects of acetate and bicarbonate haemodialysis in LV function. Kidney International 27: 768–773

Rylance P B, Gordge M P, Ireland H, Lane D A, Weston M J 1984 Haemodialysis with prostacyclin (Epoprostenol) alone. In: Davison A M, Guillou P J (eds) Proceedings of the European Dialysis and Transplant Association. Pitman London, 21: 281–286

Schetz M, Lauwers P, Ferdinande P, Van de Wall E J 1984 The use of CAVH in intensive care medicine. Acta Anaesthesia Belg 35: 67–78

Scicli A G, Carretero O A 1986 Renal kallikrein-kinin system. Kidney International 29: 120–130

Shapiro M F, Shapiro for HPPC MCP 1985 Apheresis in chronic inflammatory demyelinating polyneuropathy and in renal transplantation. Annals of Internal Medicine 103: 630–633

Simpson K, Allison M 1985 Acute renal failure, can we improve the prognosis? American Society of Nephrology (In press)

Stoff J S 1984 Non-steroidal anti-inflammatory drugs and acute renal failure. Medical Grand Rounds 3: 166–174

Sturm J A, Wisner 1985 Fluid resuscitation of hypovolaemia. Intensive Care Medicine 11: 227–230

Sweet S J, Glenny C U, Fitzgibbons J P, Friedman P, Teres D 1981 Synergistic effect of ARF and respiratory failure in a surgical intensive care unit. American Journal of Surgery 141: 492–496

Talner L B, Scheible W, Ellenbogen P H, Beck C H, Gosink B B 1981 How accurate is ultrasonography in detecting hydronephrosis in azotemic patients. Urological Radiology 3: 1–6

Thul Hupp, Mann J F E, Ritz E, Allenberg J 1986 Revascularisation of renal artery occlusion by surgery by transluminal angioplasty. Kidney International 29: 191

Vanherweghem J L, Khaene M, Goldman M, Stolear J C, Sabot J P, Waterlot Y, Serruys E, Thayse C 1986 Infections associated with subclavian dialysis catheters. The key role of nurse training. Nephron 42: 116–119

Weston M 1983 The clinical uses of prostacyclin (Epoprostenol). British Medical Bulletin 39: 285–290

Woodhead M A, Macfarlane J T 1985 The protean manifestations of Legionnaires Disease. Journal of the Royal College of Physicians 19: 224–230

Index